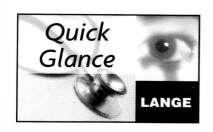

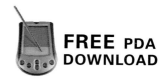

FREE PDA DOWNLOAD

PEDIATRIC EMERGENCY MEDICINE

Ghazala Q. Sharieff / Madeline Matar Joseph
Todd W. Wylie

FOLLOW THESE INSTRUCTIONS TO DOWNLOAD YOUR FREE PDA SOFTWARE

1) Use your Web browser to go to:
http://books.mcgraw-hill.com/eb.php?i=007145232X

2) Register now

3) Fill in the required fields

4) Enter your unique registration code below

5) Download the free software and sync into your handheld device

Cc

D1304560

Use this code to register ......ve your free PDA software.
See above for complete directions.

If you have any problems accessing your download,
please visit: www.books.mcgraw-hill.com/techsupport

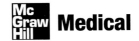

Mc Graw Hill **Medical**

p/n 0-07-146802-1

PEDIATRIC EMERGENCY MEDICINE QUICK GLANCE

NOTICE

Medicine is an ever-changing science. As new research and clinical experience broaden our knowledge, changes in treatment and drug therapy are required. The authors and the publisher of this work have checked with sources believed to be reliable in their efforts to provide information that is complete and generally in accord with the standards accepted at the time of publication. However, in view of the possibility of human error or changes in medical sciences, neither the authors nor the publisher nor any other party who has been involved in the preparation or publication of this work warrants that the information contained herein is in every respect accurate or complete, and they disclaim all responsibility for any errors or omissions or for the results obtained from use of the information contained in this work. Readers are encouraged to confirm the information contained herein with other sources. For example and in particular, readers are advised to check the product information sheet included in the package of each drug they plan to administer to be certain that the information contained in this work is accurate and that changes have not been made in the recommended dose or in the contraindications for administration. This recommendation is of particular importance in connection with new or infrequently used drugs.

PEDIATRIC EMERGENCY MEDICINE QUICK GLANCE

EDITORS

Ghazala Q. Sharieff, MD, FACEP, FAAEM, FAAP
Associate Clinical Professor
University of Florida/Shands Jacksonville
Director of Pediatric Emergency Medicine
Palomar-Pomerado Hospitals/California Emergency Physicians

Madeline Matar Joseph, MD, FAAP, FACEP
Associate Professor of Pediatrics and Emergency Medicine
Director, Pediatric Emergency Medicine Fellowship Program
University of Florida Health Science Center, Jacksonville

Todd W. Wylie, MD, MPH
Assistant Professor
Department of Emergency Medicine
University of Florida/Shands Jacksonville Health Science Center

CONSULTING EDITOR

Roger Barkin, MD, FACEP, FAAEM, FAAP
RMB Consulting, Denver
Clinical Professor of Pediatrics
University of Colorado Health Services Center, Denver
Emergency Physician, CarePoint, PC, Denver

MANAGING EDITOR

Jacqueline Mullin, RN
Department of Emergency Medicine
University of Florida/Shands Jacksonville

McGraw-Hill
Medical Publishing Division

*New York / Chicago / San Francisco / Lisbon / London / Madrid / Mexico City
Milan / New Delhi / San Juan / Seoul / Singapore / Sydney / Toronto*

Pediatric Emergency Medicine Quick Glance

Copyright © 2005 by The McGraw-Hill Companies, Inc. All rights reserved. Printed in the United States of America. Except as permitted under the United States Copyright Act of 1976, no part of this publication may be reproduced or distributed in any form or by any means, or stored in a data base or retrieval system, without the prior written permission of the publisher.

1 2 3 4 5 6 7 8 9 0   DOC/DOC   0 9 8 7 6 5

ISBN 0-07-145232-X

This book was set in Palatino by Silverchair Science + Communications, Inc.
The editors were Andrea Seils, Michelle Watt, and Penny Linskey.
The production supervisor was Catherine H. Saggese.
The book designer was Marsha Cohen.
The cover designer was Aimee Nordin.
The indexer was Pamela Edwards.
RR Donnelley was printer and binder.

This book is printed on acid-free paper.

Cataloging-in-Publication data for this title is on file with the Library of Congress.

INTERNATIONAL EDITION ISBN: 0-07-110502-6
Copyright 2005. Exclusive rights by the McGraw-Hill Companies, Inc., for manufacture and export. This book cannot be re-exported from the country to which it is consigned by McGraw-Hill. The International Edition is not available in North America.

To my dear, sweet Javaid, my beautiful daughters, Mariyah and Aleena, my mom, Afroz, and all of my family and friends who have allowed me to pursue my goals. Your never ending love, support, and encouragement mean more than words can say.

Ghazala Q. Sharieff

I dedicate this book to my husband, Michael, my children, Andrew, Christine, and Matthew for their love, patience, and support of my professional endeavors. I also dedicate this book to my parents, brothers, and all the people who during my life inspired me to pursue dreams no matter how out of reach they may seem. Thank you for your love and support.

Madeline Matar Joseph

To my wife and son, thank you for your love and support.

Todd W. Wylie

To the many talented and dedicated clinicians who serve our children in their times of urgent and emergent need, we hope that this book facilitates this care. Ghazala Sharieff's energy and enthusiasm has truly been the driving force behind this effort and we are appreciative of her commitment.

Roger Barkin

To Randy, Brian, Amy, and all my family, thank you for your unconditional love, support, and encouragement throughout this process.

Jacqueline Mullin

CONTENTS

7   LEGAL ISSUES   347

CONTRIBUTORS

Mardi Steere, MBBS

Tonia J. Brousseau, DO

Nazeema Khan, MD

Pia Myers, MD

University of Florida/Shands Jacksonville

TOXICOLOGY CONTRIBUTORS

Brian Baskin, MD

Ranaan Pokroy, MD

University of Florida/Shands Jacksonville

The inspiration for this quick guide was our fellows who were enthusiastically studying pediatric emergency medicine. We decided that the best way to learn and remember important facts was in an abbreviated, bulleted format. This led to the creation of this handbook and PDA program. We dedicate our work to all of the students, housestaff, nurses and other allied health professionals who continue to motivate us. We hope that you will find this book to be useful in your daily practice and that it will help you to feel more comfortable with the acute care of children.

Ghazala Q. Sharieff
Madeline Matar Joseph
Todd W. Wylie
Roger Barkin
Jacqueline Mullin

CHAPTER 1

PREHOSPITAL

PREHOSPITAL CARE
Prehospital Personnel

▶ **First Responders**: national course to certify community-based responders, they can provide basic life support (BLS) but usually do not immobilize or transport

▶ **Basic Life Support Providers**: often emergency medical technicians (EMTs)—assess, provide transport, spinal immobilization, ventilatory assistance (not intubation); recognize respiratory distress, altered mental status, shock, mechanism of injury, death; can triage and route

▶ **Advanced Life Support (ALS) Providers**: often paramedics—advanced resuscitation, recognize arrhythmias, drug/electrical cardioversion, intubation

▶ **Intermediate Providers**: not useful!

Equipment/Transportation Modes

▶ **Ground**: must have space for 2 patients, 60-inch head room, 2 EMTs, exterior lighting; 3 types (truck cab chassis, standard van, specialty van)

▶ **Pediatric Equipment:** all vehicles must have basic pediatric and newborn sizes of equipment

▶ **Staffing**: at least 2 persons trained in EMT; ALS units need BLS and ALS skills to manage medical and trauma emergencies

▶ **Air Transport**: two types: (1) helicopter (used in densely populated areas) and (2) fixed wing (smoother, quieter, spacious, need runway)

Medical Command

► Supervision of emergency medical services (EMS) in the community
► **Base Stations:** fire stations or hospitals
► **Levels of Control**
  • EMS director (may be physician advisory board)
  • Base station hospital medical director
  • Base hospital emergency physician
► **Types of Control**
  • **Off-line control:** physician is responsible for planning, implementation, monitoring; if more than one base station also coordinate regional prehospital care
  • **On-line control**: management of individual case by emergency physician at centralized facility—voice authorization of certain ALS procedures

Mechanics

► **Receiving**: call goes to communication center; operator routes to police/fire/medical
► **Dispatch**: first responder is immediately sent to the scene (closest personnel with BLS training), additional responders may be sent; if disaster, then multiple teams sent
► **Field Treatment**: BLS until ALS providers arrive; online assistance; command center and communication center decide on hospital
► **Completion**: receiving hospital assembles personnel/equipment while child en route

Medical Legal Issues

► Prehospital providers are responsible for actions, not protected by Good Samaritan laws.
► Prehospital providers are not required to provide care if they would be put at risk for personal injury.
► **Consent**: minors can be treated for emergencies without consent in most states. If parents refuse care, they need to sign a witnessed release; however the child must be treated if there is a life-threatening emergency, possible child abuse, or if parents are unable to understand risks of refusing care.
► **Standards of Care:** written protocols, immobilization where appropriate.

► **Documentation:** all actions should be documented, become part of the medical record, and are confidential. Providers required to report suspected abuse, gunshot wounds, and illegal drug use.

TRANSPORT MEDICINE
Transport Mode

► Should be decided by personnel availability, speed of transport required, disease process, economy of cost where practical, and weather conditions

Personnel Issues

► Transport team should have experience with critically ill neonates/children
► Pediatric critical care teams include pediatric nurses, often respiratory therapists, nonpediatric transport nurse with pediatric training or paramedic; plus drivers/pilots
► Continuing education and mortality/morbidity conferences important

Communication

► Referring hospital calls receiving facility; may request advice from receiving physician, or may be offered by receiving physician (should be dose-specific, route-specific recommendations, etc.); referring physician is under no obligation to accept advice but should consider; all should be clearly documented
► Physician-to-physician and nurse-to-nurse direct communication recommended throughout
► When transport team arrives at referring facility and en route, command physician may need to be contacted for advice; all documents, lab values, copies of radiographs should be ready for transport team
► After arrival at receiving hospital, transport team transitions care to inpatient

Patient/Team Safety

► Transport medical director responsible for continually assessing capabilities of modes of transport and personnel

Evaluation of the Team

▶ Should be able to access team through transport referral number; single referring physician; single transport command physician

▶ Follow-up to referring provider should occur regarding care of the patient

Legal Issues

▶ **EMTALA:** Transport cannot be used to avoid assessment, stabilization, or intervention, especially with regard to ability to pay. Referring physicians must do all in their power to stabilize, may not transport against patient's will unless facility cannot provide appropriate care; referring physician must advise of risks/benefits (not financial); referring physician must select means of transport; receiving hospital must accept the patient if it has the appropriate type and level of care available.

▶ If management conflicts arise, medical command physician should resolve by speaking directly with referring physician; transport team assumes total responsibility for care once they leave the referral center; the patient should be as stable as possible when they leave.

Stabilization

▶ Transport team is responsible for providing level of care provided at receiving hospital (ideally); at least maintain patient's present level of care at referring facility.

▶ Transport team should decide if further medical interventions should be performed prior to transport (if it will have a direct effect on patient outcome), and may be directed by length of time of transport.

Altitude Physiology

▶ Higher altitude = lower pressure and higher volume of gas; air is less dense with lower partial pressure of O_2 and less availability

▶ **Risks:** pneumothorax, pneumocephalus, bowel obstruction may predispose to vomiting and aspiration; endotracheal cuffs/Foley cuffs may be affected; air embolism may worsen; hypoxia

▶ Not usually an issue with helicopters (< 1000 ft); may be with fixed wing (pressurized to 5000–8000 feet which can increase gas volume)

Specific Issues

▶ **Airway:** consider elective intubation before transport; ensure airway is well secured before transport; check airway after **all** transfers (stretcher, etc.); monitor with continuous end-tidal carbon dioxide ($ETCO_2$), pulse oximetry, and cardiorespiratory monitoring. If endotracheal tube (ETT) displaced, attempt intubation. If unsuccessful, consider bag valve mask (BVM) ventilation until arrival; have adjuncts and difficult airway equipment available.

▶ **Status Epilepticus:** O_2, patent airway, accucheck to ensure not hypoglycemic. Consider giving normal saline if history suggests dehydration, or if patient was given diluted fluids (infants given strictly bottled water). Benzodiazepine (diazepam, midazolam rectal/IV/IM/IO), phenytoin/phenobarbital/fosphenytoin, if first and second line agents fail, intubate and start infusions midazolam/pentobarbital; if cannot start infusion give neuromuscular blockade (to protect team/patient).

▶ **Cardiac Arrest:** usually only transport if extracorporeal membrane oxygenation (ECMO) or other modalities at receiving facility may change outcome.

▶ **Shock:** primary and secondary IV access routes should be obtained before transport; isotonic fluids, colloid, and blood should be available

▶ **Trauma:** ABCs, immobilization crucial; blood products should be available, all radiographs and studies should be transported.

▶ **Sedation/Analgesia:** patients who already required analgesia/sedation (sickle cell, fractures); evolving sedation requirements (already intubated); transport itself increases pain/anxiety (long bone fracture); consider nonpharmacologic interventions (parent, distraction, immobilization, play); airway equipment and resuscitation medications for all patients receiving sedation (Naloxone, Flumazenil).

CHAPTER 2

RESUSCITATION

AIRWAY MANAGEMENT
Airway Anatomic Differences Between Children and Adults

► Prominent occiput can cause airway obstruction.
  • Use 1-inch towel roll below shoulders.
► Dependence upon nasopharynx patency
  • Avoid nasal airways below 1 year of age due to larger adenoidal tissue which can bleed.
► Lots of secretions
► Loose primary teeth
► Relatively larger tongues can obstruct the airway
  • May need to use an oral or nasal airway
► Epiglottis is U-shaped and floppy.
  • Use a straight laryngoscope blade to lift the epiglottis directly.
► Larynx is more anterior and cephalad.
► Cricoid area of child is smallest area of the airway.
  • Use uncuffed tubes in children < 8 years old and < size 6.0 endotracheal tube (ETT).
► Small trachea diameter and distance between rings makes tracheostomy or cricothyrotomy more difficult.
  • American Heart Association (AHA) recommends needle cricothyrotomy for difficult airways (see Appendix 2).
► Much shorter tracheal length (newborn, 4–5 cm; 18-month-old, 7–8 cm)
  • ETTs easily dislodged; re-assess position of tube frequently

▶ Large airways are more narrow than an adult airway.
  • Leads to greater resistance
▶ Ribs are more horizontal at very young age; movement is dependent on the diaphragm.
  • Decompress stomach with nasogastric (NG) tube to ventilate easier (rough guide for NG tube size is 2× the ETT size).

Indications for Airway Management

▶ Respiratory failure or impending respiratory failure
  • Respiratory rates < 12 or > 60; plus nonpurposeful or unresponsive to painful stimuli
▶ Cardiopulmonary failure
▶ Decompensated shock: helps decrease the work of breathing
▶ Emergency drug administration: lidocaine, epinephrine (dose is 0.1 cc/kg of the 1:1000 concentration); atropine, Naloxone (+ Diazepam) when no intravenous access readily accessible
▶ Neurologic resuscitation: pediatric Glasgow Coma Score (GCS) < 8 or consider in anyone with GCS < 12 and decreasing mental status; ventilate to PCO_2 of 30–35
▶ Protects the airway

Bag-Valve-Mask Ventilation

▶ Correct mask sizing: bridge of nose to cleft of chin
  • Large mask pressing on eyes can cause vagal bradycardia.
▶ Hold mask using a "C" grip: thumb and index fingers grip mask; 3rd, 4th, 5th fingers on angle of jaw "E" → "CE"
  • Avoid pushing on soft tissue below mandible: can obstruct airway
▶ **Bag Size**
  • 450 cc bag for infant or child < 5 years old
  • 750 cc bag or adult bag for older children
  • Avoid stocking ED with neonatal 250 cc bags: can cause confusion in code situation
▶ Say "squeeze/release/release" as you ventilate the child
▶ Watch for complications such as gastric distension, vomiting, aspiration, and hypoxemia

Endotracheal Intubation

▶ **Correct Endotracheal Tube (ETT) Sizing:**
- Newborns, 3.0 mm; if large newborn, 3.5 mm
- Up to 6 months, 3.5–4.0 mm
- At 1 year, 4.0–4.5 mm
- > 1 year: (16 + age years)/4 = ETT size in mm
- Length-based resuscitation tape
- Width of child's little finger nail equal to internal diameter of ETT
- Width of child's little finger equal to width of whole ETT
- Incorrect tube size can lead to inability to ventilate if too small or airway trauma if too large

▶ Depth of tube placement equals 3× ETT size appropriate for age (i.e.,: 4.0 mm ETT placed at 12 cm mark at lips) or 10 + age in years at the lips

> 1 kg = 7
> 2 kg = 8
> 3 kg = 9
> 4 kg = 10

▶ Laryngoscope blade size: rough guide, actual blade size determined by weight, body habitus, and anatomic particulars

▶ **Endotracheal Drug Delivery—LEAN:**
> **L**—**L**idocaine
> **E**—**E**pinephrine
> **A**—**A**tropine
> **N**—**N**arcan (naloxone)

- ET dosage of epinephrine is **10 times** the IV or IO dosage.
  1. Epinephrine 0.1 mg/kg of 1:1000 solution (0.1 cc/kg) given via ETT

TABLE 2-1
LARYNGOSCOPE BLADE SIZE

Age/Weight	Size (Type)
Newborn up to 2.5 kg	0 Miller
0–3 months	1.0 Miller
3 months–3 years	1.5–2.0 Miller, Macintosh or 1.5 Wisconsin
3 years–12 years	2.0–4.0 Miller or Macintosh
> 12 years	3.0 Miller or Macintosh

     a. Mix with 2–3 cc of normal saline to deliver at least 2 cc of liquid volume

     b. Can deliver with angiocath or feeding tube

     c. Aerosolize the drug by ventilating after squirting drug down ETT

     d. Other drugs ET dosages (L, A, N) are 2–3 times the IV or IO dosage

Rapid Sequence Intubation (RSI) Timelines

▶ Time to intubation 5 minutes: start preoxygenation (BVM)

▶ Time to intubation 3 minutes: give any premedication (atropine, lidocaine, fentanyl, defasciculating dose of paralytic)

▶ Intubation time: push induction and paralytic agents

▶ Apply cricoid pressure

▶ Intubate after patient is relaxed

▶ Immediately after intubation:

- Check tube placement (chest rise, confirm bilateral breath sounds, colorimetric end-tidal CO_2 detector, monitor oxygen saturation)
- Release cricoid pressure
- Secure tube
- Place NG tube

TABLE 2-2
PRETREATMENT

Drug	Dose (mg/kg)	Indication	Comments
Atropine	0.01–0.02 (min 0.1)	Prophylaxis against bradycardia with succinylcholine	Children < 10 years of age receiving succinylcholine, or any child < 5 years of age (≤ 20 kg) undergoing intubation
Lidocaine	1.0–1.5	1. Elevated ICP 2. Reactive airway disease	Mixed evidence effectiveness

TABLE 2-3
PARALYTICS

Drug	Dose (mg/ kg)	Onset	Duration of Action	Comments
Succinyl-choline	1–2	< 1 min	< 10 min	Can cause brady-cardia; pretreat children < 10 y with atropine.
Rocuroni-um	1.0	< 1 min	40–60 min	No change in potas-sium; does not cause malignant hyperthermia.
Vecuroni-um	0.1 or 0.3	2–3 min or 60–90 s	30–40 min or up to 100 min	Priming dose of 0.01 mg/kg may be given IV fol-lowed 2–3 min later by induc-tion agent and repeat vecuroni-um of 0.15 mg/ kg.

*No need to use priming defasciculating dose of non-depolarizing paralytics in children < 5 years of age as they do not have the muscle mass to fasciculate.

Source: Luten, R. Approach to the pediatric airway. In: *The Manual of Emergency Airway Management*, 2nd ed. Walls, R, Murphy, M, Luten, R, Schneider, R, eds. Lippincott Williams & Wilkins, Philadelphia: 2004.

TABLE 2-4
INDUCTION AGENTS

Drug	Dose (mg/kg)	Onset	Duration	Blood Pressure	ICP	Comments
Propofol	1–2	10–20 s	3–14″	Decrease	Decrease	Anti-epileptic effects. Do not use in patients with soy or egg allergies.
Etomidate	0.3	20–30 s	7–14″	Neutral	May decrease	Adrenal suppression, myoclonic jerks.
Ketamine	IV: 1–2 IM: 4	15–60 s	10–15″ IV	Increase	Increase	Bronchial relaxation, myocardial depression.
Thiopental	3.0–5.0	20–30 s	3–5″	Decrease	Decrease	Anti-epileptic effects, can cause broncho-spasm.
Midazolam	0.1–0.3	30–60 s	30–80″ IV	Decrease		Anti-epileptic effects.

TABLE 2-5
CLINICAL SCENARIOS

Clinical Scenario	Induction Agents
Isolated head injury	Propofol, thiopental, etomidate, *No* ketamine!
Status epilepticus	Thiopental, propofol, etomidate, midazolam
Asthma	Ketamine, etomidate, *No* thiopental!
Respiratory failure	Ketamine, etomidate, propofol

BLOOD COMPONENTS AND TRANSFUSION REACTIONS
Indications for Transfusion

▶ **Packed Red Blood Cells (PRBCs)**
- Supply O_2 delivery.
- The hemoglobin (Hgb) dissociation curve is affected by fetal hemoglobin (Hgb F) which binds less 2,3 diphospho-glycerate (2,3 DPG) than adult Hg.
- pH: low pH decreases affinity of Hgb for O_2 and the 2,3 DPG level.
- The mean Hgb is 17 mg/dL in newborns; 13 mg/dL in pre-pubertal children.
- Chronic anemia: stable vital signs with paleness due to chronic compensation (normal blood volume, increased 2,3 DPG).
- **Transfuse** if massive blood volume loss (approximately 30–35%) due to hemorrhage, splenic sequestration, severe hemolysis.
  1. PRBCs are the best choice (whole blood is better for exchange transfusion in the neonate).
     a. Maximum amount = 10 cc/kg or 1 unit, whichever is less. If Hgb < 5 mg/dL, then the Volume = Hgb level × weight in pounds.
     b. Give irradiated PRBCs if immunosuppressed to prevent graft versus host disease (GVHD). Give O-negative if urgent, otherwise type-specific and cross-matched.

▶ **Platelets**
- The cellular component that stops bleeding; normal = 150,000–450,000/mm^3; life span approximately 10 days.
- **Causes of thrombocytopenia:**
  1. Increased destruction: idiopathic thrombocytopenia purpura (ITP) rarely requires platelet transfusion—only

if life-threatening bleeding exits. Intravenous immuno-globulin (IVIG) is treatment of choice—less common adverse drug reactions.

2. Decreased production: transfuse prophylactically if platelets 10,000/mm^3 or 20,000/mm^3 with fever.
3. Acute loss.
- **Decreased efficacy** (thrombasthenias):
  1. Transfused platelets can control active bleeding, reserve for serious cases as they can form antibodies to platelet membranes.
  2. Aspirin $\rightarrow$ acquired thrombasthenia; transfusion if severe bleeding $\rightarrow$ transfused platelets release adeno-sine diphosphate (ADP) and helps aspirin-affected platelets to function.
- **Transfuse:**
  1. Pack has a minimum = 5.5×10^{10} platelets per pack with an average = 7×10^{10}.
  2. Amount to transfuse: (1 unit/10 kg weight of centri-fuged platelets) should increase platelet count by approximately 50,000/mm^3.
      a. Platelets have HLA and ABO antigens, not Rh but some contamination from RBCs and WBCs can occur.
      b. Use Rh-negative for Rh-negative pregnant women.
      c. GVHD is also possible from WBCs as filtering is not 100% effective $\rightarrow$ use irradiated for immunosup-pressed patients.

▶ **Plasma**
- **Fresh frozen plasma (FFP)** = whole blood minus RBCs, platelets. Prepared from whole blood and frozen within 8 hours, 200–250 cc/unit (1 coagulation unit per cc); large volume.
  1. Plasma concentrates
      a. Cryoprecipitate (80–100 units of factor VIII coagulant, 100–200 of fibrinogen and some factor IX, VWF)
      b. Factor VIII concentrates: give (20–30 units/kg) to stop clinical hemorrhaging in hemophilia
      c. Factor IX concentrates
      d. Prothrombin concentrates
  2. Recombinant products: factor VIII products do not con-tain VWF (except Humate-P)

Adverse Reactions to Blood Products

► Risk of transfusion reaction is 0.34–3.6% (mostly from PRBCs): 41% febrile; 58% urticarial; 1% hemolytic

► **Hemolytic Transfusion Reactions**
  • Usually ABO (human error), leukoagglutinins, or contaminants
  • Usually have history of previous transfusion, pregnancy, or other blood products
  • **Symptoms:** chills, fever, tachycardia (less often abdominal or lower back pain), if severe then hypotension, shock, renal failure
  • **Treatment**
    1. Stop transfusion
    2. Retype and recrossmatch
    3. Check for hemoglobinuria, Coombs
    4. Supportive care
    5. O-negative blood if anemia profound while awaiting typed

► Typing can be done in minutes, but crossmatching takes at least 20 minutes.

► FFP if unmatched should be given as AB Rh-positive as it contains no antibodies.

► **Delayed Transfusion Reactions**
  • Occur 3–10 days after alloimmunized patient receives compatible blood.
  • **Symptoms:** similar to immediate, may even occur weeks after (rare), usually Rh, Kidd, Duffy, Kell, MNSS system antigens (i.e., amnestic response); milder overall, usually in patients who are heavily transfused (e.g., thalassemics).

► **Nonhemolytic**
  • Usually due to WBCs or plasma protein hypersensitivity
  • **Symptoms**: fever, urticaria in 2–3% of recipients
  • **Treatment:** (1) stop transfusion; (2) antihistamines, corticosteroids; (3) epinephrine if severe (rare)
  • **Prevent** by leukocyte filters, washed/frozen RBCs

► **Anaphylaxis**
  • Rare, occurs in those with IgA deficiency after as little as 10 cc infusion of blood
  • **Prevent:** give washed, filtered, frozen RBCs

► **Donor Leukoagglutinin-Associated Transfusion Reaction**
  • Antibodies in donor blood (i.e., Rh-sensitized women, previously transfused donors; usually directed against HLA or granulocyte-specific antigens)
  • **Symptoms:** fever, neutropenia, if severe then profound respiratory distress (ARDS picture)
  • **Treatment:** supportive care
► **Complications of Massive Blood Transfusion:** i.e., replacement > total plasma volume in 24 hours (4 units of whole blood in a 30 kg child)
  • pH changes (alkalosis)
  • hypothermia
  • hypocalcemia
  • hyperkalemia
  • hyperphosphatemia
  • coagulation abnormalities
  • altered Hgb function
► **Infectious Disease:** including human immunodeficiency virus (HIV) (risk is 0.0025 per unit), cytomegalovirus (CMV), hepatitis B and hepatitis C

CARDIOPULMONARY RESUSCITATION
Introduction

► **Arrest** is usually secondary to respiratory or circulatory failure; underlying causes include:
  • Upper respiratory: croup, epiglottitis, obstruction, suffocation, trauma, strangulation
  • Lower respiratory: asthma, bronchiolitis, pneumonia, aspiration, near-drowning, pulmonary edema
  • Infection: sepsis, meningitis
  • Cardiac disorders: myocarditis, pericarditis, rhythm disturbance, congenital heart disease
  • Shock: hypovolemic, cardiogenic, distributive
  • Neurologic: meningitis, encephalitis, stroke, head trauma, hypoxia
  • Metabolic: hypoglycemia, hypocalcemia, hyperkalemia
  • Trauma/environment: hypovolemia due to hemorrhage, hypothermia, hyperthermia, submersion injury

► 10–28% of apneic and pulseless patients will return to spontaneous circulation in the ED, but only 10% of these will survive until discharge, and almost all will have long-term neurologic sequelae.

► Brain and myocardium are particularly reliant on aerobic metabolism.

► **Chain of survival** requires:
  • Early caregiver recognition
  • Early activation of EMS with initial stabilization
  • Timely ED assessment/triage
  • Early definitive care

Resuscitation Management

► **Airway/Breathing**
  • Establish unresponsiveness
  • Open airway (neutral with chin lift/jaw thrust)
  • Reassess
  • Rescue breathing (mouth/mask or bag-valve-mask [BVM]), inspiratory time 1–2 seconds, tidal volume 6–8 cc/kg

► **Endotracheal Intubation**
  • Indications: airway control, prolonged ventilation, hyperventilation, improved O_2 delivery
  • General information: **size = (age + 16)/4; length inserted = 3× ETT diameter (cm)**
  • Remember: Sellick maneuver, spinal stabilization if suspect trauma, check position (chest rise, confirm bilateral breath sounds, colorimetric end-tidal CO_2 detector, monitor oxygen saturation)
  • Cricothyrotomy (percutaneous or surgical) considered for complete upper airway obstruction

► **Foreign Bodies**
  • May impede ventilation

► **Circulation**
  • Pulse check: brachial (particularly infants < 1 year), femoral, or carotid.
  • Compressions: at least 100 compressions/min for infants, 100/min is adequate for children, compression/relaxation ratio should be 1:1.
  • Compression/ventilation ratio: 3:1 neonate, 5:1 infant/child.

Medications and Fluids

▶ **Fluids:** 20 mL/kg crystalloid (normal saline or lactated Ringer [LR] solution) for shock; repeat as indicated.

▶ **Vascular Access:** essential for all drugs (except **L**idocaine, **E**pinephrine, **A**tropine, **N**aloxone, these can be given via ETT). Intraosseous access if no IV in 60 seconds or 3 attempts.

▶ **Epinephrine:** ↑ coronary blood flow and brain perfusion, ↑ myocardial contractility, systemic vascular resistance, automaticity. Dose: 0.01 mg/kg recommended initially (1:10,000 solution). 0.1 mg/kg of the 1:1000 concentration is used through the ETT. The dose is 0.1 cc/kg of either concentration.

▶ **Atropine:** accelerates atrioventricular conduction and atrial pacemakers; for symptomatic bradycardia. Dose: 0.02 mg/kg IV/IO/ET, minimum single dose of 0.1 mg, maximum single dose 0.5 mg for infant or 1 mg in child.

▶ **Calcium: only** indicated for hypocalcemia, hyperkalemia/ magnesemia, calcium-channel blocker overdose. Dose: Calcium chloride (10%, 100 mg/mL) give 20–30 mg (0.2–0.3 mL)/kg/ dose IV.

▶ **Sodium Bicarbonate: not generally recommended in arrest,** may increase intracellular CO_2 and promote cellular dysfunction. Only indicated for hyperkalemia, tricyclic antidepressant overdose, and severe metabolic acidosis with adequate ventilation: 1 mEq/kg IV/IO, then 0.5 mEq/kg q10min.

▶ **Glucose:** if blood sugar < 40 mg/dL give 0.5–1 g/kg of $D_{25}W$ (2–4 cc/kg). Use $D_{10}W$ in 0–6 months of age.

▶ **Isoproterenol:** only for bradycardia **unresponsive** to atropine, 0.1 µg/kg/min.

▶ **Nitroprusside:** vasodilator (arterial/venous) for severe hypertension (HTN), 0.3–10 µg/kg/min (start with 0.3 µg/kg/min).

▶ **Infusions:**
  • Epinephrine: 0.05–1 µg/kg/min
  • Dobutamine: 2–15 µg/kg/min
  • Dopamine: 5–20 µg/kg/min
  • Prostaglandin E-1: 0.05–0.1 mg/kg/min

▶ **Rhythm Disturbances**
  • **Bradycardia:** treat all symptomatic patients with bradycardia
    1. Oxygenation and ventilation
    2. Compressions if heart rate < 60 beats/min in infant or child

3. Epinephrine 0.01 mg/kg IV/IO (1:10,000 solution) or 0.1 mg/kg ETT (1:1000 solution)
4. Atropine 0.02 mg/kg IV/IO (minimum dose 0.1 mg)

- **Pulseless ventricular tachycardia or fibrillation:**
  1. Immediate defibrillation: 2 joules/kg → 2–4 joules/kg → 4 joules/kg
  2. CPR, secure airway, ventilate with 100% O_2
  3. Epinephrine 0.01 mg/kg IV/IO (1:10,000 solution) every 3–5 minutes (0.1cc/kg) or 0.1 mg/kg (0.1 cc/kg) ETT (1:1000 solution)
  4. Amiodarone 5 mg/kg IV/IO or lidocaine 1 mg/kg IV/IO
  5. Lidocaine 1 mg/kg IV/IO/ETT
  6. Magnesium 25–50 mg/kg IV/IO if torsades de pointes
  7. Follow each drug with 4 J/kg defibrillation

- **Pulseless electrical activity (PEA)**
  1. Identify and treat cause:
     a. Hypoxia, hypovolemia, hyperthermia, hypo/hyper-kalemia, metabolic disorders
     b. Tamponade, tension pneumothorax, toxins/poisons/drugs, thromboembolism
  2. CPR, secure airway, ventilate with 100% O_2
  3. Epinephrine 0.01 mg/kg IV/IO (1:10,000 solution) or 0.1 mg/kg ETT (1:1000 solution)

- **Ventricular tachycardia with a pulse**
  1. Provide oxygen and ventilation as needed
  2. If patient has evidence of poor perfusion, then immediate synchronized cardioversion at 0.5–1 J/kg
     a. May double dose to 1–2 J/kg if rhythm persists
     b. Consider alternative medications: amiodarone 5 mg/kg IV over 20–60 minutes, procainamide 15 mg/kg IV over 30–60 minutes (do not administer amiodarone and procainamide together), or lidocaine 1 mg/kg IV bolus
  3. If patient has adequate perfusion then consult pediatric cardiologist, and in consult may provide synchronized cardioversion or alternative medications as in situation of poor perfusion

- **Supraventricular tachycardia (SVT)**
  1. Vagal maneuvers if stable (ice, knee-chest position, blowing on occluded straw)

2. Adenosine is drug of choice: 0.1 mg/kg IV push (half-life is 10 seconds); maximum of 6 mg first dose, may double (0.2 mg/kg) second dose with maximum of 12 mg
3. Cardioversion if unstable (and no IV access): 0.5 J/kg, then 1 J/kg
4. Other choices: amiodarone or procainamide (see above for doses)
- **Asystole**
  1. CPR, secure airway, ventilate with 100% O_2
  2. Epinephrine 0.01 mg/kg IV/IO (1:10,000 solution) or 0.1 mg/kg ETT (1:1000 solution), 0.1 cc/kg of either concentration

Pacing
▶ Indication: patients with heart block unresponsive to therapy
▶ Transvenous or transesophageal as bridge until permanent pacemaker placed

Ancillary Data
▶ CBC, electrolytes, BUN, creatinine, glucose, calcium, phosphorus, ABG, type and crossmatch blood (as indicated), chest x-ray, ECG, capnography, and monitor urine output via a Foley catheter.
▶ Remember that pulse oximetry may be unreliable in an arrest.

SHOCK
Definition
▶ Sustained, progressive circulatory dysfunction resulting in inadequate oxygen and substrate delivery that does not meet metabolic needs of tissues.

Pathophysiology
Cardiac Output
▶ **Heart Rate:** tachycardia usual response; bradycardia ominous; supraventricular tachycardia (SVT) if > 220 beats per minute (bpm) in an infant or > 180 bpm in a child
▶ **Stroke Volume**
  - **Preload:** central venous pressure (CVP) = right atrial pressure = right ventricle (RV) end diastolic pressure = myocardial

stretch = force of contraction. Normal CVP = 5–8 mm Hg; may improve output with fluids to increase (CVP) up to 10–12 mm Hg; > 12 probably not beneficial.

- **Compliance:** change in ventricular volume for a given pressure, i.e., dV/dP (mL/mm Hg).
- **Contractility:** speed and force of a contraction; measured by echocardiogram by left ventricular shortening fraction (28–44% in children) or ejection fraction, or by measuring pulmonary artery wedge pressure (PAWP) and looking at pressure/volume curve with echocardiogram ↓ with infection, hypoxia, electrolyte or acid-base imbalance; may improve with inotropes.
- **Ventricular afterload:** affected by ventricular lumen size, thickness of ventricular wall, ventricular ejection (intracavitary) pressure; usually = systemic/pulmonary pressures = blood flow/resistance. Increased with pulmonary/aortic stenosis, systemic vasoconstriction, pulmonary hypertension (hypoxia, acidosis, alveolar distension, hypothermia); may improve with vasodilators.

Oxygen Delivery

▶ Oxygen delivery = arterial oxygen content × cardiac output
▶ Arterial oxygen content = Hgb (g) × 1.34 mL oxygen/g × Hgb saturation
▶ Delivery usually = 36–40 mL/kg/min in infant; 27–30 in child; 18–20 in adolescent
▶ Consumption usually = 10–14 mL/kg/min in infant; 5–8 in child (high metabolic rate)
▶ Demand is ↑ in sepsis, hyperthermia; consumption becomes supply-dependent, causing acidosis if inadequate so treatment of shock must always include oxygen supplementation

Hypovolemic Shock

▶ **Etiology:** most common in pediatrics, usually dehydration, trauma, or distributive (sepsis, burns)
▶ **Pathophysiology:** initial adrenergic vasoconstriction (from mesenteries, renal, skin) with renin and water retention; hypotension occurs only if rapid and severe losses (20–25% blood volume loss); compensation may cause myocardial ischemia (↑consumption, tachycardia with impaired subendocardial blood flow)

► **Diagnosis**
  • History of weight loss/poor intake/increased losses
  • Physical findings: sunken fontanelle, poor skin turgor, poor perfusion, capillary refill > 3 seconds if > 10% losses
  • Laboratory/Radiology: CVP < 5–8 mm Hgb, elevated BUN/urine specific gravity, metabolic acidosis, tachycardia, small cardiac silhouette
  • Dehydration
    1. Isotonic dehydration: poor perfusion if > 10% dehydrated for young children; 5–7% in older children
    2. Hypotonic dehydration: loss of sodium, loss of osmolality, shift of fluids extravascularly, poor perfusion with 5–7% losses in young children; 3–5% for older children
    3. Hypernatremic dehydration: loss of free water, ↑ osmolality, shift of fluids intravascularly, good perfusion despite large losses, perfusion compromised when losses are > 10%, hypotension at > 15% (7–10% for adolescents)
  • Hemorrhage: normal blood volume = 90–105 cc/kg for premature infant; 85 cc/kg for term newborn; 75 cc/kg for infant; 65–75 cc/kg for children. Perfusion compromised with > 15–20% blood loss acutely (12–16 cc/kg); 10% loss causes heart rate ↑ of 20 bpm, 20% loss causes ↑ of 30 bpm, 20–25% loss causes hypotension

Cardiogenic Shock

► **Etiology**: usually after cardiac surgery, cardiomyopathy or myocarditis, severe congenital obstructive disease, drug toxicity.
► **Diagnosis**: inadequate perfusion despite adequate intravascular volume, cool extremities, poor capillary refill, mottling. CVP is often elevated with hepatomegaly and periorbital edema, may have pulmonary edema, enlarged cardiac silhouette. If postoperative, consider cardiac tamponade (pulsus paradoxus undetectable if hypotensive/tachypneic), perform echocardiogram.

Septic Shock

► **Etiology**: mortality from septic shock is approximately 25%, about half of cases are caused by Gram-negative organisms; greatest risk is at extremes of life, those with invasive catheters, surgical incisions, burns, wounds, immunocompromised, chronic antibiotics.

▶ **Pathophysiology:** infection triggers inflammatory response with several mediators—tumor necrosis factor, interleukin-1, platelet-activating factor, nitric oxide, arachidonic acid, and others. Cascading events result in vasodilation, maldistribution of cardiac output, increased capillary permeability, myocardial dysfunction, organ ischemia and failure. Endotoxin (Gram-negative cell wall component of which the active component is lipopolysaccharide) produces all the effects of sepsis, and survival is inversely related to endotoxin levels.

▶ **Diagnosis**

- **Systemic inflammatory response syndrome** (SIRS) is diagnosed by two or more of:
  1. Temperature > 38° C or temperature < 36° C
  2. Tachycardia, tachypnea, or respiratory alkalosis (Pco_2 < 32 mm Hg)
  3. White blood cell count < 4000/mm^3 or > 12,000/mm^3 or bands > 10%
- **Sepsis:** evidence of SIRS with suspected infection, does not require positive blood culture
- **Severe sepsis:** evidence of sepsis with signs of altered organ perfusion separate from the site of suspected infection, such as altered mental status, reduced myocardial ejection fraction, pulmonary failure ($\uparrow$ work of breathing and intrapulmonary shunting), gastrointestinal dysfunction (elevated liver enzymes, paralytic ileus, hemorrhage) or oliguria (< 1 cc/kg/h)
- **Septic shock:** metabolic acidosis or rise in serum lactate, decreased peripheral pulses, mottled skin, hypotension (late)

Spinal (Neurogenic) Shock

▶ **Etiology:** loss of sympathomimetic tone causes vasodilation and relative hypovolemia

▶ **Diagnosis:** signs of shock after spinal cord injury despite adequate volume replacement

- Hallmark: warm skin (due to vasodilation) + lack of tachycardia + clinical picture of shock

Management of Shock

▶ **Airway/Ventilation:** Supplemental O_2 at 3–6 L/min if breathing, bag-mask and intubation if not. Consider intubation for risk of airway obstruction (burns), hypoxemia ($PO_2 < 50$ mm Hg), hypoventilation, hypercarbia ($PCO_2 > 50$ mm Hg), ↑ intracranial pressure, evidence of intrapulmonary shunting (A-a gradient > 15 mm Hg).

- A-a gradient = PAO_2-PaO_2 = [FIO_2 × (barometric pressure $_{(B)}$ 47 mm Hg) – $PaCO_2/0.8$] – PaO_2
- ARDS = ↑ capillary permeability, pulmonary edema with progressive hypoxemia, ↑ intrapulmonary shunting, ↓ compliance; requires supplemental oxygen and positive end expiratory pressure (PEEP) (minimum amount to achieve $PO_2 > 60$ mm Hg with FIO_2 <0.5)

▶ **Circulation**
- **Heart rate**: treat bradydysrhythmias and extreme tachydysrhythmias; look for reversible causes of electromechanical dissociation (EMD)
- **Volume resuscitation**
  1. IV access: two large bore catheters, central venous catheter, intraarterial line once stabilized; consider pulmonary artery catheter if shock is unresponsive to volume and vasoactive drugs
  2. Administer IV fluids: crystalloids (initially 20 cc/kg, approximately 25% of crystalloids will remain in intravascular space so anticipate edema)
- If the patient is hypernatremic, do not allow sodium to fall more rapidly than 1 mEq/h (rapid fall decreases osmolarity and causes cerebral edema)
- Patients with sepsis may require > 40 cc/kg during the first hour and 100–200 cc/kg during next few hours
- Administer blood if there is significant blood loss (10 cc/kg packed RBC or 20 cc/kg whole RBC), type-specific if cross-matched unavailable, O-negative if profound hemorrhagic shock unresponsive to crystalloids
- If patient is coagulopathic, give blood components; evaluate response to each therapy (perfusion, heart rate, blood pressure, pulses etc.)

▶ **Base and Electrolyte Status** (see Fluid and Electrolyte Balance section for details):
- Acidosis: treat with improving perfusion, hyperventilation; use of bicarbonate is controversial and has not been shown to improve survival.

- Electrolytes: **glucose** (hypoglycemia develops in ill infants; continuous infusion preferred to bolus), **sodium** (alter slowly), **potassium** (children less sensitive to minor changes than adults, hypokalemia occurs with alkalosis due to intracellular shift and will normalize with pH restoration; hyperkalemia occurs with acidosis), **calcium** (ionized calcium precipitates with phosphate in blood products so levels will fall, alkalosis decreases ionized Ca, refractory hypocalcemia caused by hypomagnesemia; treat with CaCl 20–25 mg/kg (0.2–0.25 mL/kg) slow infusion; hypercalcemia in malignancy, if < 15 mEq/L not life-threatening; if 19–20 then renal and cardiovascular complications, treat with hydration and diuretics.

▶ **Vasoactive Drugs**
  - **Sympathomimetics**
    1. **Dobutamine** (2–15 µg/kg/min, β-1 effects with contractility and heart rate, β-2 causes peripheral vasodilatation so poor choice if hypotensive)
    2. **Dopamine** (2–5 µg/kg/min causes dopaminergic effects with ↑ renal perfusion; 5–20 µg/kg/min has β-1 effects)
    3. **Epinephrine** (0.05–0.5 µg/kg/min, β-1 β-2 and α effects, good for bradycardia or spinal shock; consider adding dopamine as it causes splanchnic/renal vasoconstriction)
    4. **Isoproterenol** (0.05–1.5 µg/kg/min, β-1 and β-2 effects with bronchodilation)
    5. **Norepinephrine** (0.1–1 µg/kg/min; α and β effects with renal/splanchnic vasoconstriction)
    6. **Amrinone** (0.75 mg/kg load then 5–10 µg/kg/min, ↑ intracellular cyclic AMP [cAMP] and delays intracellular Ca uptake causing improved contractility, arterial/venous dilation; good in cardiogenic shock)
  - **Vasodilators:** ↓ preload and afterload so requires concomitant IV fluids
    1. **Amrinone** see above
    2. **Captopril** (0.3–0.5 mg/kg PO q6–12h)
    3. **Enalapril** (5–10 µg/kg/dose IV q8–24h)
    4. **Esmolol** (50–300 µg/kg/min, β-1 blocker, effects take 30 minutes)
    5. **Labetalol** (0.25 mg/kg IV) α-1 and β-1 adrenergic blocker
    6. **Sodium nitroprusside** (0.5–10 µg/kg/min) metabolites include thiocyanate and cyanide

▶ **Gastrointestinal/Renal Support:** monitor urine output via Foley catheter, NG tube if there is a paralytic ileus, nutritional support.
▶ **Antibiotics:** cultures, broad-spectrum antibiotics, if immuno-compromised consider anaerobic, fungal, viral coverage.
▶ **Steroids:** consider treating with steroids (prior to antibiotics) if strong clinical picture of bacterial meningitis or if CSF is purulent. Steroids may improve neurologic/auditory sequelae particularly in *H. influenzae* meningitis but is otherwise controversial). Adrenal insufficiency may mimic septic shock.

DYSRHYTHMIAS

▶ **Normal Rhythm**
  • **Rate**
    1. Infant normal resting heart rate = 100–180 bpm
    2. Children < 10 years rarely have heart rate < 70 bpm, or > 140 bpm
    3. ↓ HR: vagal stimulation (breath holding, suctioning of nasopharynx), hypoxia
    4. ↑ HR: anemia, fever, pain, acute blood loss, anxiety
▶ **Premature Beats**
  • **Premature atrial contractions**
    1. **General:** premature depolarization of an atrial focus, common in infants and children, benign
    2. **Clinical:** may describe fluttering or "heart stops"
    3. **ECG:** the ectopic P wave is premature and has different morphology
    4. **Manage** with reassurance
  • **Premature ventricular contractions**
    1. **Etiology:** premature depolarization of ventricular focus or reentry
    2. **ECG:** premature QRS, different configuration, usually prolonged (infant > 0.08 seconds, child > 0.09 seconds), followed by compensatory pause, may be uniform or multiform
    3. Uniform PVCs in healthy child are generally benign
    4. PVCs in couplets, multiform, or increase with exercise should prompt evaluation for cardiac abnormality
    5. In ill children may be secondary to hypoxia, acidosis, hypokalemia, hyperkalemia, hypoglycemia

► **Tachydysrhythmias**
  • **Supraventricular tachycardia (SVT)**
    1. **General**
        a. Most common symptomatic dysrhythmia in infants and children
        b. Most commonly due to reentry circuit; associated with Wolff-Parkinson-White (WPW) conduction disturbance
    2. **ECG**
        a. Rate: infants as high as 300 bpm and usually > 220 bpm, adolescents 120–160 bpm
        b. Narrow complex QRS
        c. 25% of children with SVT have WPW on postconversion ECG
    3. **Clinical findings**
        a. Most patients uncomfortable but stable
        b. Low cardiac output and congestive heart failure (CHF) in patients with extremely fast rates
    4. **Management**
        a. If patient in shock: electrical cardioversion 0.5–2.0 J/kg
        b. If patient is stable: vagal maneuvers (unilateral carotid massage, Valsalva maneuver, diving reflex, blowing through occluded straw), adenosine (0.1 mg/kg rapid IVP) is drug of choice—maximum 6 mg. This can be followed by 0.2 mg/kg (up to 12 mg). Other choices include amiodarone 5 mg/kg over 20–60 min or procainamide 15 mg/kg.
  • **Atrial flutter**
    1. **General**
        a. Rapid atrial rates: 300 bpm
        b. Variable AV block: slower ventricular rate
    2. **ECG**
        a. Sawtooth appearance
        b. Seen best in leads II, III, aVF, V1
        c. Normal QRS morphology, but may be variable rate
    3. **Clinical findings**
        a. Symptoms related to ventricular rate
        b. Rapid conduction in AV node of infants—may cause shock or CHF

      c. Palpitations, dizziness, or asymptomatic in older children and adolescents

      d. Most older children with atrial flutter have underlying heart abnormalities

  4. **Management**

      a. Synchronized cardioversion 0.5–2 J/kg

      b. Medications under guidance of pediatric cardiologist

- **Ventricular tachycardia (VT)**

  1. **General**

      a. Defined as three successive extra systoles of ventricular origin

      b. Uncommon dysrhythmia in pediatrics

  2. **ECG**

      a. Ventricular rate usually > 120 bpm

      b. QRS duration wide in older children, may be narrow in infants

      c. Torsades de pointes: VT characterized by progressive changes in amplitude and polarity of QRS

  3. **Clinical findings**

      a. Multiple causes: acute myocarditis, congenital prolonged QT interval, metabolic (hypokalemia, hypocalcemia, hypomagnesemia), drug toxicity (quinidine, procainamide, amiodarone, sotalol, digitalis, tricyclic antidepressants, phenothiazines)

      b. Romano-Ward syndrome: prolonged QT interval; autosomal dominant; not associated with deafness

  4. **Management**

      a. Hemodynamically stable: lidocaine (1.0 mg/kg IV, then infusion of 20–40 µg/kg/min), procainamide (1 mg/kg IV q3–5min to total of 15 mg/kg or sinus rhythm), or amiodarone (5 mg/kg IV over 20–60 minutes)

      b. Hemodynamically unstable: immediate cardioversion 0.5–1 J/kg

- **Ventricular fibrillation**

  1. **General**

      a. Uncommon in children

      b. Disorganized depolarization not associated with cardiac output

  2. **ECG**

      a. Coarse or fine undulating line

3. **Clinical findings**
   a. Cardiopulmonary arrest, confirmed by absence of pulse
4. **Management**
   a. Defibrillate ×3 (2, 2–4, then 4 J/kg)
   b. Intubate, start CPR and obtain IV access
   c. Epinephrine 0.01 mg/kg of the 1:10,000 solution. May use 0.1 cc/kg of the 1:1000 solution (although high dose epinephrine is no longer emphasized by Pediatric Advanced Life Support, PALS), every 3–5 minutes
   d. Lidocaine (1 mg/kg IV), amiodarone (5 mg/kg IV to max of 15 mg/kg)
   e. Consider magnesium sulfate 25 mg/kg for refractory cases

▶ **Bradydysrhythmias**
  • **General**
    1. Definition for bradycardia: heart rate < 60 bpm
    2. Most common prearrest rhythm in pediatric patients
    3. Most clinically significant bradycardia secondary to hypoxemia
    4. Etiology: increased vagal tone, hypoxemia, hypothermia, head injury, acidosis, congenital heart block, heart transplant, toxins/drugs (β-blockers, clonidine, organophosphates)
  • **Management**
    1. Support airway, ventilation and oxygenation
    2. Epinephrine 0.01 mg/kg IV/IO (tracheal dose: 0.1 mg/kg of 1:1000 solution)
    3. Atropine 0.02 mg/kg IV/IO (minimum dose: 0.1 mg/kg)

▶ **Complete Heart Block**
  • **General:** associated with congenital heart disease, systemic lupus erythematosus (SLE), maternal connective tissue disease, Lyme disease, Rocky Mountain spotted fever, myocarditis, muscular dystrophy, myotonic dystrophy, Kearns-Sayre syndrome
  • **ECG**: no association between P and QRS waves
  • **Clinical findings:** most are asymptomatic
  • **Management**
    1. Transcutaneous pacing as bridge to transvenous pacing
    2. Sometimes improved with atropine 0.02 mg/kg IV (minimum 0.1 mg dose)

3.   Isoproterenol infusion (0.05–0.5 µg/kg/min)

FLUID AND ELECTROLYTE BALANCE

▶ Compartments: total body water (TBW) ranges from 80% weight in newborn to 60% in adult

▶ **Fluid Losses**
   • **Urine** (usually 40–60 cc/kg/d)
   • **Stool** (10–20 cc/kg/d)
   • **Fever** ($\uparrow$ insensible losses to 7 cc/kg/h for each degree [°C] rise over 37.2° C)

▶ **Dehydration**
   • Acute < 2 days (75% extracellular fluid, ECF)
   • Chronic < 7 days (50% ECF)
   • Average = 2–7 days (60% ECF)

▶ **Fluid Requirements:** calculate hourly maintenance fluid requirements according to **Table 2-7**.

▶ **Electrolyte Requirements**
   • Sodium requirement is 3 mEq/kg/d (extracellular)
   • Potassium is 2 mEq/kg/d (intracellular)

▶ **Osmolality**
   • Determines water distribution
   • Normal is 285–295 mOsm
   • Regulated by osmoreceptors in hypothalamus, which causes thirst and antidiuretic hormone (ADH) production, causing renal tubular absorption of water, which dilutes ECF, thus free water moves into intracellular fluid (ICF).
   • Plasma osmolality = $2 \times$ (Na) + (glucose/18) + (BUN/2.8)
   • Intracellular osmolality (K, PO_4, proteins) usually = plasma

TABLE 2-6
COMPARTMENTS—TOTAL BODY WATER (TBW) RANGES FROM 80%
WEIGHT IN NEWBORN TO 60% IN ADULT

ICF	75–80%
ECF	20–25%
Intravascular/plasma	
infants (80 cc/kg)	8%
adolescents (50 cc/kg)	5%
Interstitial	15%
Transcellular (secretions, peritoneal, etc.)	1–2%

ICF, intracellular fluid; ECF, extracellular fluid

TABLE 2-7
FLUID REQUIREMENTS (HOURLY)

≤ 10 kg	4 cc/kg/h
11–20 kg	40 cc + (2 cc/kg) for 11–20 kg
> 20 kg	60 cc + (1 cc/kg) over 20 kg
Examples:	
15 kg child:	40 cc + (2 cc × 5) = 50 cc/h
25 kg child:	60 cc + (1 cc × 5) = 65 cc/h

Acid Base

▶ Regulated by:
  - Kidney (response 24–48 hours) and respiratory (tidal volume or rate)
  - $(H+) + HCO_3 \rightarrow H_2CO_3 \rightarrow H_2O$ + dissolved CO_2
  - **Anion gap** = $(Na + K) - (Cl + HCO_3)$; normal: 8–12

  Wide anion gap metabolic acidosis (WAGMA) caused by **MUDPILES:**

    M—Methanol
    U—Uremia
    D—DKA
    P—Paraldehyde
    I—Iron/ibuprofen/inhalants (CO, CN)/isoniazid
    L—Lactic acid
    E—Ethanol/ethylene glycol
    S—Salicylate

▶ **Metabolic Acidosis**
  - Results from increase in hydrogen ions or decrease in bicarbonate
  - The P_{CO_2} ↑ 1.2 mm Hg for every 1 mEq/L drop in HCO_3
  - Correction of underlying condition is optimum treatment (treatment of shock)
  - Treat with improving perfusion, hyperventilation, use of bicarbonate is controversial and has not been shown to improve survival

▶ **Metabolic Alkalosis**
  - Results from increase in bicarbonate levels or a loss of hydrogen ions
  - The P_{CO_2} ↑ 0.7 mm Hg for every 1 mEq/L increase in the HCO_3
  - If symptomatic (cramps, weakness, paresthesia, tetany) or pH > 7.7, treatment = acetazolamide 5 mg/kg/24 h

▶ **Respiratory Acidosis**
  • Results from alveolar hypoventilation and CO_2 retention
  • The $HCO_3 \uparrow 0.1$ mEq/L for each 1 mm Hg increase in the P_{CO_2}
  • Treat by correcting the underlying ventilation problem
▶ **Respiratory Alkalosis**
  • May result from acute hypoxias, salicylate ingestion, or acute anxiety
  • The $HCO_3 \downarrow 0.2$ mEq/L for each 1 mm Hg drop in the P_{CO_2}
  • Treat by correcting the underlying problem

Sodium

▶ Na-K ATPase pump exchanges Na for K in 3:2 ratios.
▶ Volume sensors are in atria, RV, pulmonary interstitia, aorta, carotids, kidneys, CNS.
  • $\downarrow$ Volume causes renin/aldosterone production (vasoconstriction and resorption) and direct tubular stimulation to reabsorb water.
  • If hypervolemia is present then atria produce atrial natriuretic factor, which causes vasodilatation and inhibits Na resorption.
▶ **Hyponatremia**
  • **Causes**
    1. **Euvolemic:** polydipsia, syndrome of inappropriate secretion of antidiuretic hormone (SIADH), diuretics, CHF, hypothyroid, chronic renal failure, nephrotic syndrome, adrenal insufficiency, tricyclic antidepressants (TCAs), hypokalemia.
    2. **Hypovolemic:** vomiting/diarrhea, renal.
    3. **Pseudo:** hyperlipidemia, hyperproteinemia, hyperglycemia, mannitol. For each 100 mg/dL $\uparrow$ glucose, the Na $\downarrow 1.6$ mEq/L, i.e., true Na = (glucose − 100) /100 × 1.6 + serum Na).
  • **Treatment:** 3% NS = 4 cc/kg over 10 minutes if life-threatening.
▶ **Hypernatremia**
  • Na > 145 mEq/L
  • Usually vomiting and diarrhea cause TBW loss; or excessive salt intake leads to normal or $\uparrow$ TBW.
  • Causes CNS symptoms such as lethargy, weakness, change in mental status, seizures.
  • Intracellular dehydration means that rapid rehydration

with hypotonic fluids can cause cerebral edema. If cause is sodium overload then treatment is diuretics, oral free water.

Potassium

▶ **General Information**
- Primary control = ATPase pump and renal excretion (regulated by aldosterone).
- β-adrenergic stimulation ↑ ATPase activity and pushes K^+ into skeletal muscle.
- Insulin stimulates potassium influx into liver (glucose-independent).
- pH ↓ pushes hydrogen ions into cells, exchanging for potassium 1:1 (↓ pH 0.1 = ↑ K^+ by 0.5 mEq/L).
- Exercise releases K^+ from skeletal muscle cells.

▶ **Hypokalemia**
- Usually caused by transcellular shift (caused by alkalosis, insulin, β-adrenergic activity)
- GI losses
- Aldosterone excess (Cushing disease, renin overproduction, congenital adrenal hyperplasia [CAH], tumor)
- Hypomagnesemia (which prevents renal conservation of K^+).
- **Symptoms**: weakness, dysrhythmias (loss of T waves, U waves present), ileus, rhabdomyolysis if severe
- **Treatment**: if K^+ < 3 give 0.1–0.2 mEq KCl/kg/h IV; give $MgSO_4$ 25–50 mg/kg if dysrhythmias

▶ **Hyperkalemia**
- Due to: supplements, insulin deficiency with extracellular shift, metabolic acidosis, drugs (digitalis, succinylcholine, Aldactone, cyclosporin), renal failure (decreased excretion), CAH (most common is 21-hydroxylase deficiency)
- **Symptoms:** weakness, fatigue, ↓ deep tendon reflexes; ECG: peaked T → wide QRS/bradycardia → sine wave pattern
- If unstable patient: cardiac monitor at all times
- **Treatment:**
  1. **10% CaCl** 0.2 cc/kg bolus (**not** in digoxin toxicity)
  2. **Dextrose** 0.5–1 g/kg (2 cc/kg D25)
  3. **Insulin** 1 unit/4 g glucose (~0.1 unit/0.5 g)
  4. **Na bicarbonate** 0.5–1 mEq/kg
  5. **Nebulized albuterol** 5 mg

6. **Kayexalate** 1 g/kg with 70% sorbitol 3 cc/g
7. **Digifab** for digoxin toxicity

Calcium

▶ **General Information**
- 50% of body Ca is free ion, which is most active. $\downarrow$ pH = $\downarrow$ protein binding = $\uparrow$ free Ca ion.
- Controlled by parathyroid hormone (PTH) which:
  1. $\uparrow$ Bone resorption
  2. Stimulates kidneys to $\uparrow$ Ca reabsorption
  3. Directly $\uparrow$ PO_4 excretion.
- Also controlled by vitamin D which is converted to 1,25 dihydroxycholecalciferol which:
  1. $\uparrow$ Ca absorption in gut
  2. $\downarrow$ Urinary PO_4 loss
▶ **Hypocalcemia**
- Due to diet deficiency, hyperphosphatemia (causes negative feedback on PTH), vitamin D deficiency
- **Symptoms:** weakness, paresthesia, change in mental status, seizures, laryngospasm, dysrhythmias; if severe can cause prolonged QT
  1. Trousseau's sign: carpopedal spasm after 3 minutes of arterial occlusion
  2. Chvostek sign: facial nerve twitching with percussion
- **Treatment:** 10% Ca gluconate 0.5–1 cc/kg then 5 cc/kg/24 h
▶ **Hypercalcemia**
- Caused by endocrine derangements (PTH, vitamin D), malignancy, prolonged immobilization.
- **Symptoms:** weakness, lethargy, seizures, coma. May have abdominal cramps, dehydration (concentration defect), nausea/vomiting, polyuria/polydipsia.
- **Treatment:** 20 cc/kg normal saline (NS) bolus then run at $1^1/_2$– 2× maintenance; loop diuretics **after** hydration (Lasix). Avoid phosphates acutely as sudden death has been reported.

Magnesium

▶ **General Information**
- Co-factor for enzymes and DNA/RNA synthesis; 65% in bone, 34% protein, 1% in ECF (30% protein-bound); normal

level is 1.5–2.5 mEq/L; homeostasis parallels K^+ so if losing potassium, losing Mg.

▶ **Hypomagnesemia**
- Due to ↓ absorption (vomiting, diarrhea, short gut)
- ↑ Loss: renal (diuretics, renal tubular acidosis [RTA]), ↑ Ca, excessive bronchodilator use, endocrine (PTH, diabetes mellitus [DM])
- **Symptoms**: anorexia, nausea, weakness, psychological symptoms, hypocalcemia symptoms, bronchospasm (in β-agonist users), atrioventricular ectopy
- **Treatment:** $MgSO_4$ 25–50 mg/kg over 20–30 minutes

▶ **Hypermagnesemia**
- Usually only with severe renal failure, overdose in pre-eclampsia and excess enemas or milk of magnesia
- **Symptoms:** ↓ deep tendon reflexes, lethargy, confusion
- **Treatment:** 10% Ca gluconate 0.5–1 cc/kg if unstable (Mg antagonist); otherwise forced diuresis with diuretic and saline if normal renal function

Dehydration

▶ **Classification:**
- Hypertonic = Na > 145 (doughy skin)
- Hypotonic = Na < 130 (clammy skin)
- Isotonic = 130 < Na < 145
- **Etiology**
  1. Respiratory illness

TABLE 2-8
% DEHYDRATION

Clinical	< 5%	10%	15%
Mental status	—	Irritable	Lethargic
Eyes	—	Sunken	Glassy
Fontanelle	—	—	Sunken
Mucous membranes	—	Dry	Very dry
Tears	—	↓	Absent
Thirst	—	↑↑	Poor
Turgor	—	↓	Absent
Cap refill	< 2 s	2–3 s	> 3 s
Wet diapers	—	↓	0
HR	—	↑	↑
BP	—	—	↓

2. Emesis: pyloric stenosis causes normal Na and alkalosis, although if vomiting duodenal contents rich in HCO_3 then acidosis will be present
3. Diarrhea: toxigenic organisms cause Na and Cl losses, whereas enteroinvasive organisms cause loss of blood with Na and HCO_3
4. Viral: causes $\downarrow$ absorption of Na and H_2O
5. Renal: aldosterone deficiency, DM

- BUN is a POOR indicator of dehydration: anuria $\uparrow$ BUN by just 1 mg % per hour; a 50% $\downarrow$ in glomerular filtration rate (GFR) is required to double BUN
- $\uparrow$ Urine specific gravity of >1.030 confirms ECF depletion
- % Dehydration = (1 − [present weight/prior weight]) × 100

▶ **Treatment:**
- **Initial parenteral therapy**
  1. For patients in shock, rapidly administer initial 20 cc/kg of isotonic fluid (0.9 NS or LR).
  2. Reassess, if no clinical improvement give a second bolus of 20 cc/kg of isotonic fluid.
  3. Give third bolus (20 cc/kg of isotonic fluid) over 30 minutes if required.
  4. Monitor urine output and for signs of pulmonary edema (auscultation of chest and chest radiograph) **then** rehydrate over 24 hours.
  5. **Note:** The lactate in lactated Ringer (LR) solution is metabolized to bicarbonate in liver, which is not perfused if severe shock, so, 0.9% normal saline is more appropriate in a severe shock state.
  6. Hypotonic solutions or glucose-containing solutions should never be used for bolus resuscitation in the setting of dehydration.
- **Replacement therapy and maintenance**
  1. Calculate fluid deficit
     a. Fluid deficit (in liters) = normal weight (kg) − present weight (kg)
  2. Calculate solute deficits
     a. Sodium deficit: sodium loss = fluid deficit × percent from ECF (extracellular fluid compartment) × Na^+ concentration in ECF

TABLE 2-9
COMPONENTS OF ORAL REHYDRATION SOLUTIONS

Solution	Glucose (g/dL)	Na (mEq/L)	K (mEq/L)	Cl (mEq/L)	HCO₃/ citrate
WHO* solution	2	90	20	80	30
Rehydralyte	2.5	75	20	65	30
Pedialyte	2.5	45	20	35	30
Infalyte	1.9	50	25	45	34
Gatorade	2	50	20	50	34
Coke	10	3	0.2		13

* WHO, World Health Organization

   b. Potassium deficit: potassium loss = fluid loss × percent from ICF × K^+ concentration in ICF
 3. Calculate maintenance fluids and solutes
 4. Formulate and administer replacement fluids and maintenance fluids
   a. In the first 8 hours give $1/3$ maintenance + $1/2$ deficit
   b. In the next 16 hours give $2/3$ maintenance + $1/2$ deficit
 5. Do not forget to evaluate and replace ongoing losses (such as large watery diarrhea or frequent vomiting)

▶ **Oral Rehydration**
- Sodium is absorbed:
 1. with glucose across the cell membrane;
 2. with K^+ via ATPase pump;
 3. by solvent drag of water across ICF space;
 4. by $Na-H_2$ exchange (enhanced by intraluminal bicarbonate). It is disrupted by pathology, which causes luminal secretion of sodium. The optimal ratio for oral rehydration is 60 mEq Na: 2–2.5 g of glucose.
- Components of oral rehydration solutions: **(see Table 2-9).**
- WHO recommends 80 cc/kg over 4 hours PO, then if still dehydrated repeat again over 4 hours **or** calculate fluid deficit and replace **twice** that volume in 6–12 hours.
- Initially, try 10 cc/kg per feeding; increase amount as tolerated. If there are small amounts of emesis → cut back to 2–5 cc aliquots.
- Note: add 5–10 cc/kg for each diarrheal bowel movement.

NEWBORN RESUSCITATION

▶ **ABCs of Resuscitation**
- Do not focus on Apgar score
- Temperature control initiated at outset for all infants
- **A**—Anticipation, Assessment, Airway, **B**—Breathing, **C**—Circulation, **D**—Drugs, **E**—Extras, Evaluation

  1. **Anticipation**
     a. Recognize risk factors for depressed infant
        - **Maternal factors**
          Fetal distress, cephalopelvic disproportion, cord accident, trauma, precipitous delivery, hypotension, hypoxia, general anesthetics, opiates, sedatives, benzodiazepines, $MgSO_4$
        - **Uteroplacental factors**
          Placenta previa, abruptio placentae, vasa previa, toxemia, diabetes
        - **Fetal factors**
          Prematurity, postmaturity, congenital anomalies
     b. Assemble full team of appropriate providers for mother and infant
     c. Anticipate need for specific resources, such as O-negative blood, equipment (appropriate for premature newborn)

  2. **Assessment**
     a. Rapid general assessment of infant while initiating resuscitation

  3. **Airway**
     a. Consider a congenital malformation of the airway causing obstruction:
        - Micrognathia, macroglossia, congenital goiter, cystic hygroma, vocal cord paralysis, subglottic stenosis, subglottic tumors
     b. Excessive secretions:
        - Amniotic fluid, cervical mucous, meconium
        - Turn head to side and suction buccal pouch
        - Pharyngeal stimulation may cause vagal-mediated dysrhythmias and apnea
     c. Meconium:
        - Complicates 10–18% of pregnancies
        - Oropharyngeal suctioning before delivery
        - ET intubation for depressed infants, thick particulate meconium, or fetal distress

      d. Positive pressure ventilation:
- Start in any newborn with heart rate < 100 bpm
- Position head and neck in midline and slightly extended
- If heart rate not improved after 30–45 seconds of bag-mask ventilation, then intubate
- Estimate ETT size from birth weight

4. **Breathing**
    a. Ventilation
- Initially in depressed infant, inflate gradually to peak pressure of 20–40 cm H_2O for 3–5 seconds
- Then inflate at rate of 40 breaths/min
- If prolonged bag-mask ventilation, place orogastric tube

5. **Circulation**
    a. Bradycardia
- First priority is providing adequate ventilation and oxygenation
- Usually reverses reflex bradycardia due to hypoxia
- Bradycardia persisting > 30–60 seconds after ventilation requires cardiac massage
- ↓ Intravascular volume
- Secondary to placenta previa, abruptio placentae, umbilical cord prolapse, severe Rh isoimmunization
- Volume expanders include normal saline, residual placental blood, O-negative blood
- Administer in 10 mL/kg increments and reassess

6. **Drugs**
    a. **Indications**
- If heart rate remains below 100 bpm despite adequate ventilation and cardiac massage

    b. **Medications**
- **Epinephrine** (1:10,000 solution): dose of 0.01 mg/kg, route IV, amount 0.1 mL/kg, or (1:1000 solution): dose 0.1 mg/kg, amount 0.1 mL/kg
- **Sodium bicarbonate** (0.5 mEq/mL): dose of 1–2 mEq/kg, route IV, amount 2–4 mL/kg
- **Naloxone** (1.0 mg/mL): dose of 0.1 mg/kg, route IV, IM, or ET, amount 0.1 mL/kg
- **Atropine** (0.1 mg/mL): dose of 0.02 mg/kg (minimum dose of 0.1 mg), route IV, IM, or ET

7. **Extras**
   a. Hypothermia: dry and resuscitate under continuous radiant heat
   b. Hypoglycemia: 10% dextrose in water at 70–80 mL/kg/day continuous infusion (may need umbilical venous catheter [UVC] or umbilical arterial catheter [UAC] line)

ACUTE DISTRESS IN THE NEONATE AND POSTNATAL PERIOD
Acute Distress in the Neonate

▶ **Asphyxia Neonatorum**
  - **Predisposing factors**
    1. **Maternal factors:** hypoxia, anemia, hypotension, hypertension, prolapsed cord
    2. **Fetal factors:** placenta previa, placental abruption, fetal-maternal hemorrhage, hypotension, immature lungs
  - **Diagnostic findings**
    1. Can affect all organ systems:
       a. Common signs include hypotension, pallor, metabolic acidosis, apnea, periodic breathing
       b. Variable heart rate, may be slower than expected in presence of hypotension
       c. Acute renal failure, renal tubular necrosis
       d. **Encephalopathy**
          Stage 1: hyper-alert, easily aroused, normal respiratory pattern, jittery, excellent chances for full recovery
          Stage 2: somnolent, withdraws from painful stimuli, slowly improves over 24–48 hours, or deteriorates to seizures and apnea
          Stage 3: unarousable, seizures, signs of brain stem dysfunction
    2. Lab abnormalities include hypoglycemia, hyponatremia, hypocalcemia
  - **Management**
    1. **Stage 1** hypoxic encephalopathy: primarily observation, correct hypovolemia with 10 mL/kg of crystalloid
    2. **Stage 2 and 3** encephalopathy require intubation for apnea, periodic breathing, or seizures
    3. **Acidosis:** correct with fluid replacement

      a. Crossmatched whole blood or type O-negative blood is fluid of choice for hypovolemia

      b. Normal saline or LR if blood not immediately available

4. **Seizures**

      a. Phenobarbital (20–30 mg/kg IV) is drug of choice, additional dose (10 mg/kg) if no response

      b. Dilantin (10–20 mg/kg IV slowly) for seizures unresponsive to phenobarbital

► **Acute Respiratory Distress**

• **Respiratory distress syndrome (RDS)**

1. **General:** affects 1% of all live births in United States, occurs primarily in premature infants

2. **Pathophysiology:** underlying cause is surfactant deficiency

      a. Surfactant deficiency leads to atelectasis, alveolar hypoxia, and hypoxemia

3. **Diagnostic findings**

      a. Hallmark is decreased pulmonary compliance

      b. Intercostal, subcostal, suprasternal retractions, grunting respirations, tachypnea, nasal flaring, cyanosis

      c. Hypoxia with mixed metabolic and respiratory acidosis

      d. Hypoxia improves with supplemental oxygen

      e. Chest x-ray shows hypoinflation of lungs; severe disease may have "white out" of lungs

4. **Management**

      a. Supplemental oxygen to keep arterial PO_2 between 50 and 70 mm Hg

      b. Endotracheal intubation for severe RDS ($PCO_2 > 55$ mm Hg, or hypoxemia in presence of supplemental O_2)

      c. IV access for fluids and glucose (UAC or UVC line)

      d. Surfactant replacement (only in consultation with a neonatologist)

• **Meconium aspiration syndrome**

1. **Pathophysiology**

      a. Amniotic fluid composed of lung liquid, sloughed skin, vernix, sometimes blood and meconium

      b. Cause obstructive lung disease and chemical pneumonitis

      c. Meconium present in 10–20% of all term deliveries

2. **Diagnostic findings**
   a. Often postterm
   b. History of meconium-stained fluid, stained nail beds, umbilical cord, and meconium in ear canals
   c. Variable respiratory distress, coarse lung fields on auscultation
   d. Chest x-ray with patchy infiltrates, hyperaerated lung fields

3. **Management**
   a. Prevention: suction (with bulb) before delivery of chest, and immediately after birth
   b. If vigorous infant, do not perform tracheal suctioning even if meconium-stained amniotic fluid
   c. Tracheal intubation and suctioning if thick particulate meconium and depressed infant (poor respiratory effort, heart rate < 100 bpm, poor tone)
   d. Intubation if severe respiratory distress

- **Persistent pulmonary hypertension**
  1. **Pathophysiology**
     a. Pulmonary vascular resistance remains elevated after birth
     b. Deoxygenated blood shunted away from lungs through ductus arteriosus and foramen ovale

  2. **Diagnostic findings**
     a. Tachypnea, respiratory distress, right ventricular heave, no split second heart sound
     b. Differential oxygenation of upper and lower extremities (higher in upper)
     c. O_2 saturation monitor on right hand will have 10–15% higher saturation than right foot

  3. **Management**
     a. 100% supplemental oxygen
     b. IV fluids
     c. Echocardiogram to rule out cardiac lesions (i.e., coarctation of the aorta)
     d. Extra Corporeal Membrane Oxygenation (ECMO)

- **Upper airway obstruction**
  1. Uncommon in newborns
  2. **Etiology**: subglottic stenosis, laryngeal web, choanal atresia, posterior pharyngeal web, subglottic tumors,

micrognathia, congenital goiter, cystic hygroma, vocal cord paralysis, thyroglossal duct cysts, brachial cleft cysts

3. **Diagnostic findings**
   a. Inspiratory stridor, retractions
   b. Cyanosis at rest that improves with crying suggests choanal atresia

4. **Management**
   a. Positioning, oral or nasal airway placed, or intubation
   b. Micrognathia: obstruction from tongue, place prone on several blankets so head suspends forward

- **Lower airway anomalies**
  1. **Rare**
     a. Etiology includes tracheoesophageal fistulas, congenital lobar emphysema, bronchogenic cyst, diaphragmatic hernia, hypoplastic lungs

  2. **Diagnostic findings**
     a. Diaphragmatic hernia: scaphoid abdomen, immediate respiratory distress after birth, majority with cardiac impulse displaced to right
     b. Hypoplastic lungs: immediate postdelivery respiratory distress, generally born to mothers with oligohydramnios
     c. Chest x-ray helps diagnose almost all lower airway anomalies:
        - Abdominal contents in chest cavity in diaphragmatic hernia
        - Tracheoesophageal fistula often with air outlining esophageal pouch, or after attempted placement of oral-gastric tube confirms esophageal atresia
        - Bronchogenic cyst, congenital lobar emphysema, cystic adenomatoid, all diagnosed with chest x-ray

  3. **Management**
     a. Supportive
        - Intubation and ventilation for respiratory failure
        - Orogastric tube placement in diaphragmatic hernia (prevent gastric distension)
        - Transfer to neonatal intensive care unit

- **Narcotic depression**
  1. Narcotics like heroin, morphine, or meperidine lead to respiratory distress and apnea

      a. More common for infants receiving intrauterine narcotics within 4 hours of delivery

  2. **Diagnostic findings**
      a. Apnea, irregular breathing, decreased muscle tone
      b. If untreated, leads to cyanosis and bradycardia
  3. **Management**
      a. Naloxone 0.1 mg/kg IV or endotracheally

Postnatal Emergencies

▶ **Cardiovascular Disorders**
- **Congestive heart failure**
  1. **Etiology**
     a. Hypoplastic left heart, coarctation of the aorta, ventricular septal defect, truncus arteriosus, endocardial cushion defect, aortic stenosis, patent ductus arteriosus, arteriovenous malformations
     b. Dysrhythmias
  2. **Diagnostic findings**
     a. Signs and symptoms can be nonspecific
        - Poor feeding, tires quickly with feeding, pallor, respiratory symptoms
        - Retractions, grunting, rales on auscultation
        - Aortic stenosis and hypoplastic left heart: poor peripheral pulses in all extremities
        - Coarctation of the aorta: ↑ pulses upper extremities, absent or ↓ in lower extremities
        - Hepatomegaly
        - Chest x-ray: ↑ pulmonary vascular markings, enlarged heart
  3. **Management**
     a. Oxygen and ventilatory support, IV access
     b. Furosemide 1 mg/kg IV
     c. IV dopamine for inotropic support
- **Cyanotic heart disease**
  1. Tetralogy of Fallot, Truncus arteriosus, Transposition of the great vessels, Tricuspid atresia, Total anomalous venous return, pulmonary atresia
  2. **Diagnostic findings**
     a. Hallmark is cyanosis
        - Chest x-ray is clear or has decreased vascular markings

- Comparison of arterial PO_2 on room air and with 100% oxygen: improves in pulmonary disease, but not with cyanotic heart disease
▶ **Endocrine and Metabolic Disorders**
- **Ambiguous genitalia/congenital adrenal hyperplasia**
  1. **General information**
     a. Congenital adrenal hyperplasia is most common cause of female virilization and male precocious puberty
     b. Suspect in any infant with shock, hyponatremia, and hyperkalemia
        - Confirm diagnosis by elevated urinary excretion of 17-ketosteroids and elevated plasma ACTH
- **Hypocalcemia**
  1. **General information**
     a. Defined as plasma concentration < 7.0 mg/dL
     b. Early onset: occurs in first 72 hours of life, associated with premature infants, birth asphyxia, diabetic mothers
     c. Late onset: high-phosphate formulas, maternal hyperparathyroidism, congenital hypoparathyroidism, hypomagnesemia
  2. **Diagnostic findings**
     a. Signs: jitteriness, poor feeding, tetany ($\uparrow$ muscle activity, twitching, vomiting, carpopedal spasm, clonus), laryngospasm, clonic seizures
  3. **Management**
     a. Obtain magnesium and serum protein or ionized calcium level
     b. For hypocalcemic seizures: calcium gluconate (10%) 100–300 mg/kg IV (1–3 mL/kg at 1 mL/min) (watch for bradycardia)
     c. For hypomagnesemia: magnesium sulfate 20 mg/kg IV (watch for respiratory depression)
- **Hypoglycemia**
  1. **Definition**
     a. Premature infants: whole blood glucose < 20 mg/dL, or plasma glucose < 25 mg/dL
     b. In first 3 days of life: whole blood glucose < 30 mg/dL, or plasma glucose < 35 mg/dL
     c. After first 3 days: whole blood glucose < 40 mg/dL, or plasma glucose < 45 mg/dL

2. **Etiology**
    a. ↓ Glycogen store (prematurity, small for gestational age)
    b. Metabolic (amino acid disorders, galactosemia, glycogen storage disease)
    c. Hyperinsulinism (diabetic mother, insulin-secreting tumor, Beckwith-Wiedemann syndrome)
    d. Sepsis, asphyxia, polycythemia
3. **Diagnostic findings**
    a. Clinical findings: lethargy, obtundation, hypotonia, jitteriness, seizures, apnea
4. **Management**
    a. 0.25–0.5 g/kg of glucose IV (given as 3–5 mL/kg of 10% dextrose IV)
    b. Then start continuous IV infusion of 10% dextrose at 4 mL/kg/h
    c. If no IV access, give glucagon 0.1 mg/kg IM

► **Gastrointestinal Disorders**
  • **Abdominal wall defects**
    1. Include: omphalocele, gastroschisis, omphalomesenteric duct
    2. **Management**
        a. Orogastric tube placement
        b. Cover exposed intestines with saline soaked sterile gauze
        c. IV fluids
        d. Pediatric surgery consult
  • **Bowel obstruction/perforation**
    1. **Numerous potential causes**
        a. Hypertrophic pyloric stenosis, ileus, gastric perforation, duodenal atresia, imperforate anus, intussusception, annular pancreas, intestinal atresia, necrotizing enterocolitis, Hirschsprung disease, intestinal duplication, meconium ileus, malrotation with volvulus, peritoneal adhesions, hypoplastic left colon
    2. **Diagnostic findings**
        a. Upper intestinal obstruction: abdominal distension may be absent
            ■ Bilious emesis in neonate: assume malrotation with volvulus until proven otherwise

- Projectile vomiting and right upper abdominal mass: suggest pyloric stenosis (3–6 weeks of age)
  b. Lower intestinal obstruction
     - Abdominal distension
     - Vomiting is a late sign
3. **Management**
   a. GI decompression with orogastric tube
   b. Fluid resuscitation with isotonic crystalloid boluses of 10 mL/kg (repeat as clinically needed)
   c. Antibiotic coverage including anaerobes for possible perforation
   d. Pediatric surgical consultation

▶ **Hematologic Disorders**
- **Anemia**
  1. Hemoglobin in normal newborn ranges from 13.7–20.1 g/dL
     a. Anemia is hemoglobin < 13.0 mg/dL
     b. Hemoglobin drops over 8–12 weeks after birth to average of 11.4 ± 0.9 g/dL
  2. **Etiology**: three major categories
     a. Blood loss: (most common) premature cord clamping, fetal-maternal hemorrhage, early detachment of placenta from uterus
     b. Increased destruction of red cells: isoimmunization (ABO and Rh), inherited defects (G6PD deficiency), spherocytosis, hemolytic anemia due to infection (TORCHS, *Escherichia coli*)
     c. Impaired red cell production: (uncommon) vitamin deficiencies, congenital viral infections
- **Polycythemia**
  1. **Definition:** venous hematocrit value > 65%
  2. **Etiology**: Twin-twin transfusion, chronic *in utero* hypoxia, late clamping of umbilical cord, idiopathic
  3. **Diagnostic findings**
     a. Seizures, jaundice, renal vein thrombosis, respiratory distress, cyanosis
     b. Many are asymptomatic
  4. **Management** (for symptomatic patients):
     a. Partial exchange transfusion with isotonic crystalloid to achieve hematocrit < 60%

- **Thrombocytopenia**
    1. **Definition:** Platelet count < 100,000/mm^3
    2. **Etiology**
        a. Destruction by sepsis or congenital infections most common cause
        b. TORCHS infections, after exchange transfusion, immune thrombocytopenia, disseminated intravascular coagulation (DIC), entrapment within giant hemangioma
    3. **Diagnostic findings**
        a. Petechiae and abnormal bleeding
        b. Arterial or venous platelet count
    4. **Management**
        a. Platelet transfusion for bleeding infants or those with platelet count < 30,000/mm^3
- **Hyperbilirubinemia**
    1. **Unconjugated** (indirect) bilirubin is a normal breakdown product of hemoglobin
        a. Conjugated by enzyme glucuronyl transferase
        b. Glucuronyl transferase activity is low for several days after birth: leads to increased indirect bilirubin levels
    2. **Physiologic jaundice** is a result of elevated indirect bilirubin due to low activity of glucuronyl transferase
        a. Occurs in normal newborns
        b. Peaks on day 4–5 of life
        c. Infant appears healthy, feeding well, has no hepatosplenomegaly, and no underlying disease
    3. **Nonphysiologic jaundice**
        a. Causes include: sepsis, fetal-maternal blood group incompatibility, polycythemia, G6PD, spherocytosis, inborn errors of metabolism, hypothyroidism, direct hyperbilirubinemia
        b. Hepatosplenomegaly associated with hemolytic process, sepsis, TORCHS infections, congestive heart failure
    4. **Diagnostic findings**
        a. Physiologic hyperbilirubinemia: total bilirubin usually < 13 mg/dL, direct fraction < 10% of total
        b. Elevated reticulocyte count suggests hemolytic process

TABLE 2-10
GUIDELINES FOR PHOTOTHERAPY IN NEONATAL HYPERBILIRUBINEMIA

| | Total Serum Bilirubin (mg/dL) | | | | |
| | Postnatal Time | | | | |
Risk Category	24 h Day 1	36 h Day 1.5	48 h Day 2	72 h Day 3	96 h Day 4
High Risk (35–37 6/7 wks gestational age + risk factors)	8	9	11	13	14
Medium Risk (≥ 38 wks gestational age + risk factors, or 35–37 6/7 wks and well)	10	12	13	15	17
Low Risk (≥ 38 wks gestational age and well)	12	14	15	18	20

- For phototherapy in infants ≥ 35 weeks gestation
- Total bilirubin value is used
- Risk factors include: isoimmune hemolytic disease, asphyxia, G6PD deficiency, sepsis, acidosis, lethargy, temperature instability, or albumin < 3.0 g/dL
- Guidelines are for phototherapy use which is indicated when total serum bilirubin values exceed those values within the table

This table and the values herein are adapted from the American Academy of Pediatrics Clinical Practice Guidelines (Subcommittee on Hyperbilirubinemia) Management of hyperbilirubinemia in the newborn infant 35 or more weeks of gestation. *Pediatrics* 2004;114:297–307.

5. **Management**
   a. Phototherapy depends on gestational age, patient's age, bilirubin level, presence or lack of hemolysis, etiology of jaundice
   b. Cases of direct hyperbilirubinemia should be admitted for further evaluation. This includes obtaining urine analysis and urine culture as well as evaluation for sepsis if indicated by history and physical examination.
   c. Jaundice presenting at or beyond age 3 weeks, or sick infant: check results of newborn thyroid and galactosemia screen, and evaluate infant for signs or symptoms of hypothyroidism.

▶ **Infections**
   • **Bacterial sepsis and meningitis**
      1. **General information**
         a. Risk factors include chorioamnionitis, premature

rupture of membranes, maternal fever, maternal colonization with group B streptococcus

b. Common bacteria include: group B streptococcus, *E. coli, Listeria monocytogenes*

2. **Diagnostic findings**

a. Clinical signs and symptoms include: lethargy, temperature instability, jaundice, petechiae, poor feeding, tachypnea, vomiting, abdominal distension

b. May see neutropenia (< 2000 PMN/mm^3) or neutrophilia (> 16,000 PMN/mm^3)

c. Sepsis or meningitis confirmed by blood or CSF culture

3. **Management**

a. Hospitalization and intravenous antibiotics:
   - Combination of ampicillin (200 mg/kg/24h divided q6h) and cefotaxime (150 mg/kg/24h divided q8h)

- **Congenital infections**

1. **Etiology**

a. TORCHS: **T**oxoplasma gondii, **O** "other" rubella, **C**ytomegalovirus, **H**erpes simplex virus, **S**yphilis

b. Human immunodeficiency virus (HIV)

2. **Diagnostic findings**

a. May have no signs or symptoms early in newborn period

b. Findings may include: intrauterine growth retardation, pneumonia, hepatosplenomegaly, dermal erythropoiesis, jaundice, hearing deficits, retinopathy, encephalitis, cataracts, corneal clouding

c. Classic vesicular lesions of herpes infection only present in 50% of cases

d. Herpes simplex virus has an incubation period of 2–40 days

e. Serologic tests for syphilis, rubella, cytomegalovirus (CMV), *T. gondii*, herpes simplex virus, and HIV
   - CMV culture from urine
   - Herpes simplex virus from skin lesion scraping, CSF, and nasopharynx

3. **Management**

a. **Herpes simplex virus:** acyclovir 30 mg/kg/24 h divided TID

b. **Congenital syphilis:** benzathine penicillin G 50,000 units/kg IM single dose, if spinal tap is positive, then aqueous crystalline penicillin G 50,000 units/kg/24 h for 10 days

c. **HIV:** infants born to mother seropositive for HIV should be started on zidovudine 2 mg/kg PO q6h and referred to specialist

d. **Hepatitis B:** infants born to mother with hepatitis B, thoroughly bathe, hepatitis B immunoglobulin 0.5 mL IM and begin vaccination with hepatitis B vaccine

e. **Hydrops fetalis:** infants may require respiratory support

► **Neurologic Disorders**
- **Drug withdrawal**
  1. **Diagnostic findings**
     a. Symptoms appear 24–48 hours after delivery
     b. Irritability, fever, sweating, vomiting, diarrhea, decreased sleep time, seizures (uncommon: occur in 3%)
     c. Cocaine exposure *in utero* leads to small head circumference, irritability, jitteriness, vigorous sucking, and (rarely) seizures
     d. Drug screens are unreliable
  2. **Management**
     a. Admit to hospital
     b. Benzodiazepines, phenobarbital, paregoric may be used to treat symptoms (but only in consult with admitting service)
- **Meningomyelocele**
  1. Failure of neural tube closure
     a. Incidence approximately 1 in 500 births
  2. **Diagnostic findings**
     a. Obvious malformation over spinal column: contains neural elements and meninges
     b. Always have associated neurologic deficits
     c. Usually associated with Arnold-Chiari malformation of brain: may cause hydrocephalus
     d. Prenatal detection with α-fetoprotein and ultrasound

3. **Management**
   a. Cover meningomyelocele with saline-soaked sterile gauze
   b. Broad-spectrum antibiotics (ampicillin: 100 mg/kg/24 h and gentamicin 5 mg/kg q12h)
   c. Consult neonatologist

- **Seizures**
  1. **Etiology**
     a. Hypoglycemia, hyponatremia, hypernatremia, hypocalcemia, pyridoxine deficiency, birth trauma, asphyxia, intracranial hemorrhage, narcotic withdrawal, inborn errors of metabolism, CNS structural abnormalities
  2. **Diagnostic findings**
     a. Seizure activity may be tonic-clonic or subtle: staring spells, prolonged eye deviation, lip smacking, tongue thrusting, bicycling, apnea
     b. Microcephaly or macrocephaly denotes underlying structural brain abnormalities
     c. Bulging fontanelle indicates increased intracranial pressure (meningitis, intracerebral hemorrhage)
     d. Cataracts or corneal clouding may indicate congenital infections or inborn errors of metabolism
  3. **Management**
     a. Secure ABCs: intubate if necessary
     b. Phenobarbital 15–20 mg/kg IV load is first-line agent
     c. Phenytoin 10–20 mg/kg slow IV load or lorazepam 0.1 mg/kg IV are used for recalcitrant seizures (benzodiazepines may be used acutely if necessary)
     d. Identify underlying cause (i.e., hypoglycemia, hypocalcemia, hyponatremia, etc.) and correct
     e. IV antibiotics for suspected meningitis

▶ **Renal Disorders**
  - **Acute renal failure**
    1. **Etiology**
       a. Prerenal: hypoperfusion of kidney due to hypovolemia, hypotension, hypoxia, congestive heart failure
       b. Renal: multiple, including damage due to drugs or toxins, congenital malformations, asphyxia

  c. Postrenal: obstruction due to anatomic reasons (posterior urethral valves), or physiologic (neurogenic bladder)

 2. **Diagnostic findings**

  a. Prerenal: signs of congestive heart failure or hypovolemia

  b. Renal: history of traumatic delivery, maternal diabetes, sibling renal disorders

  c. Postrenal: inadequate stream in male neonate

  d. Should be suspected if urine output is < 0.5 mL/kg/h or BUN > 20 mg/dL

  e. Hyperkalemia is a late finding

  f. Fractional excretion of sodium < 2 in prerenal and > 3 in renal causes

 3. **Management**

  a. Place urinary catheter to rule out obstruction

  b. If prerenal cause treat accordingly (e.g., fluids for hypovolemia)

  c. Withhold potassium from fluids

▶ **Respiratory Disorders**

 • **Apnea**

  1. **Definition**: Cessation of breathing for ≥ 20 seconds; shorter if cyanosis, bradycardia, or pallor

  2. **Etiology**

   a. Central: apnea of prematurity, maternal narcotic use

   b. Infectious: meningitis, sepsis, pneumonia

   c. Metabolic: hypoglycemia, hypothermia, hypocalcemia

   d. CNS injury: hypoxic brain injury, seizures, hemorrhage

   e. Pulmonary: pneumonia, hyaline membrane disease, obstructive process

  3. **Diagnostic findings**

   a. Workup to reflect potential etiology

  4. **Management**

   a. ABCs as necessary

   b. Admission to hospital with continuous monitoring

 • **Bronchopulmonary dysplasia**

  1. **General information**

   a. Acquired chronic lung disorder

       b. Occurs in infants who required neonatal intensive care

       c. Prone to fluid overload and cor pulmonale

       d. Often require home oxygen, diuretics, bronchodilator therapy

  2. **Diagnostic findings**

       a. Hypoxemia and hypercarbia

  3. **Management**

       a. Treat hypoxemia with supplemental O_2 to keep O_2 saturation > 90%

       b. Chest x-ray to evaluate for viral or bacterial pneumonia

       c. Nebulized albuterol

       d. If fluid overload, treat with furosemide 1 mg/kg IV

- **Pneumonia**
  1. **Etiology**
     a. Group B streptococcus
     b. *Chlamydia trachomatis*
     c. Herpes simplex virus: type 2 (HSV-2)
     d. Cytomegalovirus (CMV)
     e. Respiratory syncytial virus (RSV)
  2. **Diagnostic findings**
     a. Range from mild respiratory symptoms to respiratory distress and shock
     b. Tachypnea one of most reliable signs
     c. Chest x-ray shows hyperinflation and interstitial or alveolar infiltrates
     d. Eosinophilia common with chlamydial pneumonia
  3. **Management**
     a. Admission to hospital
     b. Supportive therapy including supplemental oxygen and IV fluids
     c. Start empiric antibiotics: ampicillin (200 mg/kg/d) and cefotaxime (150 mg/kg/d)

- **Pneumothorax/lobar emphysema**
  1. **Etiology**
     a. Congenital lobar emphysema: unknown
     b. Pneumothorax may be secondary to congenital lobar emphysema
  2. **Diagnostic findings**
     a. Lobar emphysema generally presents between weeks

1 and 4 of life
- Primary symptom is dyspnea
- Respiratory distress, wheezing, hyper-resonance over affected lobe

b. Pneumothorax with similar signs, but rapid onset
c. Diagnosis of both confirmed by chest x-ray
- Lateral decubitus film differentiates between pneumothorax and lobar emphysema

3. **Management**
a. Lobar emphysema: bronchoscopy and possibly thoracotomy—urgent pediatric surgery consult
b. Pneumothorax: thoracostomy tube for moderate to severe cases, admission and observation for mildly symptomatic patients

CHAPTER 3

TRAUMA

EMERGENCY CARE OF MINOR WOUNDS

► Use nylon (Dermalon, Ethicon), Prolene, or fast-absorbing gut on the face.

► Use Dexon or Vicryl for deep layers: can take up to 40 days or more to absorb but loses tensile strength within 14 days. Lowest infection rate of absorbable suture types.

► Povidone-iodine is an excellent antiseptic with few toxic effects. Do not use any topical agents with detergent near open wounds as extensive necrosis can occur (i.e., Betadine scrub or Phisohex).

► Vermilion border laceration requires exact realignment.

► Through-and-through cheek lacerations carry a higher incidence of infection than lacerations through the external skin only; prophylactic antibiotics for 3–5 days have been shown to be beneficial.

► Puncture wounds of the foot through a tennis shoe are concerning for *Pseudomonas* infection.

► Silk sutures have a significant rate of infection.

► Plain gut sutures maintain tensile strength for approximately 7 days; they have high reactivity when compared to synthetic absorbable sutures. Good for mouth wounds.

► Chromic gut retains its tensile strength for 2–3 weeks and also has high reactivity and pyogenicity.

► Fast-absorbing gut breaks down within 5–7 days. There is a risk of ↑ pyogenicity, so it should only be used for clean wounds in well-perfused parts of the body.

► Denervated fingers do not sweat. Denervated skin will remain smooth when placed in water even after 15–20 minutes, while skin that has intact innervation will wrinkle.

TABLE 3-1
SUTURE REMOVAL TIME FRAME

Location	Suture Size	Removal Guideline
Face	Use 6.0 for skin sutures nylon or Prolene 5.0 Vicryl or Dexon for deep layers	3–5 days
Scalp	3–5.0 nylon or Prolene 4.0 or 5.0 Vicryl or Dexon for galea	5–7 days
Mouth	6.0 Vicryl or Dexon or 4.0 or 5.0 plain gut	Self-absorb
Hand	5.0 or 6.0 nylon or Prolene	7–10 days unless over a joint (10–14 days)
Trunk	4.0 or 5.0 nylon or Prolene for skin	7 days
Extremities	4.0 Vicryl or Dexon for deep sutures	7–10 days

▶ Glass fragments will be seen on x-ray > 90% of the time. CT or ultrasound can identify wood or other non-radiopaque foreign bodies.

▶ Do not blindly clamp and ligate bleeding arteries in the hands, wrists, or other major arteries.

▶ If hair needs to be removed, clip it with scissors or clippers, do not shave hair as infection can increase by 5.6%. Never shave or clip the eyebrows!

▶ Toxicity occurs if > 4 mg/kg of plain lidocaine or > 7 mg/kg of lidocaine with epinephrine is used.

▶ Lidocaine with epinephrine should never be used on the tip of the nose, fingers, toes, nipple, penis, tarsal plate of the eye, or ear.

▶ Suture removal time frame: (see **Table 3-1**)

▶ Tetanus prophylaxis guidelines: (see **Table 3-2**)

MULTIPLE TRAUMA

Overview

▶ Injury is the leading cause of death in children > 9 months of age in United States and accounts for:
- 22,000 deaths/year
- 600,000 hospitalizations
- 16 million seen in ED

TABLE 3-2
TETANUS PROPHYLAXIS GUIDELINES

Tetanus Immunizations	Administer Td	Administer Tetanus Immunoglobulin
Clean wounds		
Three or more within last 10 years	No	No
Three or more, but > 10 years	Yes	No
< three or unknown status	Yes	No
Tetanus prone wounds		
Three or more within last 5 years	No	No
Three or more, but > 5 years	Yes	No
< three or unknown status	No	Yes

► **Motor Vehicle-Occupant Injuries:** the leading cause of injury deaths among children up to 19 years of age and accounts for 47% of all injury deaths. Other causes include homicide, suicide, drowning, motor vehicle-pedestrian accidents, and burns.
► **Peak Seasons for Trauma:** spring and summer.
► Males more frequently injured than females.

Unique Pediatric Aspects

► Adult trauma usually results from penetrating injury.
► **Pediatric Trauma:**
  • It is mostly due to blunt injuries.
  • 80% of all injuries involve the head (big head with weak neck muscle supports a thin cranium) and 30% of pediatric death results from head injury despite the fact that children recover from head injury better than adults do.
  • Neck injuries: usually see contusions or hematomas; if fractured—usually C1-C2 in < 8 years of age.
  • Children have more heat loss due to higher body surface area to mass ratio.
  • Abdominal contents are more susceptible to injury due to immature musculature and less fat, especially liver and splenic injury.
  • Children are diaphragmatic breathers: more respiratory distress.
  • Skeletal system immature and children have more fractures.
  • Pediatric Trauma Score can be used to evaluate pediatric trauma patients.

TABLE 3-3
PEDIATRIC TRAUMA SCORE*

Variables	+2	+1	−1
Airway CNS	Normal Awake	Maintainable Obtunded/ LOC	Unmaintainable Coma
Body weight	> 20 kg	10–20 kg	< 10 kg
Systolic BP	> 90 mm Hg	90–50 mm Hg	< 50 mm Hg
Open wound	None	Minor	Major
Skeletal injury	None	Closed fracture	Open/multiple fractures

*A score of + 2, + 1, or − 1 is given to each variable, and then added (range –6 to 12). A score ≤ 8 indicates potentially important trauma.
LOC, loss of consciousness.

▶ **Patterns of Injury**
  • Waddell triad: child pedestrian struck by a car—fractured femur secondary to leg striking the bumper, chest or upper abdominal injury due to being thrown on the hood, contralateral head injury due to being thrown clear from car onto pavement. In the U.S., injuries usually are on the patient's left side.
  • Bicycle injuries: handlebar—blunt abdominal injuries, duodenal hematomas, head injury if not wearing helmet.
  • Shaken impact syndrome: < 1 year of age leads to severe neurologic impairment.

Primary Survey

Five Steps: ABCDE
▶ **A—Airway Management and Cervical Spine Control**
  • Inspect for foreign body, broken teeth, lacerations, jaw and tracheal deformities, and cyanosis
  • Pediatric Glasgow Coma Scale (PGCS) < 8, consider intubation to control airway
  • Place cervical collar until a physician can clear the cervical spine by examination or radiographs
  • Nasal intubation not preferred in children, optional in adolescents
▶ **B—Breathing**
  • Inspect for chest wall movement and any abnormal breathing

patterns such as retractions, grunting, flail chest, splinting, or ↓ breath sounds
- Evaluate for pneumothorax:
  1. Deviated trachea, unequal breath sounds
  2. **Diagnosis and treatment:** 14-gauge needle into 2nd intercostal space in mid-clavicular line and draw air or fluid back
  3. **Definitive treatment:** chest tube into 5th intercostal space at mid-axillary line

▶ **C—Circulation**
- Evaluate the following: capillary refill, heart rate, and blood pressure. Extremity deformities and abdominal guarding should raise suspicion of potential blood loss.
- Establish intravenous access (large-bore peripheral line). Intraosseous line can be used in children if IV access cannot be obtained due to shock.
- Fluid resuscitation for shock: LR or NS bolus 20 cc/kg. After three boluses use colloid blood products—these improve the stability of vascular volume and hemoglobin-oxygen carrying capacity → give 10 cc/kg quickly.
- Military anti-shock trousers (MAST): indicated for use only if weight is 25 to 35 kg or child > 6 years of age. Primarily used for pelvic or femur fracture stabilization but controversial as to benefits.

▶ **D—Disability**
- Neurologic responsiveness: can use Pediatric Glasgow Coma Scale (PGSC) system or AVPU (see Head Trauma)
- Pupillary size and response
- Spinal cord injury assessment

▶ **E—Exposure**
- Remove clothing to look at all possible injuries.
- It is imperative to take the temperature and cover areas not being directly examined with warmed sheets or blankets.

Resuscitation Phase

▶ Simultaneous with primary survey. It may include endotracheal intubation, needle cricothyrotomy, intraosseous access if no IV access after 3 attempts or 90 seconds.

▶ Obtain labs and radiographs as indicated by the patient's clinical status.
▶ Obtain past medical history using the mnemonic **AMPLE**:
  • **A**—**A**llergies/immunizations (tetanus status)
  • **M**—**M**edications
  • **P**—**P**ast medical and surgical history
  • **L**—**L**ast meal
  • **E**—**E**vent preceding injury

Secondary Survey

▶ The secondary survey is a detailed head-to-toe assessment.
▶ Measure all lacerations, bruises, and document them on the medical record.
▶ The back is examined as well as the front.
▶ All tubes are placed wherever they are needed.

HEAD TRAUMA
Epidemiology

▶ Leading cause of morbidity and mortality in children > 1 year of age in United States, with 250,000 hospitalizations and 25,000 deaths or permanent disability each year in children ≤ 14 years of age.
▶ Males sustain head injury twice as much as females and have 4 times the risk of suffering fatal head injury.

Pathophysiology

▶ Classified as primary versus secondary. Primary brain injury occurs at the moment of impact. It could be focal (penetration of foreign body such as knife, bullet, or skull fragment) or diffuse (nonimpact acceleration/deceleration forces). Secondary brain injury is due to neuronal death or systemic physiologic responses to the original brain injury.
▶ Autoregulation of cerebral blood flow is poorly understood but is probably dependent on interacting neurogenic, vasogenic, and myogenic mechanisms.
▶ Decreased P_{CO_2} causes cerebral vasoconstriction whereas ↑ P_{CO_2} results in vasodilatation (may be lost in ischemia).

▶ The brain swelling response of an injured brain is due to an ↑ in blood flow (cerebral hyperemia) not edema.

▶ Cerebral perfusion pressure (CPP) = mean arterial pressure (MAP) − intracranial pressure (ICP).

▶ When ICP ↑ > 15–20 mm Hg, interruption of cerebral blood flow begins.

▶ Initially ↑ in intracranial volume may be compensated for by downshift of CSF from skull to spinal dural sac.

▶ Children have more elastic skulls than adults and can tolerate ↑ ICP better, but pressure elevations are more common in children (80% of all head injuries).

▶ When sufficient ICP develops, skull contents follow the path of least resistance and herniate into spinal canal.

- **Two patterns:**
  1. **Central herniation:** clinically orderly progression of brain stem failure as the brain stem is compressed into the spinal canal.
  2. **Uncal herniation:** deterioration may be rapid and difficult to predict. Earliest signs are deterioration of consciousness, unilaterally dilated pupil (side of herniating brain from compression of CN III by temporal lobe). Later on, patient may have decerebrate posturing, contralateral extremity hemiparesis, and contralateral pupillary dilation. Finally, there is alteration of respiration, bradycardia, and hypertension (Cushing triad) followed by respiratory arrest.

Etiology

▶ Mechanism of head injury varies by age:
- Infants and children < 2 years old: fall from furniture or caregiver's arms. Consider child abuse if appropriate.
- Preschool children: falls (most), motor vehicle crashes (MVC) (~25%).
- School-age children/adolescents: equally—falls, sports, recreational activities, and MVC.

▶ Motor vehicle crashes have the highest morbidity and mortality in all age groups. Anatomically, the disproportionately ↑ head size in a child (versus adult), higher water content, and unmyelinated brain make them more susceptible to shear injuries.

However, the ability of the immature brain to "regrow" itself (inherent plasticity) accounts for better outcomes in children compared to adults.

Clinical Findings

Prehospital

▶ The history and a detailed description of the mechanism of injury is crucial in determining the extent of injury and priority of care.

▶ Suspect child abuse in:
- Any unexplained injury
- Discrepancy among caretakers as to mechanism of injury
- Explanations that are not consistent with the injury severity or the developmental level of the child
- Delay in seeking medical care
- Bruises, welts, scars, or burns on soft-tissue areas (old or new)

▶ **Past Medical History:** including any history of epilepsy, hyperactivity, hydrocephalus, bleeding diathesis, and intracranial malformations

▶ **Primary Survey:**
- Airway, Breathing, Circulation (C-spine control and immobilization)
- Neurology: pupillary examination (size and reactivity), level of consciousness (**AVPU**):
  1. **A**—**A**lert
  2. **V**—Responsive to **v**erbal stimuli
  3. **P**—Responsive to **p**ainful stimuli
  4. **U**—**U**nresponsive

▶ **Secondary Survey:** Identify potentially life-threatening situations and readdress interventions begun in the primary survey. Identify recognized patterns of injury:
- Waddell triad of injuries to the child pedestrian (chest-abdominal injury, leg injury, head injury— includes a contrecoup head injury that is serious and may not be obvious).
- Crush or impact injuries associated with parietal skull fractures should make examiner suspicious of epidural hematoma (middle meningeal artery).
- Child abuse injuries may be due to direct blows to skull or shaking injuries.
- The coup injury of shaken baby syndrome and other accel-

eration deceleration injuries may be associated with a high cervical spine injury even in the absence of external signs of trauma.

- Subdural hematoma is the most dangerous injury associated with child abuse and presents with coma, convulsions, and ↑ ICP.

- Seizures manifested after 48 hours of life are the most common presenting symptom of subarachnoid or subdural hemorrhage produced by birth trauma that may or may not be associated with external signs of trauma. Hematomas or cephalohematomas after newborn period may substantiate other findings of child abuse.

- Neurologic examination should be much more detailed than the primary survey including careful palpation and examination of the head and cervical spine, evaluation of motor and sensory functions, noting any asymmetry of function, flaccidity or spasticity, stereotyped posturing (decorticate, decerebrate), response to noxious stimuli, tests of brain stem function (i.e.,: doll's eyes), corneal reflexes, cold calorics, deep tendon reflexes, and funduscopic examination. Frequent neurologic examination is important.

- The Glasgow Coma Score (GCS) and its pediatric modification (PGCS) in younger children as well as the Pediatric Trauma Score (PTS) should be used to evaluate the child.

Complications

▶ Shock is usually not attributable to head trauma alone, so other sources should be sought.

- Exceptions include: epidural hematoma associated with a large fracture in children < 1 year of age, young children with large CSF spaces (hydrocephalus), and occasionally a large subgaleal hematoma in infants.

▶ Apnea after trauma is more common in children than adults, and is most likely related to transient impairment of the reticular activating system. This is usually transient and resolves with ventilation unless more serious brain or C-spine injury is present. Foreign body aspiration must be ruled out.

▶ Cortical blindness and migraines are thought to be variations of the same manifestation. Usually acute and resolves within hours to days.

TABLE 3-4
PEDIATRIC GLASGOW COMA SCORE (PGCS)*

Glasgow Coma Score	Pediatric Modification	
Eye Opening (≥ 1 year of age)	**Eye Opening (0–1 year of age)**	
4 Spontaneously	4 Spontaneously	
3 To verbal command	3 To shout	
2 To pain	2 To pain	
1 No response	1 No response	
Best Motor Response (≥ 1 year of age)	**Best Motor Response (0–1 year of age)**	
6 Obeys commands	6 Spontaneous	
5 Localizes pain	5 Withdraws to touch	
4 Flexion withdrawal	4 Withdraws to pain	
3 Flexion abnormal (decorticate)	3 Abnormal flexion	
2 Extension (decerebrate)	2 Abnormal extension	
1 No response	1 No response	
Best Verbal Response (> 5 years of age)	**Best Verbal Response (2–5 years of age)**	**Best Verbal Response (0–2 years of age)**
5 Oriented and converses	5 Appropriate words and phrases	5 Cries appropriately, smiles, coos
4 Disoriented and converses	4 Inappropriate words	4 Cries, irritable
3 Inappropriate words	3 Cries/screams	3 Inappropriate crying/screaming
2 Incomprehensible sounds	2 Grunts	2 Grunts/moans to pain
1 No response	1 No response	1 No response

*PGCS is the sum of individual scores from eye opening, best verbal response, and best motor response. PGCS of 13–15 indicates mild head injury; PGCS of 8–12 indicates moderate head injury; PGCS of < 8 indicates severe head injury.

► ↑ ICP must be recognized by the following signs and symptoms:
- Headache, lethargy, seizures, bulging fontanelle, pupillary dilation, Cushing triad (↑BP, bradycardia, and irregular respirations), projectile vomiting, dizziness, visual changes, unsteady gait, high-pitched cry, head tilt
- Signs of brain compression as well as Cheyne-Stokes respirations (cyclic crescendo-decrescendo respiration with a period of apnea between each cycle)

▶ Seizures are common after head trauma.
  • There is no prognostic significance of a sole seizure immediately after injury.
  • Approximately 5% of children hospitalized with head trauma have a seizure within the 1st week. 80% of them will not seize subsequently.
  • Another 5% will have a seizure after the 1st week.
  • Half will eventually stop having seizures.
  • 25% will continue to have seizures, and 25% will have > 10 seizures per year.
  • There is an ↑ risk of posttraumatic seizures in children with a PGCS of 3–8 upon presentation, patients in coma > 6 hours (almost 50%), intracranial laceration (versus concussion), subdural (versus epidural) bleeds, depressed skull fractures, and severe brain injury (GCS 3–5).
▶ **Posttraumatic Syndrome:** includes headache, irritability, nervousness, inability to concentrate, and behavioral or cognitive impairment
  • Motor skills and language function (receptive and expressive) appear to be more sensitive than intelligence.
  • Children < 3 years old at time of injury may be more vulnerable to persistent expressive language deficits.
  • Most children recover normally, although symptoms can persist for several weeks.
  • Posttraumatic syndrome may be difficult to differentiate from the premorbid state in children with previously undiagnosed attention deficit hyperactivity disorder.

Ancillary Data

▶ **Laboratory Studies:** CBC, type and cross, electrolytes, toxicology screens, blood alcohol levels as clinically indicated
▶ **Radiologic Studies:**
  • Skull x-rays: controversial but an essential part of the full skeletal survey in child abuse.
  • Computed tomography (CT): indicated in severe head trauma, instability with multiple trauma, or head trauma with focal deficit neurologic examination, posttraumatic seizures, amnesia, progressive headache, alcohol/drug intoxication, unreliable/inadequate history, vomiting > 3

times in 8 hours postinjury, loss of consciousness > 5 minutes after injury, or signs of basilar skull fracture.

- Magnetic resonance imaging (MRI): more sensitive than CT in detecting more nonhemorrhagic intracranial lesions, and is the definitive procedure to identify diffuse axonal injury. Less practical than CT for evaluating acutely injured or unstable head-injured child.

Management

▶ **Continue Primary and Secondary Surveys:** identify and correct pre-arrest syndromes (respiratory failure, shock and ↑ ICP).

▶ Osmotic agents such as mannitol are not used prophylactically but may be occasionally necessary to ↓ ICP (only after adequate fluid hydration).

▶ Anticonvulsants are only needed in certain injuries including acute subdural hematoma, open depressed skull fracture with parenchymal damage, brain contusions, or severe head injury (PGCS ≤ 8).

▶ Corticosteroids have little use in head injury (although useful in head tumors).

▶ The efficacy of barbiturate coma, hypothermia, and ICP monitoring is controversial.

▶ It is important to deliver adequate resuscitative fluids to the child in hypovolemic shock even if head injury is severe.

▶ Further management should reflect severity of injury.

Specific Clinical Entities

▶ **Scalp Injuries:** very vascular (can bleed profusely), control bleeding with direct pressure, irrigate well, rapid closure, tetanus prophylaxis.

▶ **Concussion:** transient loss of awareness and responsiveness with impaired consciousness. Amnesia is the hallmark (temporary, permanent, retrograde, or antegrade). May have headache, dizziness, vomiting, and a normal head CT. Most can be discharged unless there is loss of consciousness > 5 minutes, persistent symptoms, or inadequate home observation.

▶ **Contusion:** bruising or tearing of brain tissue, which is the most common brain injury found on CT. Symptoms include loss of

TABLE 3-5
MANAGEMENT OF HEAD INJURY

Head Injury	Description	Management	Outcome
Severe	PGCS < 8, or GCS ↓ with 2 or more (not attributable to seizures, drugs, etc.), focal signs on neurologic exam, penetrating skull injury, palpable depressed skull fracture, or compound skull fracture.	Prompt neurosurgical consultation and head CT. Intubation: (maintain C/spine immobilization) using RSI with premedication to avoid ↑ ICP. Do not hyperventilate. Keep PCO_2 about 30 mm Hg.	Poor.
Moderate	PGCS = 9–12, loss of consciousness for ≥ 5 min, progressive lethargy or headaches, post-traumatic amnesia, seizures, or signs of multiple trauma.	Injuries to other areas should be evaluated and treated, serial assessment with PGCS, CT scan, and neurosurgical consultation if patient deteriorates or no improvement.	Poor. Often associated with multiple trauma or child abuse.
Mild	PGCS = 13–15, momentary loss of consciousness (< 5 min), arrive awake, may be asymptomatic or complain of mild headache or dizziness.	Thorough physical exam. Patients with a GCS = 15 may be discharged with a responsible adult and a specific head injury instruction sheet.	Good.

RSI, rapid sequence intubation.

consciousness, disturbance in strength or sensation, visual changes, focal neurologic signs (seizures). Need neurosurgical consultation and hospitalization.

► **Skull Fractures:**
   • **Linear fracture:**
      1. Most common pediatric skull fracture (75%).
      2. Parietal bone is most common site and is associated with intracranial lesions in 48%; need neurosurgical consultation.

3. Most common complication is a subgaleal hematoma.
4. "Growing fracture"—a unique fracture in patients < 2 years of age: skull fracture with a dural tear. As the brain grows quickly, extrusion of brain or a CSF cyst (leptomeningeal cyst) through the dural defect prevents fusion of fracture margins. Needs neurosurgical correction.

- **Depressed skull fracture:** neurosurgical consultation
- **Basal skull fractures:**
  1. Clinical signs: hemotympanum, battle sign (purple color behind ear)—suggests posterior fracture; raccoon eyes (periorbital bruising)—suggest anterior fracture. May have blood or CSF drainage from nose or ears.
  2. Best diagnosed by CT.
  3. **Management:** neurosurgical consultation and symptomatic care. Prophylactic antibiotics are controversial.

▶ **Intracranial Hemorrhage**

- Most intracranial hemorrhage associated with birth trauma is subarachnoid, and most commonly manifests with seizures within the first 48 hours.
- **Epidural hemorrhage**
  1. Most commonly occurs in the lateral temporal fossa as a result of laceration of the middle meningeal artery or vein secondary to skull fracture.
  2. The classic picture of a brief loss of consciousness with a lucid interval and then clinical deterioration is more common in children but not consistent.
  3. CT scan will show a convex lens-shaped extra-axial fluid collection ($\uparrow$density).
  4. **Treatment** is surgical drainage and support.
- **Subdural hemorrhage**
  1. Caused by venous bleeding from disruption of the bridging veins across the dura.
  2. Slower time course because bleeding is not constrained by the tight dura and clot has more room to expand.
  3. Associated with underlying lacerations or contusions, and rarely with fractures.
  4. Classic feature of shaken baby syndrome, so abuse should be considered especially in child < 1 year.

5. **Physical findings:** full fontanelle, vomiting, lethargy, irritability, and occasionally retinal hemorrhages or bruising of the pinna.
6. CT scan: crescent-shaped hyperdense extra-axial fluid collection. Hematoma may be bilateral and located in the interhemispheric fissure in shaken babies.
7. **Management:** serial subdural taps in infants and burr holes in older patients.

Disposition

▶ **Criteria for Hospitalization:** documented prolonged loss of consciousness, coma, altered mental status, seizure, focal neurologic deficit, persistent vomiting, severe and persistent headache, alcohol or drug intoxication (interfering with a reliable examination), suspicion of child abuse, unreliable caregiver, infants and toddlers (difficult examinations), patients with underlying hydrocephalus or coagulopathy.

▶ Outcome is better for children than adults because they continue to improve for months.

▶ The family whose child sustains major head injury faces major stresses; early intervention by social and rehabilitation services is important.

FACIAL TRAUMA

Anatomy

▶ **Craniofacial Proportions**
- Newborn → 8:1
- 5 years of age → 4:1
- Adult → 2:1
- The peak age for face and head growth is between 3–5 years of age.
- The face is approximately 80% of the adult size at 5.5 years of age (facial fractures are rare before the age of 5 years).

Clinical Evaluation

▶ It is part of the "secondary" trauma survey.

► Associated with other injuries (cranial, cervical, spinal, thoracic, and abdomen).
► Oral airway preferred, especially with maxillofacial trauma: DO **NOT** attempt nasotracheal intubation—endotracheal tube could go into cranial vault!

Ancillary Data

► The Waters view is the most informative radiograph for fractures.
► Coned-down views of specific bones can be helpful.
► CT scan is an excellent tool for diagnosis of facial fractures along with other cranial abnormalities.
► Facial, chest, and abdominal radiographs should be considered when trying to locate a missing or an avulsed tooth.

Facial Soft-Tissue Injuries

► **Contusions and Abrasions**
  • Only the hematoma of the external ear and nasal septum must be drained to prevent cartilage deformity.
► **Burns**
  • 27% include face
  • Scald (#1), flame, flash, contact, chemical
  • Total Burn Surface Area (TBSA) in facial burns:
    1. Birth: 8.5%
    2. 1 year of age: 6.5%
    3. 5 years of age: 5.5%
    4. Adult: 3.5%
  • **Management:**
    1. Airway
    2. Consult surgeon
    3. Antibiotic cream (not Silvadene—may cause depigmentation)
    4. Wound care
    5. Corneal evaluation
  • Electrical mouth burn (cord bite)
    1. Watch for bleeding in the first 2 weeks
    2. Microstomia
    3. Admit if electrocuted
► **Lacerations**
  • **TAC** (**t**etracaine, **a**drenaline, and **c**ocaine): cocaine causes corneal abrasions, seizure, and death. Not commonly used and not recommended.

- **LET** (**l**idocaine, **e**pinephrine, **t**etracaine): the preferred agent
- Irrigate with normal saline; no Betadine in wound—impairs healing
- Suture along "wrinkle lines"
- **Lips**
  1. Align vermilion border
  2. Use buccal or submental block
- **Oral**
  1. Assess dental injuries
  2. Vicryl (if needed)
  3. Salt water gargles
- **Tongue**
  1. Most lacerations do not require any repair (make sure avulsed or fractured teeth are not embedded in the tongue).
  2. Tongue lacerations that require suturing:
     a. Deeper lacerations that go through both outer layers.
     b. Those that are $1/2$ the width of the tongue.
     c. Those that involve the tip.
     d. Those that bleed excessively.
  3. Absorbable Vicryl or gut sutures.
  4. A buried knot technique is preferred to minimize discomfort from exposed sutures.
- ▶ **Foreign Bodies**
  - **Oral**
    1. Remove (toy, wood, pencil)
    2. Assess palate and vascular structures
    3. Suture as needed
    4. Oral antibiotics and gargles
    5. Cautious if in hypopharynx: use topical anesthetic and remove
  - **Nasal**
    1. "Foul odor" purulent nasal discharge (commonly unilateral)
    2. Alligator forceps
    3. A topical vasoconstrictor such as 1% phenylephrine hydrochloride can be used to facilitate the removal.
    4. Treat sinusitis
    5. Both nares and ear canals should be inspected for other foreign bodies.

Facial Fractures

▶ Nasal (#1), mandible, maxilla, orbit, zygoma.

▶ Uncommon < 5 years of age because infants and children have a larger forehead and cranium which protects the face.

▶ Etiology: children: play and fall (bones more elastic, less brittle, less pneumatized), adolescents: motor vehicle crashes (MVC) and assault.

▶ Evaluate for CSF leak (clear or serosanguineous rhinorrhea or otorrhea). Diagnosis: test the fluid by the glucose oxidase reaction or obtaining a glucose measurement of > 50 mg/dL, step-off, crepitus.

▶ Evaluate for associated injuries to the parotid gland or duct, facial nerve (palsy or paresthesia).

▶ Plain films: Waters, Caldwell, Towne, lateral, frontal, submentovertex.

▶ CT: better for facial fracture (Panorex: best for mandibular fracture).

Frontal Bone
▶ **Basilar Skull**
  • Battle sign
  • Raccoon eyes = periorbital hematoma
  • Hemotympanum
  • CSF otorrhea or rhinorrhea
▶ **Management**
  • Linear nondepressed: observe.
  • Depressed or frontal lobe contusion, dural tear, or significant CSF leak: requires open reduction.
  • Most CSF leaks heal spontaneously within 1 week.

Frontal Sinus
▶ Uncommon (nonexistent) before adolescence.
▶ CT scan for air-fluid levels.
▶ Abscess formation is a late complication.

Orbital Floor
▶ **"Blowout" = Infraorbital Floor Fracture**
  • Upward gaze palsy (entrapped inferior rectus muscle)
  • Surgery required
  • Suspect if: lateral subconjunctival hemorrhage, infraorbital

nerve hypoesthesia, unilateral epistaxis, and abnormalities in orbital rim

Zygoma
► The arch fracture is usually the "greenstick" type.
► Suspect if:
  • Swelling, bruising, crepitus, or flattened malar area
  • Hypoesthesia in the distribution of the zygomaticotemporal branches of the infraorbital branches of cranial nerve V
  • Trismus = fracture fragments impinging on the coronoid process of the mandible.
► Surgical intervention if: depressed fracture (flattened malar area), or orbital complex is involved

Supraorbital
► Suspect if: hypoesthesia of the distribution of the supraorbital nerve, ptosis, exophthalmos, and limited extraocular movement (EOM).

Maxillary (Le Fort)
► **Le Fort I:**
  • Uncommon in children < 10 years of age
  • Includes: lower third of maxilla, palate, and pterygoid plate
  • Suspect if: flattening, edema or bruising over midface, split palate, or malocclusion.
► **Le Fort II:** through nasal bones, orbit floor, and pterygoid
► **Le Fort III:** same as II, but through zygomatic arches, with complete separation from cranium

Mandibular
► Falls on chin: symphyseal or parasymphyseal fractures associated with unilateral or bilateral condylar fracture.
► Lateral forces cause an ipsilateral angle or body fractures associated with contralateral condylar or angle fractures.
► Suspect if: facial asymmetry, malocclusion, trismus, open bite, mandibular shift.
► **Management:** plastic surgeon, otolaryngologist, or oral maxillofacial surgeon (OMFS) consult—mainly closed techniques. Open reduction is reserved for fractures resulting in malocclusion or poor jaw movement.

Nasal Contusions and Fractures

▶ More cartilaginous than adults
▶ **Septal Hematoma**
  • Evacuated immediately to prevent septal cartilage damage (saddle nose deformity, septal necrosis, perforation, or nasal obstruction)
  • Discharge with anterior packing
  • Antibiotics: always prescribe antibiotics if packing placed
▶ **Nasoethmoid Fracture:** flattened broad nose (evaluate other facial bones) and consult OMFS.

Ocular Injuries

▶ **Anatomy**
  • Enucleation: trauma (#1 cause), retinoblastoma, infection, inflammation, or congenital deformities.
  • CN III: levator palpebrae (opens eye) and pupil constrictor
  • CN IV: superior oblique muscle
  • CN VI: lateral rectus
  • CN VII: orbicularis oculi (closes eye)
  • Sympathetic fibers: pupil dilation
▶ **Eyelid**
  • Lid margin lacerations: refer to ophthalmology
  • Improper repair can result in: ptosis, entropion leaving cornea exposed
  • Rule out globe rupture and lacrimal system injuries (particularly with medial laceration)
▶ **Corneal**
  • Laceration: assess depth
  • Full-thickness corneal injury:
    1. Seidel sign: "waterfall" fluorescein—the fluorescein strip is touched directly to the site of injury. The aqueous humor dilutes the fluorescein and causes the stream of florescence at the site of injury.
    2. Pupil irregularities: secondary to globe penetration.
    3. **Treatment:** immediate ophthalmology consult, bed rest, atropine sulfate drops, an antiemetic and broad-spectrum antibiotics (IV cefazolin).
▶ **Ocular Foreign Bodies**
  • Lid eversion is essential.
  • **Treatment:** tetracaine, irrigate, and removal with a cotton tip.

▶ **Contact Lens Injury**
- Traumatic insertion: abrasions
- Lens overwear syndrome:
  1. Suspect if excessive wear of contact lens causing hypoxic corneal epithelium leading to death and sloughing of cornea over 2–4 hours causing severe eye pain.
  2. It occurs with both hard and soft lenses.
  3. **Treatment:** tetracaine, remove lens by gently touching the lens with the index finger while the patient is looking up and slide it onto the inferior conjunctiva. Here the lens is pinched and removed.
  4. Fluorescein examination with ophthalmology follow-up (no lens should be worn until then).

▶ **Blunt Ocular Injury**
- Rapid acceleration/deceleration or direct blow
- Immediate loss of vision: severe retinal or optic nerve damage
- Gradual loss: contusion of optic nerve or vascular occlusion
- Photophobia: traumatic iritis
- Diplopia: blowout fracture
- Flashes and floaters: vitreous hemorrhage or retinal tear
- Afferent pupillary defect:
  1. (Mild) hyphema, cataract, vitreous hemorrhage
  2. (Severe) retinal detachment or optic nerve injury
- Subconjunctival hemorrhage: resolve spontaneously in 2–3 weeks
- Conjunctival chemosis (swelling): rule out scleral perforation or rupture (conjunctival crepitus associated with blowout fractures)
- Hyphema: blood in anterior chamber
  1. Check intraocular pressure
  2. Late complications: glaucoma, optic atrophy, corneal blood staining
  3. Rule out sickle cell disease, hemophilia, leukemia, juvenile xanthogranuloma, and retinoblastoma
  4. **Treatment:**
     a. Cycloplegic
     b. Analgesics/non-ASA
     c. Hospitalization or close outpatient follow-up
     d. Aminocaproic acid (to prevent re-bleeding)

    e. ± Patch, steroids

    f. Consult opthalmology

- Traumatic iritis
  1. "Flare and cell"
  2. **Treatment:** homatropine
- Traumatic mydriasis
  1. Pupillary sphincter damage (transient or permanent)
  2. No ED treatment
- Traumatic cataracts: lens trauma (weeks to months later)
- Subluxation and dislocation of lens
  1. Zonules broken
  2. Present with "trembling iris"
  3. Surgical repair
  4. Rule out nontraumatic causes: Marfan syndrome, homocystinuria, and inflammation
- Scleral rupture
  1. Superonasal quadrant most frequently involved
  2. "Soft" eye
  3. Bloody chemosis
  4. ↓ Intraocular pressure (IOP)
  5. Afferent pupillary defect (APD)
  6. **Treatment: SANTA (s**hield, **a**ntiemetic, **N**PO, **T**d, **a**ntibiotics), and immediate ophthalmology consult
- Vitreous hemorrhage
  1. Poorly visible fundus
  2. Absent red reflex
  3. APD
  4. **Treatment:** elevate head, avoid Valsalva strain, ophthalmology follow-up in 24 hours
- Retinal tears
  1. Leads to detachment
  2. Associated with vitreous hemorrhage
  3. Ophthalmology consult
- Retinal detachments
  1. Can be permanent
  2. Appears as grayish flap out of focus with disk
  3. **Treatment:** immediate ophthalmology consult, bilateral patch, NPO, bed rest
- Retinal hemorrhages: suspect child abuse, ophthalmology consult

- Berlin edema (commotio retinae): appears as patchy whitening of the retina; sign of chorioretinal trauma opposite to the site of impact
- Choroidal rupture: yellow-white curvilinear scar concentric on disk (worse prognosis if macula involved)
- Fat emboli: yellow exudate "flame-shaped" hemorrhages; associated with long bone fractures
- Optic nerve injury: contusions; **treatment:** glucocorticoids or surgery
- Avulsion: permanent
- Retrobulbar hemorrhages
  1. Ocular emergency
  2. Ptosis, tense eyelids, variable vision loss, APD
  3. ↑ IOP can cause central retinal artery occlusion
  4. **Treatment:** mannitol, lateral canthotomy, digital massage, paracentesis, inhale CO_2

▶ **Penetrating Injury**
- Most frequent (BB gun, propelled glass or steel or lawn mower foreign body [FB]).
- Poor prognosis, often results in enucleation to avoid sympathetic ophthalmia affecting the nontraumatized eye.
- **Treatment:** patch; immediate ophthalmology consult; remove FB in operating room (within 24 hours); Td, antibiotics, antiemetics. Intraocular hemorrhage: vitreous or hyphema (CT for further evaluation of retina). Chorioretinal hemorrhage: poor prognosis with bleeding and scarring.
- Infection: traumatic endophthalmitis. **Treatment:** antibiotics.
- Chalcosis: sterile endophthalmitis due to copper-containing FB.

▶ **Chemical Injury**
- Acid
  1. Destructive protein precipitation limited to cornea.
  2. Better prognosis than alkali.
- Alkali
  1. Lime, lye, ammonia agents
  2. Penetrate cornea and cause coagulative necrosis
- **Treatment:** copious irrigation using Morgan lens (at least 1 liter of NS), corneal evaluation, test pH (it should be close to 7.4), contact poison center
- Ophthalmology consult if: corneal opacification, conjunctival blanching, ↑ IOP

- "Super glue": saline compresses or Neosporin ophthalmic ointment, evaluate for corneal abrasion
► **Radiation Injury**
    - Tanning booths: (ultraviolet keratitis) punctate fluorescein lesions
    - **Treatment:** cycloplegia, topical antibiotics, ± patch, analgesia
► **Thermal Injury**
    - Rare, superficial injury, like corneal abrasion (if necrosis: ophthalmology consult)

Ear Injuries
► **Foreign Bodies**
    - Lidocaine HCl: kills insects and provides analgesia
    - Avoid irrigation if food, paper (it swells)
    - Removal: alligator forceps, curette, super glue on Q-tip, suction
    - Refer to ENT if difficult
    - Rule out tympanic membrane perforation
► **External Ear Trauma**
    - Auricular hematoma: doughy mass. It needs drainage to prevent "cauliflower" caused by cartilage necrosis and formation of new cartilage (if bilateral: suspect abuse).
    - Lacerations: cartilage needs to be covered to avoid resorption.
    - Chondritis (infection of cartilage): 95% *Pseudomonas* mixed with *Staphylococcus* 50% of the time.
    - Amputations: wrap ear in moist sterile gauze; can replant.
► **Tympanic Membrane Trauma**
    - Diving, explosions, slap over ear
    - CN II, IV, V, VI, VII, VIII can be involved: requires immediate ENT consult
    - Rule out basilar skull fracture
    - Heals within 2–3 weeks, if not need ENT consult.
► **Middle and Inner Ear Trauma**
    - Tympanometry is required with ENT consult.

Dental Injuries
► **Development**
    - Primary-erupt: 6 months of age. Exfoliate: 6 years of age (imbedded in alveolar bone).

- Secondary: begin to erupt: 5–6 years of age.
- Enamel, dentin, pulp.

► **Injuries**
- Luxations: injuries to the periodontal ligament and alveolar bone. Parents must be advised of the potential for tooth discoloration.
- Concussion: tooth maintains stability with no displacement, but is tender to pressure or occlusion.
- Subluxation: tooth is mobile, 2 mm displacement but in socket.
- Intrusion: traumatic impaction, laceration of periodontal ligament.
- Extrusion: vertically dislodged.
- Avulsion: completely detached, severed periodontal ligament.
- **Treatment:** locate tooth (chest x-ray—rule out aspiration), store in Hank's Balanced Salt Solution, normal saline, milk or saliva, splint ASAP, and dental consult.

► **Fractures (Ellis Classification)**
- I: involves only the enamel (smooth edges as needed)
- II: involves the enamel and dentin (calcium hydroxide, dental referral)
- III: involves the enamel, dentin, and pulp (immediate dental consult, calcium hydroxide, composite repair)

NECK AND SPINAL CORD TRAUMA
Epidemiology

► Most frequent cause of spinal cord injury (SCI):
- 1st decade: motor vehicle crash (MVC), firearm injuries.
- 2nd decade: sports, MVC. Males have a higher incidence than females, > 2:1.

Anatomy

► **Cervical Spine**
- Most mobile joint space with greatest angular displacement is at:
  1. (C3/C4): 3–8 years of age
  2. (C4/C5): 9–11 years of age
  3. (C5/C6): 12–15 years of age

- Occipitoatlantoaxial complex
  1. C1 body (atlas)
     a. Two ossification centers at birth (usually): each center forms a lateral mass.
     b. Third ossification center appears at 1 year of age, forms anterior arch which fuses with lateral masses by 7–10 years of age.
  2. C2 (axis)
     a. Five primary ossification centers.
     b. Odontoid = dens process rests posterior to anterior arch of C1.
  3. Cruciate ligament = atlantal transverse portion + triangular ascending and descending bands.
  4. Atlantal transverse is the largest, strongest ligament: main stabilizer of atlantoaxial complex.
- C2 to C7 have up to three ossification centers
- Spina bifida occulta: retardation of the closing of the neural arches of the C-spine.

► **Thoracic Spine**
- T1-T10: considerable stability because of strong costal transverse and intertransverse ligaments
- T11-L1: more vulnerable to osseoligamentous injuries (lack of rib splinting)
- L1-L2: spinal cord terminates as the conus medullaris

► **Sacral/Coccygeal Spine**
- Relatively stable
- Innervates the perineum, bowel, bladder, and legs

► **Spinal Cord**
- Midbrain to L1/L2
- Diameter enlarges at C5-C6 (origin of brachial plexus)
- Elasticity and plasticity limited by pia mater
- Anterior spinal artery runs on ventral surface of cord
- White matter tracts: anterior and lateral corticospinal, lateral vestibulospinal, spinocerebellar, spinothalamic
- Gray matter: lies deep to white, consists of ventral and dorsal horns, central canal
- Relative hypermobility of cervical and dorsolumbar junction ↑ frequency of spinal cord injuries in these areas
- Odontoid fracture: most common osseous injury, mostly without neurologic disability.

Pathophysiology

▶ Immature spine ossifies progressively throughout childhood, therefore younger children sustain avulsions or epiphyseal separations instead of true fracture.

▶ Hypermobility with large head and weak neck musculature: ↑ risk of injuries with acceleration and torsion forces

▶ Theories on traumatic injury to cord leading to ischemia and loss of neurologic function:
  • Calcium flux causes lipid peroxidation.
  • Initiates free radical reactions, and alters spinal blood flow by arachidonic acid metabolism.
  • Calcium compromises respiratory function or neuronal mitochondria.

Mechanism of Injury

▶ **Most Common C-spine Lesions** (in children < 8 years of age):
  • Odontoid fracture
  • Atlantoaxial dislocation or subluxation
  • Hyperextension fracture of axis
  • Small % of neurologic deficits because of "large diameter of spinal canal at C1"

▶ **Flexion**
  • Hyperflexion: most common.
  • Posterior elements disrupted: ligamentum flavum, facet capsules, interspinous ligaments.
  • Clay-Shoveler fracture: avulsion of spinous process at C6, C7, or T1.
  • Flexion teardrop: triangular bony fragment displaced anteriorly from anteroinferior portion of the vertebral body. It may be associated with neurologic damage.

▶ **Extension**
  • Anterior longitudinal ligament distracted and posterior elements compressed.
  • Hangman's fracture of the posterior neuronal arch of C1 or pedicles of C2.
  • C4-5 most common.
  • Buckling of the ligamentum flavum into the posterior spinal canal can produce central or posterior cord syndromes.

▶ **Axial Loading/Vertical Compression**
- Anterior cord: compression of nucleus pulposus which compromises anterior spinal canal.
- Jefferson burst: bilateral displacement of articular mass of C1 relative to lateral margins of C2.

▶ **Rotation**
- Facet fracture or dislocation
- Unstable articular process fracture in the lumbar region

Diagnostic Findings

▶ Observe breathing patterns: loss of diaphragmatic breathing, hypoventilation, or apnea may be due to injuries to C3, C4, C5 which supply the phrenic nerve.

▶ **Spinal Shock:** bradycardia with severe hypotension with warm skin due to vasodilation.

▶ **Central Cord:** (hyperextension) "burning dysesthesias" in hands.

▶ **Motor Deficits:** purposeful and spontaneous, lower motor neuron (flaccidity), upper motor neuron (spasticity with hyperreflexia).

▶ Mass flexion withdrawal movements in response to stimulation may occur in infants with paralyzed limbs and may be indistinguishable from normal movements.

▶ Rectal tone is important prognostically; if it is present, sacral sparing is implied with subsequent partial or complete recovery in up to 30–50%. Its absence implies 2–3% chance of partial or complete recovery.

▶ Sensory/reflex level of deficit: (see **Table 3-6**).

▶ Key points to remember during the neurologic examination:
- Sensory and motor examinations should be performed bilaterally
- External anal sphincter after insertion of the examiner's finger includes testing (graded as absent or present) of the following:
  1. Perceived sensation
  2. Contractions around the examiner's finger
- The strength of each muscle is graded on a six-point scale:
  0 = total paralysis
  1 = palpable or visible contraction

TABLE 3-6
NEUROLOGIC EXAMINATION TO DETERMINE SENSORY/REFLEX LEVEL OF DEFICIT

Nerve	Sensory Examination	Motor Examination Function (innervated muscle[s])	Reflex
C2	Occipital protuberance	Breathing	
C3	Supraclavicular fossa	Spontaneous breathing (trapezius)	
C4	Top of the acromioclavicular joint	Spontaneous breathing (trapezius)	
C5	Lateral side of the antecubital fossa	Elbow flexors (biceps, brachialis)	Biceps brachialis (deep tendon)
C6	Thumb	Wrist extensors (extensor carpi radialis longus and brevis)	Brachioradialis (deep tendon)
C7	Middle finger	Elbow extensors (triceps)	Triceps (deep tendon)
C8	Little finger	Finger flexors (flexor digitorum profundus) to the middle finger	
T1	Medial (ulnar) side of the antecubital fossa	Small finger abductors (abductor digiti minimi)	
T2	Apex of the axilla		
T3	Third IS		
T4	Fourth IS (nipple line)*		
T5	Fifth IS (midway between T4 and T6)*		
T6	Sixth IS (level of xiphisternum)*		
T7	Seventh IS (midway between T6 and T8)*		Upper abdominal (superficial)
T8	Eighth IS (midway between T6 and T10)*		
T9	Ninth IS (midway between T8 and T10)*		
T10	Tenth IS (umbilicus)*		
T11	Eleventh IS (midway between T10 and T12)*		

continued

TABLE 3-6
NEUROLOGIC EXAMINATION TO DETERMINE SENSORY/REFLEX LEVEL OF DEFICIT (CONTINUED)

Nerve	Sensory Examination	Motor Examination Function (innervated muscle[s])	Reflex
T12	Inguinal ligament at mid-point		Lower abdominal (superficial)
L1	Half the distance between T12 and L2		
L2	Mid-anterior thigh	Hip flexors (iliopsoas)	
L3	Medial femoral condyle	Knee extensors (quadriceps)	Knee/patellar (deep tendon)
L4	Medial malleolus	Ankle dorsiflexors (tibialis anterior)	
L5	Dorsum of the foot at the third metatarsal phalangeal joint	Long toe extensors (extensor hallucis longus)	
S1	Lateral heel	Ankle plantar flexors (gastrocnemius, soleus)	Ankle/Achilles (deep tendon)
S2	Popliteal fossa in the midline		
S3	Ischial tuberosity		
S4-5	Perianal area (taken as one level		

*Indicates that the point is at the mid-clavicular line.

IS, intercostal space

     2 = active movement, full range of motion (ROM) with gravity eliminated

     3 = active movement, full ROM against gravity

     4 = active movement, full ROM against moderate resistance

     5 = (normal) active movement, full ROM against full resistance

     NT = not testable

- For those myotomes that are not clinically testable by a manual muscle exam, i.e., C1 to C4, T2 to L1, and S2 to S5, the motor level is presumed to be the same as the sensory level.

▶ **Incomplete Spinal Cord Syndromes**
- **Anterior cord**
    1. Contusion of the anterior cord or laceration/thrombosis of the anterior spinal artery

2. Caused by flexion or vertical compression injuries
3. Complete paralysis and hyperalgesia with preservation of touch and proprioception

- **Central cord syndrome**
  1. Caused by hyperextension
  2. Loss of spinothalamic tracts, preservation of long white matter tracts
  3. Motor weak, but able to feel; motor weakness in arms worse than legs
  4. Damage to central gray matter
  5. Variable bladder and sensory involvement
- **Posterior cord**
  1. Loss of proprioception and variable paresis
  2. Extension and buckling of ligamentum flavum into posterior spinal cord
- **Horner syndrome**
  1. Ptosis, anhidrosis, miosis, enophthalmos, and facial flushing
  2. Disruption C7-T1 sympathetic chain
- **Brown-Séquard syndrome**
  1. Penetrating injuries can produce a cord hemisection.
  2. Ipsilateral motor, proprioception, and light touch deficits.
  3. Contralateral pain and temp deficits (POT = **p**ain and **t**emp **o**pposite).

Radiographic Evaluation

▶ Alignment should assure the continuity of four continuous curvilinear lines without step-offs: The anterior and posterior vertebral bodies, spinolaminar lines, spinal canal, and spinous process tips from C2-C7.

▶ Epiphyseal growth plates may resemble fractures.

▶ ↑ C1-C2 may be observed in a normal spine (not posterior ligamentous disruption).

▶ Pseudosubluxation of C2 anterior to C3 (3 mm): the posterior cervical line is used to distinguish normal from pathologic subluxation. This includes drawing a line from the anterior aspect of the spinous process of C1 to the anterior aspect of the spinous process of C3, which should miss the anterior aspect of the spinous process of C2 by < 2 mm (1.5 mm is borderline).

▶ **Prevertebral Soft Tissue**
- Variable with flexion and extension, crying, or adenoids size
- Normal:
  1. < 7 mm at C2 or < 40–50% of the vertebral body AD diameter
  2. 5 mm at C4
  3. < 14 mm at C6 (children < 15 years of age)

▶ **Predens Space**
- Normal < 5 mm (< 8 years of age) or < 3 mm adults

▶ **Laxity of Transverse Ligament/Instability of Atlantoaxial Level:** Down syndrome, Morquio disease, and rheumatoid arthritis

▶ **Odontoid Fracture**
- Type 1: involves the apex of the dens
- Type 2: (most common) crossing the waist of the dens near its junction with body of C2
- Type 3: extend into body of C2

▶ **Indications to Obtain C-Spine Series**:
- Acute neurologic deficits
- Altered mental status second to head injury or shock
- Intoxication
- Midline neck or back tenderness
- High-risk mechanism
- Distracting injury

▶ CT scan evaluation is recommended if there are equivocal radiographs or if there is suspicion about fracture with negative radiograph.

▶ **SCIWORA** (**s**pinal **c**ord **i**njury **w**ithout **r**adiologic **a**bnormality)
- Most common cause: motor vehicle crash (MVC)
- Most common presentation: paresthesias
- Mechanism: hyperextension with inward bulging of interlaminar ligaments, reversible disk prolapse, flexion compression of the cord, longitudinal distraction of the cord, vertebral artery spasm or thrombosis
- Diagnosis of exclusion
- Paresthesias may be only clinical finding
- MRI needed to rule out spinal cord compression, or 1–3 months later may reveal atrophy of the spinal cord
- Incidence 4–66%

▶ **Missed Spinal Fracture**
- False negative rate: 1–20%

- Incomplete views, inappropriate evaluation, normal variants
▶ **Myelography**
  - Recommended for clinical signs of cord compression, neurologic deficits, or deterioration
▶ **Magnetic Resonance Imaging (MRI)**
  - To rule out spinal cord injury and the assessment of ligament integrity
  - To evaluate:
    1. Nucleus pulposus
    2. Intervertebral disk
    3. Parenchymal contusion and intracranial hemorrhage (ICH)

Specific Spine Injuries

▶ **Chance Fracture:** flexion-distraction
  - Due to hyperflexion
  - Occurs in children with lap belt injury, look for associated abdominal injuries
▶ Children are more susceptible than adults to rotational stresses resulting in unstable fracture-dislocations
▶ Disk herniation: rule out cauda equina (sphincter dysfunction, perineal sensory loss, urinary incontinence)
▶ Most fractures: T10-L4
▶ **Neck Injuries**
  - **Suspect spinal cord injury (SCI)** if:
    1. Neurologic deficit
    2. Horner syndrome
    3. Stridor or alteration in phonation (vagus nerve injury)
    4. Trapezius muscle weakness (damage to the spinal accessory nerve)
    5. Deviation of the tongue toward the injured hypoglossal nerve
  - **Types of injuries:**
    1. **Penetrating**
       a. Zone 1: below sternal notch
       b. Zone 2: sternal notch to angle of mandible
       c. Zone 3: above angle of mandible
    2. **Blunt**
       a. Extensive vascular and visceral injury with subsequent thrombosis

        b.   Can include trachea or esophagus

3. **Torticollis**
   a. Congenital: "wryneck" associated with breech, contusion of sternocleidomastoid (SCM) (**Treatment: ROM exercises**)
   b. Traumatic: mild trauma due to sports, falls, rule out rotary subluxation of atlantoaxial (AO) joint

- **Management**
  1. Immobilization with c-collar, log roll as needed, airway management with in-line stabilization, neurosurgical consult.
  2. Steroids: generally administered, long-term effects are controversial. Methylprednisolone 50 mg/kg. Start within 8 hours of injury, then infusion of 5.4 mg/kg for 23 hours.
  3. Naloxone: promise to minimize neurologic deficits in a traumatic myelopathy by improving spinal cord blood flow.
  4. Gangliosides: complex acidic glycolipid present in the CNS—may enhance recovery of motor function.
  5. Skeletal traction:
     a. Stable injuries: treated with rigid orthosis
     b. Subluxation: attempt reduction
     c. Surgical decompression: for acute neurologic decompensation, penetrating neck injuries, unable to perform "closed reduction"
     d. Unstable C-spine: halo vest, prolonged traction, operative fixation
     e. Occipitoatlantal dislocation (usually fatal): halo
     f. Hangman: halo vest
     g. Atlantoaxial dislocation (with odontoid fracture): skeletal traction, posterior fusion if translational
     h. Jefferson: halo

THORACIC TRAUMA
Epidemiology

▶ Blunt > penetrating: death is more often due to concomitant head or abdominal injuries.

► Blunt: in 50% of major blunt trauma, rib fractures and pulmonary contusions occur, < 25% have pneumothorax; approximately 10% have significant hemothorax.

► Penetrating: death usually due to massive hemothorax or hemorrhagic shock, less often due to tension pneumothorax, cardiac tamponade, or aortic interruption.

Anatomy

► Children have a very mobile mediastinum, and rib compliance causes force to be transmitted to intrathoracic organs without fracture or obvious signs of trauma.

Pathophysiology

► Children are less able to compensate for thoracic injury due to:
  • Larger oxygen consumption and smaller functional residual capacity (FRC), making them susceptible to hypoxia.
  • ↑ Chest wall compliance and ↓ pulmonary compliance, causing tachypnea in response to hypoxia.
  • Horizontal ribs with immature intercostal muscles, causing diaphragmatic breathing and fatigue.

Mechanism of Injury

► **Blunt:** 75% in motor vehicle crashes (MVC), 25% falls/bicycles/motorcycles
  • Waddell triad: femur, torso (chest/abdomen), and head injury when child versus automobile
  • Falls: head, multiple extremity and chest wall injuries; lap belt: diaphragm blowout
► **Penetrating:** 15% of pediatric chest injuries seen in the trauma center, more adolescents—gunshot wounds (GSW).

Pattern of Injury

► **Pulmonary:**
  • Contusions are a major source of morbidity, associated with great force (MVC, fall from great height); may progress to posttraumatic pulmonary insufficiency (PTPI), similar to adult respiratory distress syndrome (ARDS).

- Large lacerations show a cavity appearance on chest x-ray; requires surgery if air leak or hematoma.
- Hematomas are uncommon as there is much tissue thromboplastin in the lung and low pressure.

▶ **Cardiac:** infrequent
- Contusions: most common, self-limited unless ventricular fibrillation occurs.
- Cardiac tamponade may occur with penetrating trauma.
- Rare complications: myocardial rupture, myocardial necrosis, traumatic aortic/mitral insufficiency, pericardial laceration, and cardiac herniation.

▶ **Great Vessels:** if injured, most victims die at the scene, aortic rupture most frequent.

▶ **Ribs:** direct transmission of force without fracture occurs in up to 50% or cases. If sternal fractures or dislocations occur, they indicate severe injury.

▶ **Other (rare):** traumatic diaphragmatic hernia, tracheobronchial disruption, and esophageal injuries. Laryngeal transection is associated with a hangman fracture.

Diagnostic Findings

▶ **History:** mechanism, time of injury, "AMPLE" history, last tetanus
▶ **Examination:**
- **Primary survey:**
  1. Tracheal deviation
  2. Paradoxical chest movement (sucking chest wound)
  3. Tension pneumothorax = unilateral ↓ in breath sounds with hyperresonance; may have falsely transmitted breath sounds; may have lack of jugular venous distension if patient is hypovolemic.
  4. Hemothorax = unilateral ↓ with dullness.
- **Secondary survey:**
  1. Evaluate for hypothermia (↑acidosis)
  2. Abnormal breath sounds, rapid/shallow respirations, cyanosis, and hemoptysis
  3. Chest wall tenderness, crepitus (rib fractures, flail = multiple posterolateral)
  4. 1st/2nd rib fractures associated with lung/great vessel injury

5.   Lower ribs with liver/spleen damage
6.   Abdominal tenderness (intercostal nerve injury may mimic peritonitis)

▶ **Ancillary Data:** arterial blood gas (ABG) ($\uparrow$A-a gradient is sensitive), hematocrit < 30% indicates significant hemorrhage.

▶ **Radiology:** wide mediastinum in children is common and aortic rupture is rare, posterior anterior (PA) view helpful.

Management

▶ **Resuscitation:** humidified O_2 via non-rebreather, or BVM/intubation if respiratory failure or obstruction. Consider NG tube to decompress stomach to minimize dilation and reduce limitation of diaphragmatic motion and the risk of aspiration.

▶ **Thoracostomy:** all blood or air requires immediate drainage with chest tube.

▶ **Thoracotomy:**
   • In OR, if initial blood drainage > 10 cc/kg or > 5 cc/kg/h or uncontrolled air leak/food/saliva from chest tube, cardiac tamponade
   • In ED, if penetrating trauma causing arrest/tamponade

▶ **Disposition:**
   • PICU if respiratory insufficiency/resuscitation
   • Monitor overnight if any anatomic or physiologic derangement

Specific Injuries—Life-Threatening

▶ **Upper Airway Obstruction:** Neutral head position (padding beneath shoulders), look for foreign body (remove with Rovenstein forceps), attempt endotracheal intubation before surgical airway.

▶ **Tension Pneumothorax**
   • **Clinical diagnosis: no time for x-rays!**
      1.   It presents with respiratory distress, distended neck veins, contralateral tracheal deviation, ipsilateral hyperresonance to percussion, and $\downarrow$ breath sounds.
      2.   It may be associated with cardiovascular collapse due to mediastinal shift and superior and inferior vena cava (SVC/IVC) kinking.

- **Treatment:** Decompression—immediately using over-the-needle catheter placed percutaneously through the 2nd intercostal space mid-clavicular line just above the 3rd rib (to avoid intercostal vessels). **Definitive treatment:** chest tube.

▶ **Open Pneumothorax**
- It occurs as a result of loss of a portion of the chest wall that approaches at least the size of the bronchial lumen (such as gunshot, large knife wounds, or blast injury).
- **Diagnostic findings:** paradoxical breathing.
- **Treatment:**
  1. Temporarily close chest wall with flutter valve (three-sided dressing), put in chest tube at different site from open wound.
  2. Large defect, to close airtight may require assisted ventilation and urgent thoracotomy for repair of chest wall.

▶ **Massive Hemothorax**
- It occurs from lung (GSW/blunt trauma) or intercostals (stab), massive hemothorax **rare** in children unless high-speed MVC/extreme falls.
- **Diagnostic findings:** may have signs mimicking tension pneumothorax.
- **Treatment:** large bore chest tube with blood transfusion; consider thoracotomy.

▶ **Cardiac Tamponade**
- It is usually caused by a stab wound with sudden decompensation when pericardial blood compromises venous return.
- **Diagnostic findings:** muffled heart sounds, pulsus paradoxus (BP drops 10 mm Hg with inspiration), narrow pulse pressure, and tachycardia.
- **Treatment:** Pericardiocentesis under ECG monitoring; thoracotomy and pericardiotomy with myocardial repair by surgery unless decompensated shock, then ED thoracotomy.

▶ **Flail Chest:** parallel double fractures > two adjacent ribs, poorly tolerated by children. **Treatment:** supportive with positive end expiratory pressure (PEEP) 5–10 cm H_2O. Opioids rarely needed as pain tolerated well and can cause respiratory depression.

Specific Injuries—Potentially Life-Threatening or Serious

▶ **Pulmonary Contusion:** "traumatic wet lung", often not seen on initial x-ray as constricted circulatory state so presumptively diagnose in ED if mechanism present. Excessive crystalloids may precipitate posttraumatic pulmonary insufficiency (PTPI), give least amount of respiratory support possible (low PEEP and FIO_2).

▶ **Myocardial Contusion:** in children, ventricular tachydysrhythmias and ECG abnormalities are rare. Give IV lidocaine if arrhythmias occur.

▶ **Traumatic Bronchial Disruption:** rare but highly lethal, associated with ipsilateral tension pneumothorax with persistent air leak. Diagnosis is by bronchoscopy. If complete, needs surgical airway below level of disruption.

▶ **Traumatic Diaphragmatic Hernia:** rare, part of lap belt complex. Left > right. Right hernia presents late as large viscera herniated. X-ray may look like loculated subpulmonic pneumothorax. Can confirm fluoroscopically with water-soluble contrast. Surgical repair required.

▶ **Traumatic Rupture of Great Vessels:** Rare, higher risk in Marfan syndrome, and with 1st/2nd rib injuries. Chest x-ray with widened mediastinum, obliteration of aortic knob, apical pleural cap, deviation of trachea/esophagus. AP view in normal children often has wide mediastinum, check PA view.

▶ **Traumatic Esophageal Rupture:** EXTREMELY RARE, similar to Boerhaave syndrome (post-emetic esophageal rupture), which progresses rapidly to mediastinitis, sepsis, and death if unrecognized. It should be suspected if pain and shock out of proportion to apparent injury. Hamman sign (mediastinal crunch) is rare, chest tube with continuous bubbling throughout breathing cycle. The only cue to diagnosis could be the presence of mediastinal emphysema on chest x-ray to be confirmed by fluoroscopy. Urgent surgery is required.

▶ **Simple Hemothorax:** if it is large enough to see on x-ray, it generally needs a chest tube (at least 10 cc/kg).

▶ **Rib Fractures**: uncommon. If posterolateral, consider child abuse, narcotics not recommended.

▶ **Simple Pneumothorax:** position upright, chest tube for all patients as may have associated hemothorax.

▶ **Traumatic Asphyxia:** RARE; acute $\uparrow$ in intrathoracic pressure causes transmission of pressure to upper body/neck/head with petechial hemorrhage or conjunctivae, sclerae, scalp, skin, and brain (with associated transient neurologic findings). Requires thoracic CT.

▶ If penetrating trauma is present below the level of the 6th rib, consider abdominal trauma.

ABDOMINAL TRAUMA
Epidemiology

▶ Abdominal trauma follows both head injury and thoracic injury as a cause of traumatic death in childhood, accounting for 6% of the mortality with inadequate resuscitation remaining the leading cause of preventable deaths.

▶ Serious abdominal injuries are relatively common in childhood; 8% of children admitted to the pediatric trauma center have abdominal injuries, but < 15% require operative management; most are victims of penetrating wounds.

▶ Blunt trauma is most common (85% in children versus 50% in adults), of which motor vehicle crashes are the most lethal agent.

▶ Males > females, 2:1 ratio.

▶ Spleen is the most common solid organ injured followed by liver and kidneys.

Anatomy

▶ Children are more prone to abdominal injury than adults because:
  • Larger solid viscera (particularly the liver) and protuberant abdomen makes them more prone to multiple organ injury.
  • Flexible, thin, and poorly muscular ribs cover less of the abdomen and transmit impact to organs below.
  • Lack of abdominal musculature and subcutaneous fat.
  • In small children the bladder is an intra-abdominal structure, hence, a distended bladder is more likely to rupture after a blow to the abdomen (no protection by the pelvic bone).
  • Children may have extraperitoneal or retroperitoneal hemorrhages without bony injury due to their softer axial skeleton.

Therefore, significant internal injuries may not be accompanied by external marks.

- The presence of fractured ribs should heighten the clinician's suspicion that serious injury has occurred.

Mechanism

► **Blunt Trauma:** caused by compression of solid abdominal organs against the spine, compression of a hollow viscus, or shearing forces (as seen in rapid deceleration)
► **Penetrating:** primarily gunshot or stab wounds

Patterns of Injury

► **Motor Vehicle versus Pedestrian:** closed head injury, intra-abdominal injury, and mid-shaft femur fracture on the left (Waddell triad). Unilateral femur fracture causes about a 3–6% drop in hemoglobin, which is not enough to cause shock. Therefore, shock in the presence of a unilateral femur fracture should prompt further evaluation of other associated injuries.
► **Motor Vehicle Occupant:** unrestrained pediatric passengers are at risk for multisystem trauma; head trauma is the most common and most lethal, but the significant bleeding occurs from abdominal and pelvic injuries. Among restrained children "lap belt" injuries occur, which consist of bursting of solid and hollow viscus, flexion-extension (Chance type fractures), lumbar spine fractures, and rarely, diaphragm rupture. Lap belt injuries occur when children wear lap belts without appropriately sized booster seats or improperly fitted three-point restraints allowing the lap belt to move up and compress the abdomen.
► **Bicycle:** Head injury is most lethal. Specifically, injury by handlebars can cause laceration or contusion to any of the abdominal organs. These injuries should be considered as serious injuries despite the fact they are viewed as trivial injuries and the onset of symptoms could be delayed from few hours to days (mean time is 24 hours). Perineal straddle injury can lacerate the scrotum, rectum, or vaginal walls.
► **Inflicted Injury:** caused mainly by blunt trauma and may have no external signs of trauma (up to 50% of cases). Delay in presentation makes these injuries particularly lethal. Duodenal hematoma is the classic injury.

► **Sports Injuries and Falls:** typically isolated injury with falls being the most common mechanism in childhood. Falls from ≥ 2 stories are associated with serious intra-abdominal injury, whereas ≥ 5 stories have significant mortality because of the vertical displacement of organs and vasculature.

Key Points/Diagnostic Findings

► Clinical:
  • Gastric dilatation from air may make the examination difficult. Decompress with a nasogastric or orogastric tube and simultaneously look for blood or bile. The abdomen remaining distended after gastric decompression is an ominous sign suggesting intra-abdominal injuries particularly when it is associated with hemodynamic instability.
  • Tachypnea without retractions can be an early sign of hypovolemia; rapid, shallow breathing can result from abdominal wall or peritoneal injury.

► Laboratory Studies:
  • Laboratory tests may include: type and crossmatch, CBC, ABG, electrolytes, liver enzymes, serum/urine amylase, and urinalysis.
  • Hematocrit ≤ 30% suggests significant hemorrhage; ≤ 25% suggests massive hemorrhage in the presence of a clinical picture consistent with shock.

► Radiologic Studies:
  • X-ray findings that suggest abdominal injury:
    1. Gastric distension
    2. Medially displaced lateral stomach border (marked by the NG tube) by the spleen suggests splenic rupture or hematoma
    3. Inferiorly displaced transverse colon
    4. Ground glass appearance suggests intraperitoneal whole blood or urine
    5. Blurring of psoas shadow(s)
    6. Associated lower rib fracture(s)
    7. Signs of ileus
    8. Pneumoperitoneum suggests rupture of hollow viscus
  • Ultrasonography is useful for evaluation of pancreatic injuries and detection of intraperitoneal hemorrhage, particularly in the splenic and pelvic fossa.

- CT scan of the abdomen should be obtained whenever there are signs of internal bleeding such as abdominal tenderness, distention, bruising, or gross hematuria, as well as a history of shock in the field that responded to volume resuscitation.
- CT scan is best for evaluation of liver, kidneys, spleen injuries, and to a lesser extent GI injuries.
- Water-soluble oral contrast medium should be used for suspected gastric, duodenal, and rectal perforations.

▶ Diagnostic Peritoneal Lavage (rarely used)—it is positive if:
  - Free blood is aspirated
  - Murky fluid after instilling 10 cc/kg of an isotonic fluid
  - Fluid, or if RBC/mm^3 in effluent fluid is > 100,000
  - The integrity of the bowel is considered to have been violated if the effluent contains:
    1. Stool
    2. 500 WBC/mm^3
    3. Amylase > 175 IU/L
    4. Alkaline phosphatase > 6 IU/L

Management

▶ Triage guidelines for emergency management of abdominal trauma: (see Table 3-7)
▶ Indications for emergency operation:
  - Penetrating
    1. All gunshot wounds
    2. All suspected thoracoabdominal injuries
    3. All stab wounds associated with:
       a. Physical signs of shock or peritonitis

TABLE 3-7
TRIAGE GUIDELINES FOR EMERGENCY MANAGEMENT OF ABDOMINAL TRAUMA

Condition	Indications for CT*	Results of CT	Response to Volume	Disposition
Stable	(−)	NA	NA	Acute Care Area
Stable	(+)	(−)	NA	Acute Care Area
Stable	(+)	(+)	NA	PICU versus OR
Unstable	(+)	(−)	Yes	PICU versus OR
Unstable	(+)	(+)	Yes	PICU versus OR
Unstable	NA	NA	No	OR

*See text for clinical indications.
PICU, Pediatric Intensive Care Unit; OR, operating room

      b. Evisceration
      c. Blood in stomach, urine, or rectum
      d. Radiologic evidence of intraperitoneal or retroperitoneal gas

- Blunt
  1. Decompensated shock or physical signs of peritonitis on admission
  2. Hemodynamic instability despite adequate volume resuscitation
  3. Transfusion requirement > 50% of estimated blood volume
  4. Radiologic evidence of pneumoperitoneum, intraperitoneal bladder rupture, or renovascular pedicle injury

▶ Specific Injuries
- Immediate exploration of all gunshot wounds is recommended since 85% penetrate the peritoneum and 95% directly or indirectly injure an organ
- Selective management of penetrating injuries is acceptable because two thirds do not penetrate the peritoneum if:
  1. There are no signs of shock or peritonitis
  2. No blood in stomach, rectum, or urine
  3. No free or retroperitoneal air on x-rays
  4. Serial examination by an experienced surgeon who is familiar with selective management

GENITOURINARY (GU) TRAUMA
Epidemiology

▶ Of children with multiple injuries, GU tract injury is second in incidence to brain injury.

▶ Approximately 10% of trauma patients seen in the ED have GU injuries.

▶ The majority of patients are males and two thirds are over the age of 10 years.

Retroperitoneal Structures

Renal Injuries

▶ The kidney is injured more often than any other GU structure in children due to the large kidney size in relation to body size, ↓ perirenal fat and fascia, more flexible thoracic cage, weaker anterior abdominal muscles, and presence of more lobulations.

► > 80% of renal injuries are due to blunt trauma or deceleration injury. The majority of renal injuries are due to motor vehicle accidents, followed by falls, sports injuries, direct blows to the flank, and penetrating trauma. 85% are minor. Hematuria occurs in 96% of cases.

► It is important to note that 50% of patients with renal pedicle injury may not have hematuria.

► Preexisting renal abnormalities may be found in up to 15% of patients evaluated for renal trauma.

► **Classification for Renal Injuries:**
  • **Grade I:** Contusions or hematomas that are small, subcapsular, and nonexpanding.
  • **Grade II:** Hematomas confined to the retroperitoneum and lacerations < 1 cm in depth that do not result in urinary extravasation.
  • **Grade III:** Lacerations into the perirenal fat > 1 cm in depth but not involving the collecting system. There is no urinary extravasation.
  • **Grade IV:** Deep lacerations into the collecting system and renal vascular injury with contained hemorrhage.
  • **Grade V:** Shattered or fractured kidney and renal pedicle injuries resulting in renal devascularization.

► Radiographic evaluation of the kidney is warranted if:
  • Hematuria of > 20–50 RBCs/HPF
  • Microscopic hematuria with shock
  • Gross hematuria
  • Penetrating trauma to the abdomen
  • Physical findings consistent with renal injury such as flank pain, tenderness, or hematoma (Grey Turner sign) or periumbilical ecchymosis (Cullen sign) may indicate urologic trauma or retroperitoneal hemorrhage. In addition, lower rib or pelvic fractures can be associated with GU tract trauma.
  • A significant mechanism that warrants GU tract evaluation.

► CT scan of the abdomen is considered the diagnostic test of choice for the detection of renal injury in the stable patient.

▶ Ultrasound can detect perinephric and intra-abdominal fluid collections as well as locate shotgun pellets in the renal parenchyma or collecting system.

▶ X-ray findings associated with renal injuries include lower rib or transverse process fractures, loss of the psoas shadow (indicates retroperitoneal blood), and an abnormal spine curvature concave toward the side of the injury.

▶ In patients with blunt trauma and Grade I–III injury, observation is the only treatment that is necessary. Grade IV–V injuries may require operative intervention. Patients with mild injury who are discharged home should have a 24-hour re-evaluation. If the hematuria has not resolved, then an intravenous pyelogram (IVP) should be performed.

Ureteral Injuries

▶ Injury to the ureter occurs in < 5% of patients with GU tract injury. Penetrating trauma is the most common external mechanism with gunshot wounds accounting for 90% of cases.

▶ Signs and symptoms of ureteral injury may be absent immediately after the injury. Nonspecific complaints such as fever, hematuria, ileus, and flank or abdominal pain that follows may appear as evidence of ureteral injury.

▶ Hematuria is not reliable as it is absent in up to 40% of patients with ureteral injury.

▶ Exploration of the ureter may be the only reliable way to detect ureteral injury.

▶ ED management of the patient with ureteral injury is focused on associated life-threatening injuries, followed by surgical repair.

Bladder Injuries

▶ Bladder injuries account for 22% of all urologic injuries (approximately 25% of patients < 18 years of age). Associated injuries are present in 90% of patients, with pelvic fractures occurring in 73–84% of patients.

▶ The bladder tends to be intra-abdominal in children, placing them at greater risk for injury. There is an ↑ in the incidence of bladder rupture with anterior arch pelvic fractures.

▶ > 90% of patients with bladder rupture have hematuria. BUN levels can result from urine absorption from extravasation.

▶ The cystogram is the radiographic method of choice in evaluating bladder injury.

▶ Indications for a cystogram include:
- Penetrating trauma with a suspected GU tract injury
- Pelvic fracture with hematuria, lower abdominal pain, or inability to void
- Lower abdominal or perineal trauma with hematuria
- Gross hematuria
- Inability to void

▶ Patients with bladder contusions and associated injuries or small extraperitoneal ruptures can be managed with urethral or suprapubic drainage for 7–14 days.

▶ Patients with intraperitoneal bladder ruptures require surgical repair with bladder drainage. Patients with large extraperitoneal ruptures with extravasation may need surgical debridement of a bone spicule from the pelvic fracture and bladder laceration repair.

▶ Patients with bladder contusions without associated injuries can be discharged with close follow-up.

External Genitourinary Structures

Urethral Injury

▶ The anterior urethra is injured in males by direct blows to the perineum by straddle injuries.

▶ The posterior urethra is injured more frequently and injuries occur when the bladder is pulled upward causing tension on the posterior urethra. Motor vehicle collisions with direct blow to the perineum account for 79% of cases, and straddle injuries are responsible for the remainder of injuries. The female urethra is rarely injured.

▶ Pelvic fractures are present in > 90% of cases of posterior urethral injury, and urethral injury is present in 4–25% of patients with pelvic fractures.

▶ Blood at the urethral meatus is present in > 90% of patients with urethral injury. Other signs of urethral injury include a high-riding, floating, or boggy prostate, scrotal or penile ecchymosis.

▶ Retrograde urethrogram is the radiologic method of choice for diagnosis of urethral injury. If there is no extravasation, then the urinary catheter can be advanced into the bladder and a cystogram should be performed to rule out bladder injury.

Scrotal and Testicular Injuries

▶ Testicular dislocation occurs when the testicle is forcibly displaced from its anatomic position manifesting as an empty hemiscrotum or a testis palpated in another location.

▶ Testicular torsion can occur after trauma.

▶ Testicular rupture is caused by the testicle being forced against the pubic bone, with tearing of the tunica albuginea and resulting extrusion of seminiferous tissue.

▶ Patients with significant blunt trauma to the testis should first undergo an ultrasound, followed by a radionuclide scan to rule out testicular torsion.

▶ Testicular torsion is treated with reduction and bilateral orchiopexy. If the testicle is necrotic, then orchiectomy and contralateral orchiopexy are performed. Testicular rupture is treated with excision of the necrotic seminiferous tubules and suturing of the torn tunica albuginea. Orchiectomy may be needed in 6–33% of patients.

Penile Injury

▶ The most common cause of injury to the penis is from circumcision complications. Other causes are falls, sports injures, direct blows to the perineum, tourniquet syndromes, and zipper entrapment. Most injuries are minor abrasions and symptomatic treatment is all that is necessary.

▶ If there is marked penile swelling, ecchymosis, blood at the meatus, or the patient is unable to void, then a retrograde urethrogram should be performed.

▶ Penile fracture occurs at the corpora cavernosa and rarely involves the urethra.

▶ Zipper entrapment of the foreskin occurs in uncircumcised males, typically between the ages of 3 and 6 years. The zipper is removed by splitting the median bar of the zipper with a bone cutter or soaking the zipper with mineral oil.

▶ Small vulvar hematomas from straddle injures can be treated with ice packs. Large hematomas should be incised, the clot should be removed, and the area should be loosely packed. Prophylactic antibiotics are recommended, and sitz baths should be initiated. If the patient cannot void, then a urethrogram, followed by a cystogram, are indicated.

CHAPTER 4

ENVIRONMENTAL EMERGENCIES

ANIMAL AND HUMAN BITES
Overview

▶ Boys are bitten by dogs twice as often as girls.

▶ The most common dog involved in bites is the German shepherd.

▶ The pit bull is implicated in over 70% of dog bite fatalities.

▶ Up to 60% of dog bites in children involve the head and neck region.

▶ Less than 5% of dog bites become infected.

▶ Cat bites and scratches cause less tissue damage than dog bites but are infected more often than dog bites. Girls are involved more often than boys.

▶ Deep tissue penetration can occur with cat bites due to their sharp teeth. Tendon sheaths of the hand or finger joints may be involved.

▶ For human bites, measure the distance between the center of the canine teeth (3rd tooth on each side of the lateral incisor). If the distance is > 3 cm, the biter has permanent teeth.

▶ Intracranial involvement can occur with animal bites to the head, particularly in infants.

▶ Wound infections are more common on the extremities. Puncture wounds account for up to 40% of infected wounds.

▶ The most common flora involved in dog and cat bite infections are *Pasteurella multocida* (most common) and *Staphylococcus aureus,* with signs of infection developing within 72 hours of the injury.

▶ *Pasteurella* infections are more virulent and symptoms occur within 12–24 hours of the bite, while *S. aureus* infections occur later.

▶ Cat scratch disease occurs 3–50 days after a scratch and is accompanied by regional lymphadenopathy.

▶ The human mouth has many organisms including *Eikenella corrodens,* streptococci, anaerobes, and *S. aureus.*

▶ Human mouth bites of the hand often involve puncture of the joint space or extensor tendon of the hand by an incisor and are accompanied by high rates of infection.

Management

▶ Radiographs should be obtained if there is a deep wound or puncture of a joint space is suspected. Skull films should be considered in children with significant wounds on the scalp.

▶ Most bites should be left open; however, for cosmetic reasons bites on the face are often sutured after copious irrigation and within 6 hours of the bite. Deep puncture wounds especially from cats should not be closed.

▶ Td should be updated and the wound should be copiously irrigated using a high-pressure system.

▶ Bites involving the periorbital area should be referred to ophthalmology. Up to 40% of cat wounds close to the eye involve a corneal abrasion.

▶ Prophylactic antibiotics are typically given for: hand wounds, deep puncture wounds, wounds that have sutures placed, and wounds in immunocompromised patients. Copious irrigation is essential.

▶ *Pasteurella* is penicillin-resistant and therefore treatment requires either a combination of penicillin and cephalexin or Augmentin (amoxicillin/clavulanate). Trimethoprim/sulfa can also be used to cover for *Pasteurella* in patients with penicillin allergies.

▶ Patients with wounds that are not responding to outpatient management, or those who appear toxic on initial evaluation should be admitted and treated with IV antibiotics (nafcillin and penicillin).

VENOMOUS ANIMAL BITES AND STINGS

▶ See **Table 4-1**.

TABLE 4-1
VENOMOUS ANIMAL BITES AND STINGS

Type	Description	Clinical Presentation	Management	Other
Crotalidae (pit vipers) Rattlesnakes Copperheads Moccasins	Vertical elliptical pupils Triangular head Pit between eye and nostril Venom = peptides + enzymes	**Local:** Tissue damage to vascular endothelial cells Progressive edema and subcutaneous hemorrhage at bite site RBC hemolysis and muscle cell necrosis **Systemic:** ↓ Fibrinogen ↓ Platelets ↑ FSP DIC **Severe envenomation:** Hypotension Acute renal failure Pulmonary edema Serum sickness	No tourniquet Mark level of edema Transport to nearest medical facility **Labs:** CBC + differential Coagulation studies FSP Fibrinogen CK (if severe) Observe 6–8 h if asymptomatic If envenomation confirmed; give antivenom If antivenin = Wyeth-Ayerst, then test for horse serum sensitivity. If local swelling and no system symptoms, give 5 vials.	Copperhead is least toxic If skin test +, dilute vials H1 and H2 blockers If anaphylactic shock: Fluids Colloids Td updated Snakes hibernate in winter (90% of bites occur between April and October) 40% nonaccidental (snake handlers)

continued

TABLE 4-1
VENOMOUS ANIMAL BITES AND STINGS (CONTINUED)

Type	Description	Clinical Presentation	Management	Other
Elapidae (coral snakes)	Round pupils Yellow/red rings "Red on yellow, kill a fellow."	**Neurotoxin:** Cranial nerve palsies Mild bite site swelling	If moderate systemic symptoms, give 10 vials. If severe systemic symptoms, give 15 vials. If antivenin = Crofab, then no sensitivity testing. Give 4–6 vials initial dose Antivenom is always required for any confirmed bite regardless of presence or lack of presence of symptoms Supportive care: i.e., (ETT); volume	Found in Arizona and southern Gulf states

Latrodectus Black widow spider	Black with red hour glass 2 small fang marks Venom: releases ACH	HA, nausea/vomiting Severe muscle cramps—paralysis Systemic HTN **Upper extremity bite** Can cause respiratory distress **Lower extremity bite** Abdominal pain/rigidity	No labs indicated Supportive care: Valium Analgesics Antivenin if: Severe cramps HTN Children <6 years of age	Severe in children due to higher dose of venom relative to body size
Loxosceles reclusa Brown recluse	Brown with violin-shaped mark Usually painless bite Venom: (Sphingomyelinase D): Damages endothelium RBC hemolysis Activates platelet thrombosis	Causes local infarction/necrosis	**Mild:** Resolves 5–7 d Treatment: corticosteroid cream **Severe:** Systemic—nausea, vomiting, fever, chills, muscle tissue; necrosis DIC (rare) Treatment: dapsone debridement, plastic surgery repair	HBO is experimental
Scorpions (Centruroides)	Venom: releases ACH and nor-epinephrine	Cardiotoxic Marked local hyperesthesia	**Mild:** Cold compresses Local injection of anesthetic	No narcotics, may worsen dysrhythmias

continued

TABLE 4-1
VENOMOUS ANIMAL BITES AND STINGS (CONTINUED)

Type	Description	Clinical Presentation	Management	Other
Sculptured scorpion is only species dangerous to humans. All others are harmless.	Lives in southwestern U.S. and Mexico		Monitor for several hours **Severe:** ↑HR CNS stimulation, convulsions; **Treatment:** barbiturates Muscle twitching and incoordination can cause respiratory compromise HTN; **Treatment:** hydralazine, nifedipine	Antivenom experimental in Arizona
Triatoma Kissing bug Texas bedbug	Feed on vertebrate blood Black: 2.5 cm length long probosas	Symptoms range from itching to severe anaphylaxis	Cool compress Corticosteroid cream (oral if moderate symptoms are present) Oral antihistamines	Sensitization increases with subsequent bites
Centipedes	Cytolytic venom: Phosphatase Histamine Serotonin	Superficial necrosis Nausea Dizziness	Symptomatic care Tetanus prophylaxis	Venom not toxic, but can cause rhabdomyolysis and acute renal failure

Millipedes	No venom apparatus	Toxin causes contact dermatitis "Mahogany discoloration" Blepharospasm, conjunctivitis, periorbital edema, corneal ulceration may develop	Copious irrigation; treat as 2nd degree chemical burn Refer eye injury to ophthalmologist
Coelenterata Jellyfish Anemones Corals	Venom apparatus composed of nematocysts Venom: proteins, histamines, catecholamines, heat stable	**Mild:** Local reaction Burning Paresthesias: may progress to necrosis/ulceration **Severe:** CNS: HA, vertigo, seizure, coma, paralysis	Bathe in salt water (fresh activates!) Vinegar inactivates nematocysts Scrape off with razor/knife **Treatment:** topical corticosteroids, analgesics Td update	Cardiac dysrhythmias, respiratory failure (rare) No antivenom for North American jellyfish, Portuguese man-of-war, or sea-anemones
Echinodermata Starfish Sea urchin	Spines may have venom	**Local:** Burning pain Rapid swelling Redness Pain **Systemic:** Weakness Syncope Facial muscle paralysis Respiratory failure	X-ray: localize spine Removal technique—controversial (cautious of multiple small spines with invisible sheath) **Treatment:** may need antibiotics if infection develops	Must remove spines as they cause a foreign body reaction and infection If spine penetrates joint: removal in operating room is necessary

continued

TABLE 4-1
VENOMOUS ANIMAL BITES AND STINGS (CONTINUED)

Type	Description	Clinical Presentation	Management	Other
Stingrays	Venomous organ is on dorsal tail Punctures feet Venom: contains serotonin, PDE, nucleotides	**Local:** Barb pieces imbedded Pain Edema Hemorrhage **Systemic:** Muscle cramps Nausea/vomiting Weakness ↑ HR ↓ BP	Copious irrigation Hot water immersion: inactivates venom Foreign body removal Debridement Supportive care	Death (rare)
Scorpaenidae Sculpin Lionfish Stonefish	Coastal waters (CA, FL, HI) Venomous spine: heat labile protein: cardiotoxic	**Local:** Ischemic and cyanotic (immediately) Edema Paresthesias Necrosis **Systemic:** GI CNS CV	Copious irrigation Hot water immersion: inactivates venom Foreign body removal Debridement Supportive care	Antivenom for stone fish

ACH, acetylcholine; BP, blood pressure; CBC, complete blood count; CK, creatine kinase; CNS, central nervous system; CV, cardiovascular; DIC, disseminated intravascular coagulation; ETT, endotracheal tube; FSP, fibrin split products; GI, gastrointestinal; HA, headache; HBO, hyperbaric O₂; HR, heart rate; HTN, hypertension; PDE, phosphodiesterase; RBC, red blood cell

NEAR DROWNING

- Drowning is the second most common cause of unintentional injury death in those between the age of 5–24 years.
- It's the third most common cause of unintentional death in children 0–4 years.
- The peak incidence occurs between 1–4 years of age and between 15–24 years (often due to alcohol/drugs).
- Males > females (teenage girls have one fifth the drowning rate of teenage boys).
- Of those who require cardiopulmonary resuscitation (CPR) in the ED, 60–100% of survivors are severely brain damaged.
- 7–10% of drowning deaths are "dry drownings" in which aspiration of water does not occur.
- In 85% of drowning deaths < 22 cc/kg of water is aspirated.

Definitions

- **Drowning:** death from asphyxia within 24 hours of submersion; sometimes further classified into "classic white cases" (loss of consciousness from seizure/head trauma/stroke prior to submersion) and "classic blue cases" (panic and struggle resulting in pronounced catecholamine release).
- **Secondary Drowning:** death occurring 24 hours after submersion due to complications. These patients seem well initially.
- **Immersion Syndrome:** sudden death after contact with cold water (vagal discharge causes cardiac standstill or ventricular fibrillation).
- **Submersion Injury:** any submersion resulting in hospital admission or death.

Pathophysiology

- **Injury:** initially occurs in the lung. The secondary effects are due to hypoxia, which leads to brain injury.
- **Freshwater:** surfactant is diluted → basement membrane damaged → alveolitis, pulmonary edema, alveolar collapse.
- **Seawater:** hypertonicity of water → intravascular water moved into alveolar space → surfactant is inactivated and washed out of alveolar space and resultant basement membrane damaged.

▶ **"Shallow Water Blackout":** occurs because swimmers hyperventilate before swimming leading to a ↓ P_{CO_2} and lower stimulus to breathe. This in turn causes a loss of consciousness.

▶ **Chlorine:** does not affect prognosis, but the presence of mud, vomitus, sand, and over 20 human pathogens found in saltwater can cause a pneumonitis.

▶ **Hypothermia:** the rate of heat loss in water is 32 times > in air, children have greater body surface area and therefore are at ↑ risk.

  • **Symptoms:** loss of coordination, ↑ muscle rigidity, clouded sensorium, ↓ duration of breath holding, dysrhythmias, and exhaustion

  • **Benefits of hypothermia:** ↓ O_2 consumption, metabolic rate, cerebral metabolism

▶ **Diving Reflex:** face exposed to cold → reflex shunting of blood to heart and brain with bradycardia. Probably has little influence on ultimate patient outcome.

Etiology

▶ 90% of drowning deaths occur in freshwater (50% swimming pools, of which 90% are residential—mostly weekends, summer, 4–6 p.m.; teenagers are more involved in lake, river, and beach drownings).

▶ 10–20% of residential drownings occur in bathtubs. (Risk factors: unattended child, seizure disorder, consider nonaccidental trauma.) Infants (7–15 months of age) can drown in 3–5 gallon buckets filled or partially filled with water.

▶ Two-thirds of boating-related drownings occur due to boats capsizing or flooding.

▶ Children with seizure disorders are 4–5 times more likely to drown than the general population.

▶ Adolescents are most likely to be involved in diving accidents, 70% have water depth < 4 feet.

Diagnosis

▶ History should include:

  • Time of submersion

- Time until CPR began
- Preceding trauma
- Loss of consciousness
- Seizure history
- Medications
- Drugs/alcohol
- Prehospital treatment, if given

▶ **Potential Complications:** hypoxia causing respiratory insufficiency, aspiration pneumonia, acute respiratory distress syndrome (ARDS), disseminated intravascular coagulation (DIC), hemolysis, renal failure, brain injury, cardiac dysrhythmias, and cardiogenic shock.

▶ **Laboratory Studies:** ABG (arterial blood gas) are most important ± arterial line → may be needed for ongoing monitoring; complete blood count (CBC), electrolytes, liver function tests (LFTs), coagulation studies, and baseline urinalysis.

▶ Chest x-ray looking for associated injuries, infiltrates, barotrauma, and endotracheal tube (ETT)/nasogastric (NG) tube placement. The initial chest x-ray may not show the classic fluffy infiltrates of aspiration.

Management

▶ **Prehospital**
- Call 911, early CPR (directly affects prognosis)
- C-spine immobilization
- If hypothermic: (see section on Hypothermia if temperature is < 35° C)
   1. Do not aggressively over-manipulate as this may precipitate arrhythmias
   2. Remove wet clothing
   3. Keep patient warm and dry
   4. Establish IV access
   5. Treat hypotension with normal saline (NS) 20 cc/kg boluses

▶ **ED**
- **Respiratory**
   1. If hypoxic, O_2 via 100% non-rebreather mask
   2. If persistent hypoxemia and self-ventilating, continuous positive airway pressure (CPAP)

3. If no improvement with CPAP, intubate with positive end expiratory pressure (PEEP) starting at 5 mm Hg; (PO_2 < 60 mm Hg or PCO_2 > 50 mm Hg are probable indicators for intubation)
4. Use albuterol for bronchospasm
- **Cardiac**
    1. IV access: hypotension can be due to cardiomyopathy, acidosis, central shunting, CNS injury, blood loss with trauma, spinal shock, or hypothermia
    2. Treat initially with 20 cc/kg NS or lactated Ringer (LR) solution and repeat as needed
    3. Monitor central venous pressure (CVP). The patient may require vasopressors (dobutamine or dopamine 5–20 µg/kg/min) if normovolemic
- **Hypothermia** (see section on Hypothermia)
    1. Profound hypothermia requires active rewarming with warmed NS, consider peritoneal/thoracic lavage, warmed O_2 in circuit

▶ **Cerebral Edema**
- Raised intracranial pressure (ICP) is related to mortality but is not predictive of neurologic sequelae.
- Treatment of ICP does not change mortality.
- ICP does not usually ↑ until hours after the anoxic event.
    1. In the ED events raising ICP should be minimized.
        a. Maintain PCO_2 at 30 mm Hg
        b. Elevate head to approximately 30 degrees
        c. Minimize procedures (such as NG tubes, Foley catheter placement)
        d. Restrict fluids to 50–60%; maintenance after blood pressure (BP) stabilized
        e. Keep CVP 8–10 mm Hg
        f. Keep urine output between 0.5–1 cc/kg/h
        g. Consider Lasix 1 mg/kg or mannitol 0.5 g/kg q3–4h if needed for raised ICP
        h. Barbiturates do not affect outcome: consider pentobarbital 3–20 mg/kg IV then 1–2 mg/kg/h infusion; if seizures occur, control with diazepam 0.3 mg/kg or phenytoin 10–20 mg/kg
▶ Prophylactic antibiotics and steroids are not recommended.

Disposition

▶ Admit all with hypoxia, tachypnea, retractions, wheezing, rales, congestion, tachycardia, cyanosis, confusion.

▶ ICU for those with hypothermia < 32° C, depressed mental status, persistently abnormal ABGs, requiring CPAP, unstable cardiovascular status.

▶ Consider admission for all significant near-drowning patients as secondary drowning phenomenon occurs in 5% of near-drowning patients.

Prognosis

▶ Survival: 75–93%; intact neurologic survival 58–93%; affected by length of submersion, water temperature, presence of respirations or pulse, pupillary response, level of consciousness, blood pH, immediate CPR, length of time CPR given, response to CPR.

▶ Poor outcome is associated with the necessity of cardiotoxic drugs, submersion over 9 minutes, CPR over 25 minutes, ↑ ICP or cerebral perfusion pressure (CPP), elevated blood glucose level.

ELECTRICAL AND LIGHTNING INJURIES
Pathophysiology

▶ 300 injuries/100 fatalities per year in the United States.

▶ Two thirds of lightning strike survivors have permanent sequelae.

▶ The fetus is at higher risk of injury than the mother due to the 200-fold less resistance of fetal skin and also because the hyperemic pregnant uterus and amniotic fluid also conduct electricity well.

▶ Extent of injury is determined by:
  - **Tissue resistance**
    1. ↑ Resistance generates greater heat and resultant thermal injury
    2. (**Highest**) Resistance bone> fat > tendon > skin > muscle > vessels > blood > nerves (**lowest**)
  - **Intensity of current**
    1. Skin with lower resistance (i.e., thin, high H_2O content, newborn) allows for deeper tissue damage

2. Pregnancy: (fetal death) alternating current (AC) > lightning > direct current (DC)
- **Pathway of current flow:** contact to "ground"
  1. **Hand to hand:** ↑ mortality due to transection of the spinal cord from C4-C8
  2. **Hand to foot:** causes dysrhythmias
  3. **Foot to foot:** mortality is < 5%
- **Types of current**
  1. **AC:** Causes tetany, "lock on" phenomenon
     a. Commercial high voltage
     b. Household low voltage
  2. **DC:** Massive energy, but brief contact resulting in a single strong contraction
     a. Lightning (direct strike, side, stride potential, flashover phenomenon)
     b. Defibrillation

Definitions

▶ **Direct Strike:** most serious type, major current flow is through the victim's body.
▶ **Side Flash:** lightning passes from the primary strike area through the air to a nearby victim.
▶ **Stride Potential:** current hits the ground, enters one leg of the victim and exits through the other leg. Mortality rate of 30% in patients with leg burns due to stride potential.
▶ **Flash Over Phenomenon:** lightning energy flows outside the body of the victim usually via wet clothes. Pathognomonic featherlike skin burns may be present.

Clinical Manifestations

▶ **Cardiac**
- Primary cause of death (dysrhythmias, myocardial damage, secondary to respiratory arrest)
- AC current results in ventricular fibrillation
- DC current results in asystole
- Lightning is direct current (asystole)
▶ **Pulmonary**
- Respiratory center paralysis or forced tetanic contractions of respiratory muscles.

- Aspiration, ARDS, pulmonary edema.
- Duration of apnea appears to be the critical factor in patient survival, so aggressive management in the clinically dead is indicated.

▶ **Central Nervous System**
- Most frequently involved system
- Immediate effects are loss of consciousness, paralysis, visual disturbances, amnesia, intracranial hematoma, Horner syndrome
- Later complications include: paraplegia, brachial plexus injury, syndrome of inappropriate secretion of antidiuretic hormone (SIADH), diabetes insipidus (DI), hearing loss, neuropathy, seizures

▶ **Renal**
- ↑ Injuries with high-voltage electrical injury
- Hypoxic renal injury is a direct effect of current on tissue
- Myoglobinuria (most common, especially with "lock on" tetany)

▶ **Oral**
- "Child bites cord" or "sucks on live cord."
- Intense heat causes coagulation necrosis and liquefaction: lesions are painless because the nerves are destroyed.
- Lip commissure burn/eschar complication "delayed bleeding of labial artery" 5–14 days later.
- Long-term effects: microstomia, speech problems, adhesions, abnormal dentition/arch formation.

▶ **Ocular**
- Cataracts, optic neuritis/neuropathy, extraocular muscle paralysis

▶ **Fractures/Compartment Syndrome**

Management

▶ **Prehospital**
- Extrication, removal from source, cut wires with wooden cutters
- Cervical spine immobilization

▶ **Hospital**
- IV: NS or LR 20 cc/kg bolus. Titrate to urine output > 1 cc/kg/h.
- Intubate for intracranial injuries.

- Minimal fluid resuscitation for lightning injuries due to CNS effects.
- CBC, chemistry panel, urinalysis, myoglobin, creatine phosphokinase (CPK), electrocardiogram (ECG), x-rays as needed.
- Myoglobinuria: keep urine pH > 7.45, Lasix (1 mg/kg), mannitol (0.5 mg/kg).
- Aggressive respiratory management even if patient seems "dead."
- Cardiac arrest from lightning injury have higher survival rates.
- Dysrhythmias: ACLS/PALS protocol.
- Fasciotomy may be needed for compartment syndrome.
- Admit all children (except those with minor burns and those who are asymptomatic after a minor household injury).
- Admit all lightning injuries.
- Tetanus booster.

THERMAL INJURIES
Epidemiology

▶ Second most common cause of death (motor vehicle crashes #1) in children < 3 years of age.
▶ House fires cause 75% of all fire-related deaths.
▶ 5% are due to clothing ignition.
▶ Tap water scalds account for 25% of scald injuries with 50% occurring in children < 5 years of age.

Pathophysiology

▶ **Total Body Surface Area (TBSA):** "rule of 9's" applies to children > 9 years old: each lower extremity: 18%; each upper extremity: 9%; head and neck: 9%.
▶ Smaller children: larger heads and smaller extremities so the Lund/Browder chart should be used. The critical areas of involvement are the eyes, ears, face, hands, feet, and perineum.
▶ For children < 5 years of age, patient's palm area is approximately 1% TBSA.

Management

▶ **Prehospital**
  - Smother flames, place patient supine to avoid facial burns, hair ignition, and inhalation

TABLE 4-2
CLINICAL CLASSIFICATION OF BURNS

Depth/degree of burns
Superficial (1st degree): epidermis
Partial thickness (2nd degree): epidermis and dermis with blisters
and scar
Full thickness (3rd degree): epidermis, dermis, and subcutaneous tissue,
leathery skin that is insensate
Severity:
Major:
Partial thickness > 15–20% (adult > 25%)
Full thickness > 10% TBSA
Moderate:
Partial 10–15% (adult: 15–25%)
Full thickness 2–10% TBSA
Minor:
Partial thickness < 10% TBSA
Full thickness > 2% TBSA

TBSA, total body surface area

- Cool/iced solution for pain but only in patients with < 20% TBSA burns
- Cover burn with a clean or sterile sheet
- Do not break intact blisters unless they are in flexion creases
- NPO
- Transfer to a burn center: (see Burn Center Evaluation Criteria below)
- O_2
- Cardiac monitoring
- Blankets: prevent cooling
- Two intravenous lines
- Morphine for pain

▶ **Inpatient (Major Burns)**
- Admit: > 15% TBSA burns, or burns involving the critical areas

TABLE 4-3
FLUID MANAGEMENT FOR BURN INJURIES

Most common fluid replacement formula is the Parkland formula:
$4 \text{ mL} \times \text{kg} \times \%$ TBSA over 24 h (LR or NS) + maintenance IV (D_5W $1/2$
NS)
Administered as:
1st $1/2$ over 8 h, 2nd $1/2$ over the next 16 h

TBSA, total body surface area

- Second or third degree burns > TBSA 10% need IV fluids, 40% need central line
- Keep urine output > 1 mL/kg/h
- Nasogastric tube, NPO
- Debridement: BID, whirlpool, Silvadene
- Complications: *Pseudomonas,* staphylococcal infections
- No antibiotics indicated: unless Group A strep colonization
- Peptic ulcer disease (PUD) prophylaxis

▶ **Burn Center Evaluation Criteria**
- Second- and third-degree burns on the hands, feet, or perineum
- Second- and third-degree burns over 10% body surface area in a child < 10 years of age
- Second- and third-degree burns over 20% body surface area in children over the age of 10 years
- Second- and third-degree circumferential burns
- Electrical and lightning burns
- Inhalation burns

▶ **Outpatient (Minor Burns)**
- Silvadene for > 5% burns, otherwise bacitracin is sufficient
- Lotion/lanolin/sunscreen
- Td prophylaxis if > 7 years of age

HEAT-INDUCED ILLNESSES
Overview

▶ Neonates and infants < 2 years lack good thermoregulatory control, have greater surface area/mass ratio, and have a high metabolic rate.
▶ Older children differ from adults in that they do not sweat as much, have greater surface area/mass ratio; do not instinctively replace losses or limit exertion in extreme heat.
▶ Teenagers exercise in the heat and athletes push themselves to their limit, may not adequately replace losses, especially over consecutive days of exertion.
▶ Chronic diseases such as cystic fibrosis (CF), quadriplegia, and anhidrosis may ↓ ability to sweat.

▶ Drugs causing heat production include amphetamines and cocaine; phencyclidine (PCP) and D-lysergic acid diethylamide (LSD) ↓ sweating, as do antihistamines, phenothiazines, anticholinergics, diuretics, β-blockers, and alcohol.

Pathophysiology

▶ **Endogenous** heat production due to physical activity, thyroid activity, epinephrine, and fever (pyrogens stimulate prostaglandins, resetting the hypothalamus).

▶ **Exogenous** heat is environmental.

▶ **Usual core temperature** is 37° C ± 0.6 (98.6° F ± 1)

▶ **Heat illness:**
- Results when heat cannot be dissipated by:
  1. Conduction
  2. Convection
  3. Radiation (usually 60% of losses)
  4. Evaporation (25%)

▶ **Hypothalamus**
- Controls heat by:
  1. Dilation of cutaneous blood vessels by inhibition of sympathetic stimulators in the posterior hypothalamus (maximal at 40° C)
  2. Stimulation of sweating via sympathetic stimulation
  3. Inhibition of heat production by stopping shivering, which causes ↓ release of thyrotropin-releasing hormone

▶ **Temperature > 40° C**
- Causes splanchnic vasoconstriction resulting in:
  1. Nausea, vomiting, diarrhea.
  2. ↓ Urine output, ↑ liver enzymes, blood urea nitrogen (BUN), creatinine.
  3. Hypocalcemia, hyper/hypokalemia.
  4. Changes in blood sugar level.
- Acute renal failure commonly occurs in severe heatstroke, rhabdomyolysis being a major contributing factor.
- Persistent temperature > 42° C causes CNS disturbances (disorientation, seizures, coma) with cellular injury possible.
- Death occurs due to circulatory or respiratory collapse, disseminated intravascular coagulation (DIC), electrolyte imbalance, or cerebral edema.

Types of Heat Illnesses

▶ **Prickly Heat**
- (Miliaria) acute inflammatory skin eruption with sweat gland blockage caused by heat and humidity. Rash is maculopapular with erythema and vesicles.
- **Treat** by wearing light loose clothing and maintaining a cool environment; avoid talcs and powders.

▶ **Heat Edema**
- Dependent swelling of hands and feet with sudden changes in temperature. Self-limited and resolves spontaneously; probably caused by aldosterone production.
- **Treat** by being in a cool environment.

▶ **Heat Syncope**
- Seen during early heat acclimation, associated with postural hypotension and dehydration, worsened by prolonged standing or vigorous activity.
- **Treat** by removing from heat, supine position, oral rehydration, rest.

▶ **Heat Cramps**
- Occur in active muscle groups with spasms during or after activity, sometimes with ↑ body temperature. Etiology thought to be salt depletion and drinking hypotonic fluids.
- **Treat** by removing from heat, oral (1 teaspoon of salt in 500 cc water) or IV rehydration depending on severity of dehydration.

▶ **Heat Exhaustion**
- Temperature is < 40° C and mental status is **normal**
- **Two types:**
  1. **Water-depletion** with quick onset after high temperatures and insufficient fluids.
  2. **Salt-depletion** with onset over several days in children rehydrating with inadequate salt; more in those who are not acclimatized whose sweat contains more salt.
- **Laboratory studies:** ↑ hematocrit (HCT), ↑ BUN, ↓ glucose, hypernatremia or hyponatremia
- **Caused by:**
  1. High temperatures
  2. Excessive sweating
  3. Inadequate water and salt replenishment
- **Symptoms:** headache (HA), nausea, vomiting, lethargy, irritability, thirst, anorexia

- May be a precursor to heat stroke
- **Treat** with removal from heat, fluid replacement (oral if mild, IV if severe), rest

▶ **Heatstroke**
- Medical emergency with temperature > 40.6° C (105° F), neurologic dysfunction, and often anhidrosis
- Loss of thermostatic control with uncontrolled rise in temperature causing:
    1. Cellular injury (edema, vacuolization, hemorrhage) including rhabdomyolysis
    2. Renal failure
    3. Hepatocellular necrosis
    4. Myocardial damage
    5. Cerebral edema
- **Classic:** non-exertional, infants/elderly, develops over days during a heat wave
- **Exertional:** develops rapidly in young, vigorously exercising individuals who are not acclimatized to a hot environment
- **Laboratory studies:** show electrolyte disturbances, evidence of liver and renal injury
- Disseminated intravascular coagulation (DIC) may develop
- For each degree > 37° C, adjustments need to be made for: pH ↓ 0.015, PCO_2 ↑ 4.4, PO_2 ↑ 7.2
- **Treat** by airway stabilization, remove clothing, ice packs to axillae, groin, and neck; spray with water and fan until temperature is < 39° C; IV rehydration with normal saline 20 cc/kg, consider central venous monitoring if considering further fluids

ACCIDENTAL HYPOTHERMIA AND FROSTBITE
Hypothermia

▶ **Definition:** core body temperature ≤ 35° C (95° F)
▶ **Moderate Hypothermia:** core temperature = 30–32° C (86–89° F)
▶ **Profound Hypothermia:** core temperature < 28° C (82° F)
▶ **Afterdrop:** continued ↓ in core temperature; even after the patient is removed from the cold stress
▶ **Aftershock:** state of depletion of intravascular volume that occurs with rewarming

► **Complications of Hypothermia:**
- Gastrointestinal (GI) bleeding
- Acute renal failure
- Pancreatitis
- Deep vein thrombosis (DVT)
- Disseminated intravascular coagulation (DIC)
- Pulmonary edema
- Dysrhythmias

► **Factors That Influence Thermoregulatory Balance in Infants and Children:**
- Large surface area/body weight ratio
- Minimal subcutaneous fat
- Thin skin with ↑ permeability
- Delayed shivering and inefficient ability to generate heat
- Immature or inappropriate behavioral response to environment
- Infants and young children have specialized body cells called "brown fat cells": these allow for a tripling of heat production by infants—mostly found in neck and shoulder region.

► **Mechanisms of Heat Loss**
- **Radiation:** 65% of heat loss
- **Conduction:** transfer of heat from one object to another
- **Convection:** heat flow from one object to a moving object
- **Evaporation:** heat transfer as matter changes form

► **Signs and Symptoms of Hypothermia**
- 35° C (95° F): maximal shivering and slurred speech
- 32° C (89° F): altered level of consciousness (ALOC), dilated but reactive pupils, shivering stops
- 30° C (86° F): resuscitation drugs may be inactive, ↓ respiratory rate
- 28° C (82° F): bradycardia refractory to atropine, Osborne (J) waves; pupils nonreactive
- 25° C (79° F): fixed and dilated pupils, maximum risk of ventricular fibrillation (V. Fib), areflexia
- 20° C (68° F): cardiac asystole common

► **Poor Prognostic Indicators:**
- Core temperature < 15° C (59° F)
- Potassium >10 mEq/L
- Fibrinogen < 50

- Exposure > 24 hours
- Absence of cardiac rhythm

► **Management**
- **Prehospital:**
  1. Avoid rewarming of frozen limbs until cardiovascular and metabolic problems are under control.
  2. No first-line resuscitation drugs if core temperature < 30° C.
  3. Volume re-expansion is a key aspect to therapy for hypothermic patients: administration of IV saline before rewarming reduces mortality rate from 75% to 17%.
- **Hospital:**
  1. Primary consideration: return to normothermia
  2. Use pre-warmed normal saline (NS); thoracic, peritoneal, gastric cavity lavage with heated IV fluids

► **Resuscitation Attempts**
- V. Fib: try 1 J/kg, then initiate resuscitation drugs when core temperature is > 30° C.
- No need for intubation prophylaxis.
- Atrial arrhythmias more common and usually respond to rewarming.
- Use NS **not** lactated Ringer (LR) solution, since cold liver does not metabolize lactate.
- Rewarm frozen extremities after core temperature is 32–34° C (89–93° F), then use 40° C water immersion.
- Antibiotics recommended in patients with moderate to severe hypothermia.
- Rewarm patient to 30° C (86° F) prior to declaring the patient dead; prefer 32° C (89° F) if possible, "no one is dead, until they are warm and dead."
- Laboratory studies: potassium, glucose (may be ↑), prothrombin time (PT)/partial thromboplastin time (PTT), fibrinogen, CBC, electrolytes, ABG.
- Classic ECG finding is the Osborne wave, seen at 30° C.

Frostbite

► Associated with tissue freezing and vascular disruption, caused by significant environmental cold stress associated with ↓ in blood flow to the involved skin and body area.

▶ **Superficial Frostbite:** involves skin and immediate underlying layers of subcutaneous tissue; no pain or sensation before rewarming. Usually have blister formation.

▶ **Deeper Frostbite:** involves skin, subcutaneous tissues, and deeper structures—muscles, tendons, nerves, bones. No pain while frozen or even during rewarming process: usually no blister formation.

▶ **Treatment:**
  • Rewarm for 20–30 minutes for superficial and up to 1 hour for deep. Do not rewarm if there is a chance that additional freezing injury may occur.
  • Give IV pain medications prior to rewarming.
  • Use water that is 38–43° C for immersion therapy.
  • Td booster.
  • Delayed amputation until tissue demarcation lines are determined.

HIGH-ALTITUDE ILLNESS AND DYSBARISM
Acute Mountain Sickness (AMS)

▶ Most common type of altitude sickness.

▶ Highest incidence in 1–20-year-old group.

▶ Onset: 6–24 hours after ascent and lasts up to 4 days.

▶ Starts at 8000 feet, most people affected at 10,000 feet.

▶ Predisposing factors: rapid ascent, exercise, preexisting lung disease or infection, previous episode of high-altitude sickness.

▶ **Physical Examination Findings:** ataxia, tachycardia, oliguria, and localized rales in 25–35%.

▶ **Symptoms:** nausea, vomiting, fatigue, HA, irritability, shortness of breath (SOB).

▶ **Treatment:** usually self-limited, high-carbohydrate diet, rest, hydration, no alcohol (EtOH) or smoking.

▶ **Prevention:** when climbing between 10,000–14,000 feet, take 1 day to ascend each 1000 feet. Take 2 days for each 1000 feet above 14,000 feet.
  • Diamox: 5–10 mg/kg/24 h BID (adults 250 mg BID); start medications 24 hours before climb and continue for 2–3 days after reaching altitude.
  • Decadron: 4 mg PO q6h starting 48 hours before climb.
  • Combination of the two agents.

High-Altitude Pulmonary Edema (HAPE)

▶ Symptoms: fatigue, nonproductive cough with dyspnea on exertion (DOE) → productive cough with pink, frothy sputum, fever, confusion.

▶ Occurs 24–96 hours after arrival at altitude.

▶ Affects 10% of people above 14,500 feet.

▶ **Predisposing Factors:** more common in children (38%) and young adults, rapid ascent, exercise.

▶ **Laboratory Studies:** ABG: respiratory alkalosis; urinalysis: proteinuria and high-specific gravity; CBC hemoconcentration.

▶ **Radiology/Cardiac Studies:** chest x-ray—diffuse patchy infiltrates; ECG-RV strain

▶ **Treatment:** Descent—as little as 1000–2000 feet can improve pulmonary status, rest, O_2, end expiratory positive pressure (EPAP) via Down mask: works via alveolar recruitment and can ↑ hemoglobin (Hgb) O_2 saturation by 10%. Diuretics, digoxin, theophylline, steroids are not effective.

▶ **Prevention:** nifedipine may prevent HAPE and can also be used acutely. Other measures to prevent HAPE include the prophylactic use of acetazolamide or dexamethasone.

High-Altitude Cerebral Edema (HACE)

▶ Most severe form of acute mountain sickness (AMS). Hypoxia → cerebral vasodilatation.

▶ Symptoms: severe HA, ataxia, hallucinations, lethargy, coma, death.

▶ Rare below 12,000 feet.

▶ Onset 2–3 days after ascent.

▶ **Diagnosis:** Head CT reveals slitlike ventricles.

▶ **Treatment:** Rapid descent, O_2, elevate head of bed (HOB), intubate using vecuronium, pentothal, lidocaine. Decadron 4 mg q6h. Diamox not helpful.

High-Altitude Retinal Hemorrhages

▶ Painless

▶ 50% of climbers above 16,000 feet and 100% above 21,000 feet.

▶ **Symptoms:** ↓ visual acuity (VA) may imply macular involvement, retinal hemorrhages. May be a warning sign of HACE.

▶ **Treatment:** descent if there are visual changes.
▶ **Prevention:** 2–4-day stay at 5000–7000 feet for ultimate ascent to 8000–14,000 feet; for ascent to 14,000–22,000 feet additional 2–4-day stay at 10,000–12,000 feet. For >14,000 feet, only ascend 1000 feet per day with rest every other day.

Air Travel

▶ **Do not fly if:**
- Unstable congestive heart failure (CHF)
- Cyanotic heart disease
- Acute pneumonia with borderline O_2 saturations at sea level
- Pneumothorax or recent thoracic surgery ≤ 3 weeks
- Abdominal or eye surgery ≤ 2 weeks
- Newborns < 24 hours of age
- Scuba diving ≤ 24 hours of flight

▶ **Relative Contraindications:**
- Sickle cell disease (SCD) or sickle cell-thalassemia: 20% will have vasoocclusive crisis at cabin pressures of 5000 feet.
- Anemia with Hgb < 7 g/dL
- Acute otitis media (AOM) or sinusitis
- Patients with cardiopulmonary disease can fly if sea level PaO_2 is 67 mm Hg.

Dysbaric Diving Injuries

▶ **Drowning** is the leading cause of death in sport scuba divers (65%).
▶ **Barotrauma Definitions:**
- Barotrauma of descent (squeeze): occurs if air is unable to enter air-filled structures such as bowel
- Barotrauma of ascent: re-expansion of gases in the body
▶ **POPS:** **p**ulmonary **o**ver-**p**ressurization **s**yndrome
- Lung rupture secondary to ascent
- Occurs within minutes of surfacing
- Symptoms: subcutaneous emphysema, hoarseness, dyspnea, hemoptysis
- Treatment: O_2, chest tube, early recompression in dive chamber, air transport at < 1000 feet
▶ **Arterial Gas Embolization**
- Occurs ≤ 10 minutes of resurfacing and is secondary to breath-holding during ascent

- **Laboratory studies:** prothrombin time (PT)/partial thromboplastin time (PTT), CBC, ECG, CK—correlates with degree of neurologic deterioration
- **Treatment:** supine, neutral position, 100% O_2, intubation, endotracheal tube (ETT) cuff and Foley cuff filled with H_2O, IV fluids at two-thirds maintenance, dopamine
- Recompression is the definitive treatment. 2.8 atmosphere absolute (ATA) (60 feet of seawater [FSW]) with 100% O_2 for 20-minute periods alternating with room air (RA) for 20 minutes. After 75 minutes ↓ to 30 FSW with alternating O_2 and RA. If no improvement after first 20 minutes, then ↑ to 6 ATA to ↓ size of bubble.

► **Nitrogen Narcosis**
- **Symptoms:** loss of coordination, acute loss of consciousness (ALOC), obtundation
- **Treatment:** ascent, if no improvement check ABG, ECG, electrolytes, drug screen
- **Prophylaxis** for deep dives: substitute helium for nitrogen

► **Decompression Sickness: "The Bends"**
- Results from liberation of inert gas bubbles (nitrogen) from saturated tissues when environmental pressure is ↓. Deeper and longer dives ↑ the amount of nitrogen absorbed.
- Onset is 1–6 hours after resurfacing.
- Risk factors: dives < 10 meters, recent travel by plane within hours
- **Type I:** cutaneous, lymphatic, musculoskeletal (CLM)
  1. **Symptoms:** pruritus, lymph node pain and swelling, tinnitus, deafness, periarticular pain
- **Type II:** pulmonary, cardiac, CNS
  1. **Symptoms:** HA, shock, chest pain, paralysis, amnesia, behavioral changes
  2. Although rare in children, this type is more common when it does occur
- **Treatment:** 100% O_2, chest tube for pneumothorax, IV fluids 20 cc/kg bolus of NS or LR then titrate to urine output of 1–2 cc/kg
  1. Decompression
     a. Type I: 60 FSW (2.8 ATA) with 100% O_2 and RA at 20-minute cycles. After 45 minutes, transition to 30

FSW, and the patient is gradually brought to sea
level pressure. No diving for 4–6 weeks.

b. Type II: 60 FSW for 75 minutes then 30 FSW. 80–90%
recovery. No diving for 4–6 months.

INHALATIONAL INJURIES

▶ **Types of Inhalants:**
- Categorized by gases, smokes, volatiles, and vapors
- The most common agents abused are: glues, adhesives, nail
polish removers, paints, gasoline, deodorants.

▶ **Stages of Pulmonary Injury after Smoke Inhalation:**
- Respiratory insufficiency and bronchospasm at 1–12 hours
after exposure
- Pulmonary edema at 6–72 hours after exposure
- Bronchopneumonia at > 60 hours after exposure

▶ **Specific Inhalation Injuries:**
- **Smoke**
  1. Thermal and toxic gases including carbon monoxide
(CO) and cyanide.
  2. Most house fires occur at night between December and
March.
  3. Mortality ranges from 45–78%.
  4. Toxicity is affected by heat (as low as 150° C may cause
injury), particulate matter, and toxic gases (most common is CO).
  5. The upper and lower airways may be affected, resulting in
respiratory failure, asphyxiation, and systemic poisoning.
  6. Evaluation should include an ABG with co-oximetry
to check the carboxyhemoglobin level. The initial chest
x-ray is an insensitive indicator of smoke injury.
  7. Management is supportive with humidified O_2, suctioning, and early airway support.

- **Carbon Monoxide**
  1. An odorless, tasteless, and colorless gas.
  2. Toxicity is associated with smoke injuries, heating
equipment, and automobile exhaust.
  3. CO binds hemoglobin 230–270 times stronger than O_2
and children may have symptoms of syncope or altered
mental status from levels as low as 18–24%.

4. Although the child may have cyanosis or paleness, the classic presentation is the cherry-red color of the skin and mucous membranes.

5. Retinal hemorrhages are occasionally seen with this poisoning. Immediate death may occur at levels of 70–80%.

6. Long-term complications involve neuropsychiatric problems.

7. Must measure with co-oximetry

8. Comparisons of levels with symptoms are not reliable in children.

9. The PaO_2 may be normal despite cyanosis in a patient.

10. **Management:**
    a. Delivery of 100% O_2, which ↓ the half-life of carboxyhemoglobin from 4–6 hours to 46–60 minutes.
    b. Alternatively, a hyperbaric oxygen (HBO_2) chamber reduces the half-life to 20–30 minutes; if available HBO_2 should be used for symptomatic patients, pregnant patients, levels > 25–30% or symptoms that fail to resolve with 100% O_2.

- **Hydrocarbon aspiration**
    1. Most hydrocarbons are derivatives of petroleum, but common childhood ingestions include kerosene and gasoline products that are left in nonsecure containers.
    2. Toxicity is primarily dependent on the viscosity.
        a. The lower the viscosity, the higher risk of aspiration.
        b. Mineral oil has a low viscosity.
        c. Mineral seal oil and kerosene have moderate viscosity.
        d. Gasoline and naphtha have high viscosity.
        e. Patients with low-viscosity hydrocarbon ingestion should not undergo gastric emptying due to the higher risk of aspiration.
    3. **Side effects include:**
        a. Aspiration pneumonitis (most common).
        b. CNS effects, dysrhythmias, and cardiomyopathy.
        c. An ABG will demonstrate a normal $PaCO_2$ with significant hypoxemia.
        d. CBC may demonstrate a leukocytosis with a left shift ≤ 1 hour of ingestion.

    4. **Management:**
       a. Supportive with O_2 and cutaneous decontamination.
       b. All children with ingestion and suspicion of aspiration should be admitted for observation.

- **CHAMP mnemonic for hydrocarbons that should undergo GI decontamination:**

  C—**C**amphor-containing compounds

  H—**H**alogenated hydrocarbons

  A—**A**romatic hydrocarbons such as benzene

  M—Heavy **m**etals such as lead, cadmium, and selenium

  P—**P**esticide-containing hydrocarbons

- **Chlorine gas**
  1. A yellow-green gas that destroys the mucous membranes on contact.
  2. Diagnostic findings include:
    a. Lacrimation
    b. Rhinorrhea
    c. Conjunctival irritation
    d. Cough
    e. Sore throat
    f. Laryngeal edema
  3. Onset may occur within minutes of the exposure
  4. **Management** is supportive and decontamination

- **Solvent abuse**
  1. Patients present with:
    a. Euphoria
    b. Headache
    c. Nausea/vomiting
    d. Slurred speech and ataxia (drunk appearance)
  2. **Management** includes O_2, skin decontamination, and screening for methemoglobinemia

- **Ammonia**
  1. Alkaline, colorless, and lighter than air.
  2. Most home products are 5–10% aqueous ammonia solutions and side effects are mostly local irritation and superficial mucosal membrane burns.
  3. Ammonia causes liquefactive necrosis and therefore high concentrations can result in airway irritation (upper airway edema, bronchospasm), chemical burns of the eyes, and partial or full-thickness skin burns.

4. **Management:**
   a. Supportive with humidified O_2 or emergent intubation for severe cases.
   b. Some ENT physicians recommend steroids for the laryngeal edema.
   c. Skin and eye irrigation should be performed and an ophthalmologist should be consulted for eye burns.

RADIATION EXPOSURE

▶ Children are more vulnerable to radiation due to larger quantity of rapidly dividing cells.
▶ **Types of Radiation:**
   • **Nonionizing:**
     1. Solar rays, microwaves, radio waves
     2. Can be harmful
     3. Do not cause radiation sickness or radioactive contamination
   • **Ionizing:**
     1. Nuclear weapons/reactors, x-ray machines
     2. Penetrating or nonpenetrating
     3. Damage by exposing DNA to free radicals
▶ **Clinical Effects on CNS, GI, Genetic, Hematopoietic Depend on:**
   • Type and amount of radiation exposure
   • Length of exposure
   • Distance from radiation source
   • Type of shielding
   • Continuous versus intermittent exposure
▶ **Definitions:**
   • **Irradiation**
     1. Exposure to a source of radiation
     2. Does not cause patient to be overreactive
   • **Contamination**
     1. Deposition of radioactive material in or on the body
     2. Alpha, beta, and neutron effects
▶ **Diagnostic Findings:**
   • The earlier the onset of symptoms, the greater the amount and length of exposure.
   • Nausea, vomiting, malaise, depression of white cells/platelets.

TABLE 4-4
RADIATION

Types	Characteristics	Examples	Effects of Radiation
Alpha	+ Charge Limited to epidermis Not harmful Travel few centimeters	Plutonium Uranium Radium	Generally not harmful
Beta	Electrons Travel few meters Cause burns	Tritium C14 Phosphorus	Generally not harmful
Gamma	Penetrate deeply Main cause of radiation syndrome	X-rays	75–125 rads: minimum dose that produces nausea/vomiting in 20% 125–200 rads: lymphocyte depression of 50% by 48 h 240–340 rads: lymphocyte depression of > 75% by 48 h 500+ rads: GI complications, death, and bleeding 5000+ rads: CNS, GI, and CV involvement with death by 24–72 h
Neutrons	No electrical charge Penetrate deep layers	Nuclear reactors Accelerators Weapons	

- Absolute lymphocyte count 48 hours after exposure to whole body irradiation is the best estimator of ultimate prognosis:
    1. If count > 1200, prognosis good
    2. If count = 300–1200, prognosis fair
    3. If count < 300, prognosis poor
▶ **Complications:**
- ↑ Incidence of cancer (leukemia, thyroid, breast, head/neck), cataracts
- ↓ Life span

- Genetic mutations
▶ **Management:**
  - Airway, breathing, circulation (ABCs)
  - Minimize internal contamination
  - Minimize spread of unsealed radioisotope contamination
  - Evaluate and treat acute radiation syndrome
  - Enter emergency room by separate door
  - Cover patient with sheet
  - Close ventilation to room
  - Wear protective gear
  - Maximum exposure allowed per contact: 5 rems
▶ **Contamination:**
  - **External contamination**
    1. Removing clothing results in 70–90% decrease in radiation
    2. Wash patient with warm water and soap, shampoo hair
    3. Irrigate eyes, trim nails
    4. Treat open wounds first
  - **Internal contamination**
    1. Gastric lavage or emesis followed by antacids
    2. Use of cathartics recommended
    3. Remove inhaled contaminants with bronchopulmonary lavage
    4. Chelation ethylene diamine tetraacetic acid (EDTA), diethylenetriamine pentaacetic acid (DTPA)
       a. Aluminum phosphate gel-star, $BaSO_4$ or $MgSO_4$ is used for S++Ra
       b. Prussian blue for cesium, rubidium, and thallium
       c. Potassium iodide for radioactive iodide
       d. EDTA and penicillamine for radioactive lead
       e. DTPA for transuranic metals
▶ **Disposition:**
  - **Survival probable**
    1. No symptoms or mild symptoms that subside in few hours
    2. Exposure < 200 rads
    3. Normal initial leukocyte count
  - **Survival possible**
    1. Exposure to 200–800 rads
    2. Nausea and vomiting brief: 24–48 hours

3. Asymptomatic after nausea/vomiting
4. Later: thrombocytopenia, granulocytopenia, lymphopenia
5. Admit for fluid and electrolyte monitoring
- **Survival improbable**
    1. Exposure $\geq$ 800 rads
    2. Rapid onset of fulminant nausea/vomiting/diarrhea
    3. Dismal prognosis
    4. Death within 2–10 days

► **Basis for Estimating Exposure Dose and Prognosis:**
1. Type of exposing radiation (alpha, beta, gamma, neutron)
2. Duration of exposure
3. Distance between exposing agent and victim and amount of exposing agent present
4. History of exposure
5. Rapidity of onset of symptoms
6. Type of symptoms
7. Initial leukocyte count

TOXICOLOGY

TABLE 5-1
TOXICOLOGY

Drug	Antidote
Acetaminophen	N-acetyl cysteine
Anticholinergic (atropine)	Physostigmine
Benzodiazepines	Flumazenil
β-blockers	Glucagon
Calcium-channel blockers	Calcium chloride, glucagon
Carbon monoxide	Oxygen, hyperbaric chamber
Clonidine	Naloxone
Cyanide	Amyl nitrite, sodium nitrite, sodium thiosulfate
Digoxin	Fab fragments (Digibind)
Ethylene glycol	4-Methylpyrazole (fomepizole)
Organophosphates	Atropine, pralidoxime
Carbamate insecticides	Atropine
Iron	Deferoxamine
Methanol	Fomepizole
Opiates	Naloxone
Oral hypoglycemic agents (sulfonylureas)	Octreotide
Tricyclic antidepressants	Sodium bicarbonate

OVERDOSE

► In general, two types of overdose (OD):
  • Unintentional ingestions; ages: ± 1–5 years
  • Purposeful ingestions; adolescents
► **Methods to Aid Excretion**
  • Alkalinization of the urine
  • Dialysis
  • Hemoperfusion
  • Multidose-activated charcoal (MDAC)

▶ Obtain multiple drug levels during management in order to determine a trend and ensure a cessation of absorption (i.e., extended release formulations).

▶ All obtunded patients with possible OD should receive the "coma cocktail". A useful mnemonic is **DON'T**: **D**extrose, **O**xygen, **N**arcan, **T**hiamine.

▶ Check for toxidromes, including opiates, tricyclic antidepressants, anticholinergics, and sympathomimetics.

▶ Calculation of both the anion gap and the osmolar gap aids in narrowing the differential of toxic exposures.

▶ Medications may be seen on abdominal x-rays.

▶ Drug packages may also be seen. Radiopaque medications may be remembered with the mnemonic **CHIPS**: **C**alcium salts, **C**hloral hydrate, **H**alogenated **H**ydrocarbons, **H**eavy metals, **I**ron, **P**henothiazines, **S**low release medications and **S**alicylates.

▶ ECG may provide clues in diagnosis and is important to obtain in any potential OD, specifically to look for bradyarrhythmias or tachyarrhythmias and conduction abnormalities.

▶ Methods to prevent gastrointestinal (GI) absorption (GI decontamination) include:
  • Forced emesis with syrup of ipecac: rarely needed
  • Gastric lavage
  • Whole bowel irrigation
  • Activated charcoal

▶ *The sooner the GI decontamination is initiated, the better.*

▶ Activated charcoal (MDAC) is recommended for toxins within 1–2 hours of ingestion, unless it is being used to aid in excretion.
  • The main complication is aspiration and subsequent chemical pneumonitis, so use caution in those patients with impaired gag reflex, seizures, or decreased level of consciousness (LOC).
  • Substances for which activated charcoal is ineffective include:
    1. Ions (i.e., lithium, irons, lead)
    2. Acids/bases (i.e., HCl/NaOH)

▶ Whole bowel irrigation involves rapid administration of an electrolyte lavage solution (i.e., GoLytely).
  • Indications include:
    1. A large amount of toxin (i.e., cases in which charcoal will have a limited benefit)

2.   Ingestions of slow release formulations
3.   Substances not absorbed by activated charcoal
4.   Packers or stuffers
- An NG tube is recommended with a goal rate of 1.5–2 L/h in adolescents and 500 cc/h in toddlers. The end point is production of a clear rectal effluent. Contraindications include ileus, GI obstruction, and GI perforation

SPECIFIC TOXINS
Acetaminophen (APAP)

▶   140 is the major number to recall. This is the toxic dose, the level in the blood at 4 hours for which toxicity is suggested and treatment is initiated. It is also the dose of N-acetyl-cysteine in mg/kg.

▶   **Pathophysiology:**
- Rapid absorption usually within 4 hours. This is why a 4-hour level is recommended.
- 90–95% metabolized by liver via sulfate and glucuronide pathway and excreted in the urine:
  1.   The remaining drug is metabolized via cytochrome P-450 into a toxic intermediate compound.
  2.   At therapeutic doses, this compound is conjugated by glutathione into a nontoxic metabolite.
  3.   At toxic doses, the glutathione stores are depleted, leaving the toxic-metabolite to accumulate in the liver and causing centrilobular necrosis.
  4.   Children < 5 years may be less vulnerable to the toxic affects of APAP.

▶   **Clinical Findings:**
- Four distinct stages in APAP OD:
  1.   **Stage I:** Usually in the first 0.5–24 hours, patients may develop nausea/vomiting, anorexia, malaise, and diaphoresis. Nonspecific and often subtle findings.
  2.   **Stage II:** 24–48 hours after ingestion, symptoms usually resolve, further confusing the presentation. RUQ pain may be present.
  3.   **Stage III:** 48–96 hours post-ingestion, hepatic damage occurs, identified by marked increase in hepatic enzymes, abdominal pain, nausea/vomiting, anorexia, jaundice, bleeding, and mental status changes.

4. **Stage IV:** Resolution of hepatic dysfunction or fulminant hepatic failure.

▶ **Management:**
- GI decontamination (activated charcoal) if patient presents within 1–2 hours post-ingestion.
- NAC (Mucomyst) is the mainstay of therapy.
    1. IV and oral routes available.
    2. 100% efficacious if administered within 8 hours, but still indicated after this time frame.
    3. **Loading dose** is 140 mg/kg × 1 dose and then 70 mg/kg for 17 additional doses.
    4. Indications for therapy include an acute ingestion of > 140 mg/kg, a 4-hour level > 140, or a level suggestive of hepatic injury as plotted against the Rumack-Matthew nomogram.
- Supportive care and therapy directed at correcting hemodynamic issues, electrolytes, and bleeding complications.

Anticholinergic Poisoning

▶ Toxicity appears in many forms, including plants and mushrooms, and many medications, including antihistamines, phenothiazines, and antispasmodics.

▶ **Pathophysiology:**
- Well absorbed by the GI tract, eyes, and skin; elimination in children is usually longer than in adults.
- Competitively blocks acetylcholine, causing both central and peripheral nervous system manifestations (peripheral effects dominate in the majority of cases).

▶ **Clinical Findings:**
- Classically presents with the often used mnemonic, "hot as a hare, blind as a bat, red as a beet, dry as a bone, and mad as a hatter".
- More specifically broken down into peripheral and central nervous system effects.
- Peripheral nervous system effects include: blurred vision with dilated, unresponsive pupils, hot and dry flushed skin, and urinary and GI slowing (↓ bowel sounds).
- Tachycardia (one of the more reliable findings), hypertension, dysrhythmias, and fever may be seen.
- Central nervous system effects include: convulsions, delirium, hallucinations, seizures, respiratory depression, and coma.

▶ **Management:**
- Activated charcoal should be given in cases of recent exposure.
- Treatment is predominantly supportive, including continuous ECG monitoring.
- Benzodiazepines are used for severe agitation and seizures.
  1. The specific antidote is physostigmine, a reversible inhibitor of acetylcholinesterase.
     a. Physostigmine may cause adverse effects such as bradycardia, heart block, or seizure.
     b. A dose of 0.02 mg/kg (max 2 mg) should be used with effects expected in ≤ 20 minutes.
     c. Physostigmine is contraindicated in cases of suspected tricyclic antidepressant overdose (TCA OD), GI obstruction, severe asthma, and severe coronary artery disease (CAD), among others.

THE ALCOHOLS
Ethanol

▶ Common sources of ethanol ingestion include mouthwashes, colognes and perfumes, and cold remedies.
▶ **Pathophysiology:**
- Well absorbed in GI tract, usually within 30–60 minutes.
- Serum levels ↓ at a rate of 25–30 mg/dL/h.
- Hypoglycemia is of concern in children due to inhibition of gluconeogenesis.
- Lethal doses in children may be half of that for adults (3 g/kg).
▶ **Clinical Findings:**
- Euphoria, disinhibition, ataxia, slurred speech, and visual disturbance may be present at low doses.
- Obtundation, ↓ respiratory drive (leading to hypoxia and arrest), and coma
- Convulsions and seizures may be present secondary to hypoglycemia.
- Nausea/vomiting is common.
- Lactic acidosis may be present.
▶ **Management:**
- Rule out other causes of CNS depression and other toxic alcohols.
- Correction of electrolytes, dehydration, and acidosis.

- Correct hypoglycemia with 2–4 cc/kg $D_{25}W$ solution followed by $D_{10}W$ drip for persistent hypoglycemia.
- Thiamine replacement is not important in pediatric ODs except in chronic ingestions (adolescents) to correct for possible Wernicke encephalopathy.
- Dialysis useful only for unstable patients with extremely high levels.

Isopropanol

▶ Toxicity can occur by inhalation, ingestion, or skin absorption.
▶ Common sources include rubbing alcohol (most common), glass cleaners, windshield deicers, and acne remedies.
▶ **Pathophysiology:**
  - Rapidly absorbed by the GI tract.
  - CNS depressant, generally considered twice as toxic as ethanol in equal doses.
▶ **Clinical Findings:**
  - Prolonged CNS depression (up to 24 hours) without the euphoric affect and disinhibition can be seen with ethanol.
  - GI irritation, manifested by abdominal pain, nausea/vomiting, and possible hematemesis (with subsequent hypotension) may be present.
  - Hyperglycemia or hypoglycemia has been described.
  - Tachycardia, mild hypothermia, and fruity breath may be present.
  - Hypotension and coma may occur at high doses.
  - An osmolar gap without a metabolic acidosis is the hallmark of isopropanol ingestion.
▶ **Management:**
  - Supportive care with attention to blood sugar levels is the mainstay of therapy.
  - Dialysis should be considered in severely intoxicated patients, or those with levels > 150 mg/dL.

Ethylene Glycol

▶ Frequently found in antifreeze solution, brake fluid, and windshield deicers.
▶ **Pathophysiology:**
  - Rapidly absorbed by GI tract, with $1/4$–$1/2$ excreted

unchanged in the urine and the remainder metabolized to toxic intermediates.

- Metabolized by alcohol dehydrogenase (ADH) (100× greater affinity for ethanol) into glycoaldehyde and then into glycolic acid (which causes a wide anion gap metabolic acidosis). Glycolic acid is directly nephrotoxic and is further oxidized into oxalic acid (which may precipitate as calcium oxalate and deposit in various tissues like the brain, kidneys, and lungs).
- The minimum lethal dose is 1.5 cc/kg, but 0.1 cc/kg may be potentially toxic.

► **Clinical Findings:**
- Three chronologic stages have been described, a CNS stage, a cardiopulmonary stage, and a renal stage:
  1. **Stage I:** within 0.5–12 hours, CNS depression resembling ethanol toxicity, but without the odor, is the most significant finding. Cerebral edema from calcium oxalate crystal deposition may result in coma, hyporeflexia, and seizures. A wide osmolar gap is noted on laboratory evaluation.
  2. **Stage II:** cardiopulmonary findings occur 12–36 hours postingestion, and include hypertension, dysrhythmias, and pulmonary edema, progressing to multiple organ failure and shock. Death is most common during this stage. A progressive metabolic acidosis without evidence of ketoacidosis or lactic acidosis will occur, and the osmolar gap may normalize.
  3. **Stage III:** 24–28 hours postingestion, renal insufficiency will develop in 70% of cases, presenting as oliguria and costovertebral (CVA) tenderness.
- Hypocalcemia, as a result of chelation by oxalate, may be seen, and may cause myocardial suppression and tetany.
- Urinalysis may reveal the pathognomonic finding of calcium oxalate crystalluria (envelope-shaped), and may glow under a Wood lamp (due to fluorescein addition).

► **Management:**
- Similar to that of methanol therapy.
- Activated charcoal if ingestion is within 1–2 hours.
- Inhibit metabolism of ethylene glycol by ADH by ethanol or fomepizole therapy.

- Correction of electrolyte abnormalities, including hypocalcemia, and correction of acidosis with sodium bicarbonate therapy.
- Pyridoxine and thiamine administration will ↓ production of oxalate production.
- Hemodialysis will remove ethylene glycol and glycolic acid, as well as correct acidosis and electrolyte abnormalities.

Methanol

▶ Sources in the household include Sterno, window washer fluids, solvents, and multiple other products, including the by-product of contaminated illegal distillation.

▶ **Pathophysiology:**
- Rapidly absorbed from the GI tract; cases of inhalation have also been described.
- In general, 1 g/kg is considered lethal, and **1 swallow should be considered potentially toxic.**
- Majority of molecule is oxidized to formaldehyde and then to formate via ADH.
- Formate, the main contributor to methanol toxicity, is metabolized to CO_2 using folate as a co-factor.
- Formate accumulates in the eye causing visual disturbances.
- ADH has a 30× higher affinity for ethanol and fomepizole (Antizol).
- Methanol has a shorter half-life in children.

▶ **Clinical Features:**
- Delayed effects (12–24 hours) due to toxicity of intermediate products. Methanol itself may have only mild intoxicating features; more delayed symptoms if ethanol is co-ingested.
- The clinical triad of GI distress, visual effects, and metabolic acidosis is seen.
- Nausea/vomiting, abdominal pain, or GI bleeding may be seen.
- Formate accumulates in the eyes, initially causing blurred vision, yellow spots, or a snowstorm appearance, followed by poorly reactive dilated pupils and blurred disk margins.
- Various other organ systems can be involved in severe toxicity including the brain (cerebral edema), kidneys (acute renal failure, ARF), and heart (myocardial depression and shock).

- A severe wide anion gap metabolic acidosis associated with an osmolar gap is seen.
► **Management:**
  - Activated charcoal if ingestion is within 1–2 hours.
  - Serum ethanol concentrations of > 100 mg/dL will fully inhibit alcohol dehydrogenase's metabolism of methanol.
  - Initiate a drip by using a loading dose of 10 cc/kg of 10% ethanol over 30 minutes followed by a maintenance dose of 1.4 cc/kg/h. Obtain frequent ethanol levels to assure adequate therapy with a goal of 100 mg/dL; watch for hypoglycemia.
  - A newer, easier therapy, which is also more expensive, is fomepizole therapy. It has no intoxicating effects and does not require a drip, but is only FDA-approved for ethylene glycol poisoning.
  - Bicarbonate therapy to ↓ the amount of undissociated formic acid.
  - Folinic acid (metabolically active folic acid) should be given (1 mg/kg q4h) to ↑ metabolism by folate.
  - Hemodialysis should be considered in cases of visual disturbance, uncontrolled acidosis, methanol level > 50 mg/dL, or a lethal ingestion of > 1 g/kg.

Carbamezapine

► **Pathophysiology:**
  - Slow absorption by the GI tract with delayed peak concentrations, usually in 4–8 hours (up to 36–72 hours have been reported).
  - Toxicity may result with ingestions of 20–30 mg/kg, with life-threatening complications seen in ingestions of 140 mg/kg.
  - Carbamazepine is an antiepileptic that may **induce** seizure activity at high levels.
► **Clinical Findings:**
  - CNS and cardiac manifestations predominate.
  - Confusion, agitation, ataxia, drowsiness, nystagmus, followed by coma and seizures may occur. Neuromuscular changes including tremor, myoclonus, hyperreflexia, hemiballismus, and choreiform movements have been reported. Pupils may be fixed and dilated with a disconjugate gaze.

- Cardiac changes are usually seen in elderly patients and those with preexisting heart disease; they include hypotension, conduction abnormalities, and dysrhythmias; the classic ECG findings are a prolongation of the PR, QRS, or QTc intervals, although frequent PVCs and AV blocks can be present.
- Anticholinergic symptoms may also be seen.
- Coma may be present at levels > 20 mg/L, and death has been reported at levels > 40 mg/L, although levels do not accurately predict degree of toxicity.
- Effects may be delayed (days), owing to delayed absorption, active metabolites, and slow metabolism.

► **Management:**
- Supportive care with attention to ABCs
- Serial drug levels to ensure a trend
- Activated charcoal
- MDAC for patients with significant symptoms and concentrations > 20 mg/L
- Hemoperfusion in cases of severe coma, refractory seizures, severe hypotension, or life-threatening cardiac manifestations

CAUSTICS

► Acids and bases account for the majority of caustic exposures.
► **Pathophysiology:**
- Upon exposure, acids cause a "coagulation necrosis" of the involved tissue, which after initial damage, actually limits deep injury due to eschar formation. With ingestion, stomach injury is most common.
- Alkalis cause a "liquefaction necrosis", leading to substantial tissue destruction. Injury to the oropharynx and esophagus is most likely seen with ingestion.
- Depth of injury depends on the type of chemical involved, the concentration of agent, the quantity, the duration of exposure, the presence of food in the stomach, and the tone of the pyloric sphincter, among others.

► **Clinical Findings:**
- Upon caustic ingestion, intense pain, followed by nausea/vomiting, drooling, abdominal pain, cough, dysphonia, odynophagia, or respiratory distress may be present.

- The oropharynx is typically red, and may progress to ulceration and edema within 72 hours. Viscous perforation and stricture formation may follow.
- Respiratory complications due to either oropharyngeal edema or bronchospasm may be rapid and fatal.
- Esophageal carcinoma has been reported years after initial caustic ingestion.

▶ **Management:**
  - As always, ABCs and supportive care, but decontamination is the priority. All areas of exposure should be well irrigated and all potentially exposed clothes removed.
  - Therapy with ingestion includes drinking water or milk, if able, and is aimed at preventing further burns, and subsequent stricture formation.
  - Neutralization is contraindicated due to substantial exothermic reaction and potential further damage.
  - Emesis and lavage is contraindicated secondary to risk of repeat exposure of the esophagus and oropharynx.
  - NG tube with aspiration of residual caustic is controversial and may cause perforation. It is considered relatively safe in acid ingestion due to coagulation necrosis and eschar formation.
  - Early surgical/GI consultation is important to dictate further management (i.e., need for antibiotics, timing of endoscopy, steroids, etc.).
  - Asymptomatic children, who are able to swallow, may be safely discharged after 4–6 hours of observation, ensuring close follow-up.

TRICYCLIC ANTIDEPRESSANTS (TCAs)

▶ **Pathophysiology:**
  - TCAs are "dirty drugs" that act on a variety of receptors within the body, but adverse symptoms are predominantly due to:
    1. Anticholinergic properties
    2. α-blockade
    3. Excessive postganglionic norepinephrine re-uptake
    4. Quinidine-like effects on the heart
  - Children are more sensitive to the adverse effects of TCAs and exhibit effects at relatively lower doses.

- Certain TCAs have varied effects, (i.e., amoxapine toxicity may cause status epilepticus without cardiovascular effects).

▶ **Clinical Findings:**
- Symptoms are usually seen within the first 6 hours after ingestion.
- CNS stimulation or depression may be seen, presenting as agitation, fasciculation, tremulousness and seizures, to drowsiness, lethargy, or coma.
- Life-threatening cardiac effects include cardiac conduction delays, dysrhythmias, and hypotension.
- The characteristic ECG findings include tachycardia, a widening of the QRS interval, and a widening of the terminal 40 milliseconds of the frontal plane axis (manifested by a large R wave in lead AVR and a deep S wave in lead I)
- A QRS duration > 100 milliseconds is associated with seizure activity; > 160 milliseconds is associated with ventricular dysrhythmias.
- Anticholinergic symptoms are usually present.

▶ **Management:**
- GI decontamination with activated charcoal if recent exposure (1–2 hours) and active bowel sounds.
- **Sodium bicarbonate** (1–2 mEq/kg bolus, followed by continuous infusion) is the antidote of choice and is indicated if QRS duration is > 100 milliseconds or cardiac dysrhythmias are present.
  1. The goal serum pH is 7.45–7.55. Changing the pH alters protein binding of the active drug and enhances excretion. The sodium infusion also counteracts the quinidine-like effects on the heart. **Lidocaine** is the second-line antidysrhythmic of choice. **Class IA, IC, III, IV** agents are contraindicated.
- Hypotension is treated initially with isotonic fluids and then with a norepinephrine (preferred over dopamine) drip. Norepinephrine (0.05–0.1 µg/kg/min) counteracts the α-blockade and norepinephrine re-uptake blockade at the postganglionic junction.
- Seizures are best treated with benzodiazepines and then barbiturates. Neuromuscular blockade with continuous

EEG monitoring may be necessary. Phenytoin is contraindicated.

- Physostigmine is no longer given due to an increased likeli-
hood of seizure activity.

CHOLINESTERASE INHIBITORS

▶ The two main classes of cholinesterase inhibitors are organophosphates and carbamates.

▶ **Pathophysiology:**
- Rapidly absorbed from the GI tract, skin, and eyes.
- Both classes of drug inhibit the enzyme acetylcholinesterase, potentiating the action of acetylcholine and causing
overstimulation of muscarinic and nicotinic receptors found
in the central and peripheral nervous systems.
- Carbamates **reversibly** bind to the enzyme with spontaneous hydrolysis in 24–48 hours. They poorly penetrate the
blood-brain barrier.
- Organophosphates **irreversibly** bind to acetylcholinesterase
resulting in deactivation of the enzyme. Most insecticides
"age" in 24–48 hours, but the potent nerve agents may age
within minutes. Treating with the antidote (2-PAM, see
below) may prevent this process from occurring. These
agents easily penetrate the blood-brain barrier.

▶ **Clinical Findings:**
- Symptoms may occur within minutes to hours depending
on the type, quantity, and route of exposure.
- The classic symptoms of muscarinic over-stimulation usual-
ly predominate, and can be remembered using the mne-
monic DUMBBBELS:
  D—**D**iarrhea
  U—**U**rination
  M—**M**iosis
  B—**B**ronchospasm
  B—**B**ronchorrhea (the major cause of mortality; patients lit-
      erally drown in their own secretions)
  B—**B**radycardia
  E—**E**mesis
  L—**L**acrimation
  S—**S**alivation

▶ These symptoms may be difficult to distinguish in children < 3 years of age.
- Nicotinic over-stimulation may cause muscle fasciculation, cramping, and weakness leading to paralysis (including respiratory muscles).
- CNS symptoms include headache, anxiety, lethargy, stupor, coma, and seizures.
- A garlic-like odor of the breath is classically described.
- A distinct polyneuropathy characterized by paresthesias, weakness, and muscle cramping, has been described occurring 1–3 weeks after exposure, and persisting for months.

▶ **Management:**
- Decontamination.
- ABCs and supportive care is initiated as necessary.
- Gastric aspiration, followed by decontamination via activated charcoal should be considered after ensuring proper airway control.
- RBC cholinesterase levels may confirm diagnosis and predict the degree of toxicity.
- **Atropine** competitively blocks acetylcholine at muscarinic receptors, thus reversing the muscarinic (DUMBBBELS) and central symptoms (a varied effect at treating seizures and altered mental status).
  1. It does not antagonize nicotinic over-stimulation; thus, muscle weakness or paralysis will not be reversed.
  2. High doses of atropine, owing to its short half-life, and should be titrated to combat respiratory secretions.
  3. Mortality may be a function of under-dosing with atropine.
- **Pralidoxime** (2-PAM, dosed 20–40 mg/kg bolus over 30 minutes, followed by repeat dosing every 1–2 hours as fasciculations persist, and then in 6–12-hour increments for 24–48 hours) is the antidote for organophosphate exposures and should be given as soon as it is available. It will reverse some nicotinic symptoms and is synergistic with atropine at muscarinic receptors.
- Seizures are best treated with benzodiazepines and/or barbiturates, and antidote therapy.

IRON

▶ Iron is the leading cause of childhood accidental poisoning in the United States, owing to its "candy-like" appearance and taste in many preparations.

▶ **Pathophysiology:**
  • Toxicity may occur with ingestion of 20–60 mg/kg of elemental iron.

▶ **Clinical Findings:**
  • Classically divided into five stages:
    1. **Stage I** (0–6 hours) consists of abdominal pain, vomiting ± diarrhea (often bloody). If these symptoms do not occur within 6 hours, iron toxicity may be excluded.
    2. **Stage II** (6–24 hours) may not always be seen. Patients may progress directly to stage III. If present, it consists of resolution of GI symptoms (and a false sense of security). However, continued absorption and tissue deposition may occur, causing hypovolemia and acidosis.
    3. **Stage III** (24–72 hours) is characterized by systemic toxicity. CNS dysfunction, renal failure, cardiovascular collapse, and ARDS may occur secondary to overwhelming acidosis and fluid losses.
    4. **Stage IV** (2–5 days), or the hepatic stage, is manifested by increasing aminotransferases, coagulopathy, and frank hepatic failure.
    5. **Stage V** (approximately 4–6 weeks) may occur rarely if the patient survives. Gastric outlet and small bowel obstruction.

▶ **Management:**
  • ABCs and supportive care. Symptomatic patients are usually profoundly dehydrated. Asymptomatic patients observed for 6 hours may be discharged.
  • **Activated charcoal** is ineffective as a GI decontaminant, unless co-ingestion is suspected.
  • Whole bowel irrigation is recommended, unless severe vomiting is present.
  • **Deferoxamine** is the antidote. It is most often given parenterally (15 mg/kg/h as tolerated, with rates as high as 45 mg/kg/h reported), and is safe for use in children and pregnant patients. Indications for therapy include severe

signs and symptoms in any suspected iron ingestion (regardless of the serum iron level: do not wait for the level, just treat) or a serum iron level of > 300–350. **Deferoxamine** bound to iron may cause a *vin rose* color to the urine, but the absence of such a color does not exclude a toxic ingestion.

CLONIDINE

▶ **Pathophysiology:**
  • Clonidine is rapidly absorbed in the GI tract with a 9-hour half-life. Symptoms usually occur within 1 hour of ingestion.
  • Clonidine is a peripheral and central acting α2-agonist. Central effects (CNS depression, bradycardia, and hypotension) predominate, whereas peripheral (tachycardia and hypertension) effects are usually transient.

▶ **Clinical Findings:**
  • Children are most sensitive to the CNS depressive features of the drug. A "periodic gasping" or sighing, agonal-like respiratory effort may be seen.
  • Bradycardia, hypothermia, miosis, hypotension, or transient hypertension may occur.
  • Seizures may occur at high doses.

▶ **Management:**
  • Activated charcoal as a GI contaminant can be used, but rapid somnolence may reduce the gag reflex and lead to aspiration and chemical pneumonitis.
  • Large doses of Narcan may reverse somnolence; it has been used to avoid intubation in children.
  • IV fluids and low-dose dopamine for symptomatic hypotension.
  • Atropine is used for symptomatic bradycardia.

OPIATES

▶ Opiate ODs can result in respiratory compromise, pulmonary edema, and status epilepticus.
▶ **Pathophysiology:**
  • The activation of mu, kappa, sigma, and delta opiate receptors has various effects in both the central and peripheral nervous systems.

- **Mu** receptor effects include analgesia, euphoria, respiratory depression, and miosis.
- **Kappa** receptor effects include analgesia, miosis, respiratory depression, and sedation.
- **Sigma** receptors mediate dysphoria, hallucinations, and psychosis.
- **Delta** receptor activation results in euphoria, analgesia, and seizures.
- The opiate antagonists (naloxone, naltrexone) bind to and inhibit the above effects at all four opiate receptors.
- Opioids ↓ the perception of pain, they do not eliminate the source. By inducing euphoria, they ↓ the sensitivity/awareness to exogenous stimuli.
- Absorption is efficient from both the GI tract and the respiratory mucosa, however, in some cases, toxic effects may be delayed secondary to prolonged absorption because of restricted gastric emptying and slowed gut motility (both effects of the opiates).
- Although most opioids are inactivated in the liver to metabolically inactive compounds that are excreted in the urine, **normeperidine**, is a metabolite of meperidine (Demerol), which can accumulate and cause seizures in excess.

▶ **Clinical Findings:**
- Depressed level of consciousness; should be suspected when the triad of CNS depression— respiratory depression, and miosis—are present.
- Street users commonly use heroin and morphine by SC ("skin popping") and IV ("mainlining") injection, both visible on detailed skin inspection.
- Miosis is absent with some opiate preparations, and in multidrug ingestions, as well as in severe narcotic ODs; the resulting global hypoxia will lead to hypertension and mydriasis.
- Opioids slow gut motility and cause ↑ GI transit time for enhanced, albeit slower, adsorption of co-ingestants.
- Generalized seizures occur most commonly in infants and children from the initial CNS excitation. In contrast, seizure activity in adults is suggestive of meperidine or propoxyphene ingestions, because of their toxic metabolites.
- Pontine hemorrhage is the classic misdiagnosed disorder as

it also presents with altered mental status, shallow breathing, and pinpoint pupils.
- In the pediatric population, both hypoglycemia and diabetic ketoacidosis (DKA) can present mimicking an opiate ingestion.

▶ **Management:**
- A KUB may be helpful if suspecting a body stuffer or body packer, but keep in mind negative x-rays do not rule out potentially life-threatening ingestions.
- Adequate airway control (endotracheal intubation) is, as always, indicated for patients who are unable to protect their airway, or in those who need to receive activated charcoal and in whom subsequent airway compromise is likely.
- Naloxone (a pure competitive antagonist of opioid receptors) is the antidote for opiate toxicity, and should only be used to alleviate respiratory depression or to confirm the diagnosis. Caution should be maintained and only small doses that are slowly titrated to effect should be administered, as a patient can quickly become agitated/combative.
- The half-life of naloxone is roughly 20–60 minutes, with a duration period of 2–3 hours. Since some of the opiates have much longer half-lives, a Narcan drip may need to be titrated to the desired effect (adequate respiratory effort).
- In pediatric patients < 20 kg the dose of naloxone is 0.1 mg/kg.
- A naloxone drip may be instituted, administering two thirds of the initial successful dose over 1 hour in a continuous infusion.

CARBON MONOXIDE POISONING

▶ Carbon monoxide (CO) inhalation is the leading cause of death by poisoning for all age groups in the United States.
▶ Neonates and the *in utero* fetus are more vulnerable due to the naturally leftward shift of the dissociation curve of fetal hemoglobin, resulting in ↑ tissue hypoxia at similar carboxyhemoglobin levels.
▶ **Pathophysiology:**
- CO reversibly binds hemoglobin resulting in a state of functional anemia.

- CO binds hemoglobin 250 times more avidly than does O_2; thus, even small concentrations can result in significant levels of carboxyhemoglobin (COHgb).
- The binding of CO to hemoglobin causes ↑ binding of O_2 molecules at the other three O_2 binding sites, causing a leftward shift in the oxyhemoglobin dissociation curve and ↓ the availability of O_2 to the already hypoxic tissues.
- CO binds to cardiac myoglobin with an even greater affinity than to hemoglobin. The resulting myocardial depression and hypotension exacerbates the tissue hypoxia. CO is eliminated through the lungs. The half-life of CO at room air is 3–4 hours. Exposure to 100% O_2 reduces the half-life to 30–90 minutes, and HBO_2 at 2.5 atmospheres with 100% O_2 reduces it to 15–23 minutes.

▶ **Clinical Findings:**
- CNS manifestations of CO toxicity vary from irritability to coma. CO poisoning can be classified as:
    1. **Mild** (< 20% COHgb): slight dyspnea, ↓ visual acuity, and deterioration of higher cerebral functions.
    2. **Moderate** (20–40% COHgb): irritability, nausea, visual disturbances, impaired judgment, agitation, and ↑ fatigue.
    3. **Severe** (40–60% COHgb): displayed as confusion, hallucinations, ataxia, seizures, and coma.
- On ophthalmologic exam, flame-shaped retinal hemorrhages, bright red retinal veins (a sensitive early sign), and papilledema can be seen.
- On the ABG, the PO_2 should remain normal.
- Venous COHgb levels predict arterial levels with a high degree of accuracy and, therefore, children with suspected CO poisoning can be screened with the use of venous blood without the need for arterial puncture.

▶ **Management:**
- If suspected, both cyanide and methemoglobin levels should be ordered with the co-oximetry portion of the specialized ABG.
- O_2 should be delivered at the highest possible fraction of inspired oxygen (FIO_2), typically a non-rebreather mask and cardiac monitoring should be instituted.
- O_2 needs to be continued until COHgb levels return and patients are asymptomatic.

- COHgb levels ≥ 40%, any cardiovascular or neurologic impairment, or persistent symptoms after 4 hours of normobaric O_2 therapy require transfer to a hyperbaric chamber.
- Currently, universal treatment criteria do not exist; however, the following are the most common selection criteria regardless of COHgb level:
  1. Coma/transient loss of consciousness
  2. Ischemic ECG changes/arrhythmias
  3. Focal neurologic deficits/seizures
  4. Abnormal neuropsychiatric testing
- Admitted patients generally require monitored settings such as the PICU.
- Asymptomatic patients with COHgb levels < 10% may be discharged. The possibility of delayed neurologic complications, though much more common in admitted patients, should be relayed.

THEOPHYLLINE TOXICITY

▶ **Pathophysiology:**
- Theophylline metabolism is inhibited by drugs that affect the cytochrome P-450 system such as cimetidine, macrolides, and fluoroquinolones.

▶ **Clinical Findings:**
- **Cardiovascular (CV):** stimulates β1-receptors and can cause atrial tachydysrhythmias (sinus and supraventricular tachycardia) even at therapeutic levels. At ↑ levels, can cause atrial fibrillation and multifocal atrial tachycardia in patients with chronic obstructive pulmonary disease (COPD). Hypotension (refractory to fluids) occurs in severe ODs secondary to β2-receptor–stimulated vasodilatation.
- **CNS:** tremor, restlessness, and agitation also can occur at therapeutic levels. Seizures which are refractory to standard treatments occur at levels > 90 μg/cc in acute OD, and as low as 20 μg/cc in chronic toxicity.
- **GI:** nausea, vomiting, abdominal pain, and diarrhea can occur. Sustained-release preparations can form concretions and leach out over a long period.
- **Metabolic:** hypokalemia, hyperglycemia, and metabolic acidosis can occur.

▶ **Management:**
- Theophylline levels should be drawn every 2 hours until levels decline and every 4 hours until 2 successive findings are below therapeutic levels.
- Check electrolytes for metabolic acidosis, hyperglycemia, calcium, magnesium, and phosphate levels. CBC, prothrombin time (PT)/international normalized ratio (INR), and partial thromboplastin time (PTT) abnormalities indicate a severe OD that may require hemoperfusion or hemodialysis.
- NG tube placement may be required to deliver MDAC.
- Hemodialysis or charcoal hemoperfusion may be required in cases of severe toxicity and a nephrologist and clinical toxicologist should be consulted.
- **Treatment of CV effects:** the use of a short-acting β-blocker, or calcium-channel blockers for rate control of supraventricular tachydysrhythmias. Observe for hypotensive effects. Theophylline toxicity is refractory to adenosine. Give isotonic fluids for hypotension. If unresponsive to fluids, consider the use of β-blockers (to reverse theophylline stimulation of β2-receptor vasodilation). Refractory hypotension requires administration of α-agonist pressor agents, such as norepinephrine.
- Seizures should be treated with benzodiazepines and phenobarbital if necessary. Phenytoin may worsen theophylline-induced seizures.
- **Decontamination:** administer activated charcoal (1–2 g/kg). Consider whole bowel irrigation for massive ingestion of sustained-release preparations. MDAC is beneficial. Vomiting may be treated with Reglan or Zofran. Phenothiazines are contraindicated.
- **Extracorporeal elimination:** hemoperfusion is more effective than hemodialysis in theophylline elimination. Consider if the theophylline level is > 90 µg/kg in acute ingestions, or in a symptomatic patient (seizures, hypotension that is unresponsive to fluids, unstable dysrhythmias) with a level > 40 µg/kg. Patients with two consecutive ↓ theophylline levels (< 30 µg/cc), obtained 2 hours apart, and have minor symptoms, may be considered for discharge after cleared by psychiatry.

FURTHER FACTS

▶ Other common drugs that may produce seizures are easily remembered with the mnemonic "**OTIS CAMPBELL**": Organophosphates, TCAs, Iron, Insulin, INH, Sympathomimetics, Camphor, Amphetamines, Beta-blockers, Benzodiazepine withdrawal, Ethanol withdrawal, Ethylene glycol, Lead, Lithium, Lindane, Lidocaine.

▶ Special attention must be given to ingested button batteries, which may be a source of alkali exposure, and may cause damage by leakage or pressure necrosis. If x-ray demonstrates the disk is in the esophagus or airway, the disk must be removed immediately. If it has passed the gastroesophageal junction, the patient may be discharged with follow-up x-rays in 24–48 hours to ensure adequate passage.

▶ Hydrofluoric acid, although a relatively weak acid, has a potential for causing severe toxicity. The free fluoride ion may bind with calcium or magnesium and cause direct cellular death. Hypocalcemia, hypomagnesemia, and hypokalemia may cause refractory ventricular dysrhythmias. With dermal exposures, wounds may initially appear benign, but pain is severe. Treatment, after intense irrigation, is with calcium gluconate gel until pain is gone. Oral ingestion is serious, necessitating intense cardiac monitoring and electrolyte replacement.

SPECIFIC DISEASES

ALLERGIC AND IMMUNOLOGIC DISORDERS
Anaphylaxis

Pathophysiology

► Anaphylaxis is a multisystem syndrome involving cutaneous, respiratory, cardiovascular, and GI systems: need involvement of two or more systems to diagnose anaphylaxis.

► The components of anaphylactic response are:
- A sensitizing antigen
- IgE-class antibody response resulting in systemic sensitization of mast cells and basophils.
- Re-introduction of the sensitizing antigen.
- Mast cells degranulation with mediator release and their effect on the tissues of the system involved such as blood vessels, bronchi, or mucous glands.

Etiology

► Anaphylaxis is commonly an iatrogenic disorder related to drug therapy, particularly protein-based substances.

► Approximately 75% of fatal anaphylactic reactions are the result of penicillin administration (IV twice as often as orally).

► In contrast, aspirin, local anesthetics, and NSAIDs are non–IgE-mediated, therefore causing anaphylactoid reactions (the same clinical picture, different mechanism by which the mast cells are activated).

► Most common foods causing anaphylaxis: peanuts, milk, eggs, and shellfish.

▶ The venom of Hymenoptera (wasps, bees, and yellow jackets) causes allergic reactions at a range from 0.8% (in children) to 3.3% (in adults).

▶ Exercise-induced anaphylaxis syndrome = ingestion of particular food + exercise occurring 2–6 hours after eating.

▶ Cold urticaria = anaphylactic reaction in response to sudden cold exposure (such as diving in a swimming pool).

▶ Hypersensitivity disorders are listed in **Table 6-1**.

Diagnostic Findings

▶ Symptoms occur within 30 minutes and may include: urticaria, pruritus, airway obstruction, shock, angioedema, shortness of breath, wheezing, and GI symptoms, which are seen more in children (nausea, vomiting, and cramps).

▶ Many patients will also manifest a feeling of impending doom.

Management

▶ **ABCs of Resuscitation**
▶ **Epinephrine:**
  - Dose: (1:1000 solution) = 0.01 mL/kg SubQ/IM (minimum of 0.1 mL and a maximum of 0.5–1 mL)
  - The epinephrine dose can be repeated every 10–15 minutes if needed to a total of 3 doses.

▶ Epinephrine relaxes bronchial smooth muscles, supports blood pressure, and reduces subsequent release of mediators from mast cells and basophils.

▶ If hypotension continues: use fluid boluses (20 cc/kg NS). IV fluids may be run at rates 1.5–2 times that of maintenance (after 2–3 boluses as clinically indicated). In addition, epinephrine drip can be infused at a rate of 0.1–1.5 μg/kg/min.

▶ Diphenhydramine (Benadryl): 1–2 mg/kg initially, then followed every 4–6 hours to treat urticaria.

▶ Steroids: hydrocortisone 4–8 mg/kg IV every 6 hours; cimetidine: 5–10 mg/kg IV every 6 hours.

▶ For patient taking β-blockers: use nebulized atropine—0.05–0.075 mg/kg every 4 hours or glucagon 1–5 mg IV (has positive inotropic and chronotropic effects).

Disposition

▶ Severe reaction: admit because recurrent anaphylactic reactions may occur 12–24 hours after initial reaction.

TABLE 6-1
HYPERSENSITIVITY DISORDERS

Type	Onset	Type of Mediation	Causative Agent	Mechanism	Examples
Type I	Anaphylactic Immediate: < 30 min Late: 2–12 h	IgE	Pollen, fruit, insects	Histamines, leukotrienes	Anaphylaxis Allergic rhinitis Urticaria
Type II	Cytotoxic: variable interval	IgG, IgM	RBC, lung tissue	Complement	Immune hemolytic anemia, Goodpasture syndrome, Rh hemolytic disease
Type III	Immune complexes: 48 h	Antigenic Antibody	Vascular endothelium	Complement Anaphylatoxin	Serum sickness Poststreptococcal glomerulonephritis
Type IV	Delayed 24–48 h	Lymphocytes	Mycobacterium Tuberculosis Chemicals	Lymphokine	Contact dermatitis TB skin test

Juvenile Rheumatoid Arthritis (JRA)

Epidemiology
► JRA: the most common rheumatic disease of childhood.
► Females are affected twice as often as males, with the exception of the systemic onset subtype (Still disease).
► JRA has low mortality rate (1%), but it is an important cause of disability.

Diagnostic Criteria
► Onset < 16 years of age
► Arthritis in one or more joints: swelling, effusion, or limitation of range of motion, tenderness or pain
► Duration: 6 weeks–3 months
► Type of onset of disease during the first 4–6 months classified as:
  • Polyarthritis: ≥ five joints
  • Oligoarthritis: ≤ four joints or less
  • Systemic disease
    1. Prolonged fever
    2. Pericarditis
    3. Macular rash
    4. Hepatosplenomegalies, lymphadenopathy
    5. These systemic symptoms may precede the development of overt arthritis by weeks, months, or rarely years. Leukocytosis, elevated erythrocyte sedimentation rate (ESR), nonhemolytic anemia are common.
► Cervical spine involvement such as atlantoaxial subluxation should be considered when evaluating a patient with JRA presenting with neck pain, stiffness, torticollis, or paresthesias and other neurologic manifestation due to the risk of atlantoaxial instability.

Management
► Initial treatment: NSAIDs.
► Steroids are indicated in life-threatening complications, such as pericarditis, and are frequently used topically as ophthalmic preparations for uveitis and via the intra-articular route to treat an acutely inflamed joint.
► Physical and occupational therapy follow-up is very important.

TABLE 6-2
JUVENILE RHEUMATOID ARTHRITIS, SUMMARY OF FINDINGS

Presentation	Systemic (fever, salmon rash, hepatosplenomegaly, serositis, myalgia, arthritis)	Polyarticular (symmetric arthritis involving large and small joints, ≥ 5 joints affected)		Pauciarticular (asymmetric arthritis, few joints; usually large joints; < 5 affected; usually only 1 joint)	
		RF−	RF+	Type I	Type II
% of patients	20%	25–30%	10%	25%	15–20%
Age of onset	5 years	3 years	> 8 years	2 years	10 years
Sex distribution	M = F	F > M	F > M	F > M	M > F
Rheumatoid factor (RF)	Negative	Negative	Positive	Negative	Negative
ANA	Negative	Positive in 25%	Positive in 75%	Positive in 50%	Negative
Course	Self-limited; arthritis might become chronic.	Majority do well; 10% develop severe sequelae, especially hip and TMJ problems.	Severe destructive arthritis: 50% of cases.	Mild arthritis; morbidity associated with ocular problems (iridocyclitis).	Variable; may develop ankylosing spondylitis pattern.

ANA, antinuclear antibodies; TMJ, temporomandibular

Source: Edwards K, Johnston C. Allergic and immunologic disorders. In: Barkin R, ed. *Pediatric Emergency Medicine Concepts and Clinical Practice.* St. Louis: Mosby, 1997, pp 619–630.

Acute Emergent Complications

► **Uveitis**
  - Red, painful eye with or without visual disturbance.
  - It is usually insidious in onset.
  - It requires mandatory ophthalmology follow-up.
  - Its prevalence is lowest with systemic JRA and highest in children with type I pauciarticular disease with positive antinuclear antibodies (ANA).

► **Cardiovascular:** pericarditis (most common), followed by myocarditis and endocarditis.

► **Pulmonary:** pneumonitis.

Serum Sickness

► Type III hypersensitivity reaction.

► Most common cause is penicillin.

► Immune complex deposition and the inflammatory response are the basis for the vasculitic lesions.

► Fever, rash, arthritis involving large joints: knees, elbows; abdominal pain, nausea, vomiting, and generalized malaise; limited to a few days to weeks.

► Other rare manifestations: myocarditis, pericarditis, and peripheral neuritis (classically brachial plexus).

► **Laboratory Studies:** leukocytosis or leukopenia, ↑ elevated sedimentary rate (ESR), urinalysis: may reveal hyaline casts, slight proteinuria, and microscopic hematuria; should also obtain electrolytes, BUN, creatinines, and glucose.

Management

► Symptomatic and supportive treatment

► **NSAIDs:** to control joint symptoms

► **Corticosteroids:** in severe cases: renal, cardiac, or severe joint complaints

Disposition

► Generally full recovery within 2–4 weeks.

► Admit patients with:
  - Systemic involvement of the cardiovascular, neurologic, or renal systems
  - Ill patients with high fever or severe joint pain

CARDIOVASCULAR DISORDERS

▶ **Chest Pain**
- In contrast to adults, chest pain in children and adolescents generally has a benign connotation.
- Pain may be derived from any of the structures within the thorax or may be referred from other adjacent visceral structure. Abdominal pathology may cause chest pain. This is due to the innervations of the posterior and lateral portions of the diaphragm by intercostal nerves.
- **Differential consideration:**
  1. Chest wall: costochondritis, musculoskeletal, breast development
  2. Pulmonary: asthma, pleurisy, pulmonary embolus, pneumothorax
  3. Traumatic: bruise, abrasion, overuse
  4. Psychogenic: hyperventilation, anxiety, depression, conversion reaction
  5. Miscellaneous: cardiac, esophagitis, gastritis, upper respiratory infections (URI), tonsillitis, or unknown
- **Causes of myocardial infarction in children:**
  1. Coronary artery anomalies: aneurysm (Kawasaki disease), and single left or right coronary artery
  2. Congenital cardiac disease: such as stenosis or atresia of any of the valves, transposition of the great vessels, and tetralogy of Fallot
  3. Primary endocardial or myocardial disease: endocardial fibroelastosis, cardiomyopathy
  4. Collagen disorders: systemic lupus erythematosus, rheumatic fever
  5. Primary cardiac tumors: rhabdomyosarcoma, myxoma, teratoma
  6. Hematologic/oncologic: hemoglobinopathy (S-C, SS), polycythemia, and leukemia
  7. Neuromuscular diseases: muscular dystrophy, Friedreich ataxia
  8. Miscellaneous: cocaine use
- **Laboratory studies** should be considered in the presence of the following:
  1. **Historical indicators:**

a. Acute onset of pain, pain on exertion, associated fever, syncope, palpitations, and dizziness
b. Significant medical problem such as heart disease, asthma, diabetes, Marfan syndrome, Kawasaki disease, or systemic lupus erythematosus
c. Others: drugs (cocaine, contraceptive pills, tobacco), trauma, or foreign body aspiration

2. **Physical examination indicators:**
   a. Abnormal vital signs including fever
   b. Respiratory distress or decreased breath sounds
   c. Cardiac findings (murmurs, rubs, clicks, dysrhythmias)
   d. Subcutaneous emphysema, large contusions, laceration, or signs of penetrating trauma

► **Murmurs**
- **Pathologic:** systolic or diastolic, holosystolic, continuous, > 3/6, S2 fixed, click, thrills, dysmorphic features, associated with vomiting/feeding, difficulty/shortness of breath/failure to thrive/fatigue/cyanosis
- **Nonpathologic:**
  1. Still disease: systolic, vibratory, **LLSB** to apex, > 2 years of age
  2. Pulmonary flow: systolic, **LUSB**, blowing high pitch
  3. Venous hum: continuous, neck base, hum
  4. Peripheral pulmonary stenosis (PPS): systolic, LUSB back and axilla, blowing high pitch
  5. < 6 months of age

► **Congenital Heart Disease**
- Cyanotic heart diseases (The Terrible Ts)
  1. Tetralogy of Fallot
  2. Transposition of great arteries with pulmonary stenosis
  3. Transposition of great arteries with or without VSD
  4. Tricuspid atresia
  5. Truncus arteriosus
  6. Total anomalies of pulmonary venous return
  7. Ebstein anomaly of tricuspid valve with R to L shunt
  8. Eisenmenger complex
  9. Hypoplastic left heart disease

TABLE 6-3
CONGENITAL HEART DISEASE

Disease	Pathophysiology	Diagnostic Findings	Management
Tetralogy of Fallot (TOF)	Right ventricle outflow obstruction Overriding aorta VSD RVH	Cyanosis with crying CHF Clubbing of the nail beds, harsh systolic ejection murmur heard maximally in the pulmonic area Hypercyanotic spell: metabolic acidosis and hypoxemia Chest x-ray: boot-shaped heart ECG: RVH, right axis deviation	Hypercyanotic spell: oxygen, morphine, PGE (newborn to keep the ductus arteriosus open) Squatting Definitive = shunts (Blalock-Taussig, Waterston), closure of VSD, relief of right ventricle outflow obstruction.
Transposition of the great arteries (TGA)	Aorta from right ventricle Pulmonary artery from left ventricle There may be a concurrent VSD, ASD, patent foramen ovale and less commonly, left ventricular outflow obstruction due to pulmonic stenosis.	1. Intact VSD Newborn: cyanosis within the first day of life 2. Large VSD Newborn: mild cyanosis 2-6 wks: CHF 3. Left ventricle outflow obstruction Newborn: severe cyanosis at birth Chest x-ray: egg-shaped cardiac silhouette, CMG ECG: Right axis deviation $PO_2 = 35$ (unchanged with O_2)	PGE infusion CHF: reduce preload Definitive = Mustard or Senning repair, arterial switch Polycythemia ↑risk of stroke, abscesses (brain, lungs, kidneys)
Ventricular septal defect (VSD)	Small-moderate: left to right shunt	Harsh 4/6 holosystolic left lateral sternal border	Small: cardiology follow-up

continued

TABLE 6-3
CONGENITAL HEART DISEASE (CONTINUED)

Disease	Pathophysiology	Diagnostic Findings	Management
Secundum atrial septal defect (ASD)	Eisenmenger complex: right to left shunt (pulmonary vascular resistance is high) 60% of VSDs close spontaneously in 1st year Usually isolated, but can be associated with mitral valve prolapse ± mitral valve regurgitation. Minimal right to left shunt.	CHF: 1st–3rd month (large VSD) ECG: small defect—normal Moderate: RVH, LVH Large: bilateral ventricular hypertrophy, left atrial hypertrophy Fixed splitting of the second heart sound Ejection murmur at the left upper sternal border Mid-diastolic murmur at the left lower sternal border ECG: normal, some have junctional rhythms (atrial flutter)	Definitive (moderate–large) patch closure Elective surgery 4–5 years old: sooner if heart failure or pulmonary hypertension is developed Patch closure, valve construction
Complete atrio-ventricular (AV) canal	Large AV septal defect Common AV valve from both atria (usually regurgitant) Defective ventricular septum	Holosystolic mitral insufficiency murmur Loud first heart sound Systolic ejection murmur at the left upper sternal border, mid-diastolic at the left lower sternal border ECG: prolong PR, RVH and right atrial, left atrial or bilateral atrial enlargment Chest x-ray: cardiomegaly Present with: frequent URI, pneumonia, CHF, failure to thrive, and infective endocarditis	Definitive: patch closure, valve construction Treatment: CHF—digoxin, diuretics

Patent ductus arteriosus (PDA)	Incidence: 8/1000 total live births, 1/2000 full-term live births Functional closure: 10–15 hours Ligamentum arteriosum: 2–3 weeks	Small PDA in full term: no symptoms Moderate left to right shunt: poor feeding, tachypnea, irritability over 2–3 mos of age Older children: harsh continuous machinery murmur, fatigue upon exertion. Can develop left heart failure. Chest x-ray and ECG: normal	Premature: indomethacin Surgical ligation if persistent left heart failure Complication: aneurysm formation
Coarctation of the aorta	Occurs with patients with Turner syndrome and neurofibromatosis. Refers to constriction of the aorta at junction of PDA and the aortic arch just distal to the left subclavian artery.	Weak or absent lower extremities pulses, systolic hypertension in upper extremities particularly on the right, hepatomegaly Irritable, tachypnea, tachycardia In the severely ill baby: weakness of pulses in all limbs ECG: RVH Chest x-ray: cardiomegaly, rib notching	Resection and end-end anastomosis, patch and subclavian flap angioplasty

VSD, ventricular septal defect; RVH, right ventricular hypertrophy; CHF, congestive heart failure; PGE, prostaglandin-E; ASD, atrial septal defect; CMG, cardiomegaly; LVH, left ventricular hypertrophy; AV, atrio-ventricular; URI, upper respiratory infection; PDA, patent ductus arteriosus; PR, P–R interval.

▶ **ECG Findings in Patients with Congenital Heart Disease**

Typical ECG and Radiographic Findings in Cyanotic Congenital Heart Disease Based on Age of Presentation

Age		ECG	X-ray
Birth–First week of life	Transposition of the great vessels	RVH	PBF (↑)
First week of life	Total anomalous pulmonary venous return	RVH	PBF (↑)
1–4 weeks of life	Tricuspid atresia	LVH	PBF (↓)
	Severe pulmonic stenosis	RVH	PBF (↓)
1–12 weeks of life	Tetralogy of Fallot	RVH	PBF (↓)
Anytime in infancy	Truncus arteriosus	BVH	PBF (↑)

LVH, left ventricular hypertrophy; RVH, right ventricular hypertrophy; BVH, biventricular hypertrophy; PBF, pulmonary blood flow; dec, decreased; inc, increased

Age of Presentation, ECG Findings, and Pulmonary Blood Flow Patterns with Acyanotic Congenital Heart Disease

		ECG	X-ray
First week of life	Hypoplastic left heart	RVH	PBF (inc)
	Coarctation of the aorta	LVH	PBF (nl)
First 2–3 weeks of life	Complete AV canal	BVH or LVH	PBF (inc)
1–4 weeks of life	Patent ductus arteriosus	LVH	PBF (inc)
2–12 weeks of life	Ventricular septal defect	LVH	PBF (inc)

LVH, left ventricular hypertrophy; RVH, right ventricular hypertrophy; BVH, biventricular hypertrophy, PBF, pulmonary blood flow; dec, decreased; inc, increased; nl, normal

▶ **Congestive Heart Failure**
- CHF: defined as cardiac output not adequate to meet metabolic demands of patient
- Majority result from congenital defects
- CO = SV × HR
- **Etiology:**
  1. Birth: it occurs as a result of asphyxia, sepsis, hypocalcemia, hypoglycemia, or myocarditis. Structural abnormalities that may play a role at this age include tricuspid and pulmonary regurgitation, or systemic arteriovenous fistula. Contributing arrhythmias include paroxysmal SVT or congenital complete heart block.
  2. 1st week: hypoplastic left heart (shocklike state with the closure of PDA), aortic stenosis, total anomalous pulmonary venous return, and pulmonary stenosis.
  3. 1–6 weeks: coarctation of the aorta (when PDA closes), large VSD, AV canal.
  4. Infancy: (all above) + myocarditis, endocrine abnormalities (hypothyroid, adrenal insufficiency).
  5. Childhood/adolescence: valvular regurgitation, tachydysrhythmias, myocarditis.
- Clinical: cardiac wheezing, slow weight gain, difficulty feeding, tachycardia, hepatomegaly, JVD (peripheral edema: rare).
- Ancillary data:
  1. Chest x-ray: CMG, pulmonary edema, ↑ pulmonary vascularity
  2. ECG: nonspecific chamber enlargement
  3. Echo: evaluate EF/chamber sizes/response to treatment and rule out vegetations/effusions/myxoma
- **Management:**
  1. ABCs: O_2, assist ventilation if patient is in respiratory failure, IV access.
  2. Supportive: monitor vital signs, semi-Fowler position, sedation PRN, NPO or salt restriction, I/Os, correct severe anemia (hematocrit < 20%) to ↑ O_2 carrying capacity.
  3. Drug therapy: determined by patient's condition.
     a. Inotropic:
        - Digoxin

- ■ Dopamine: cardiogenic shock
- ■ Dobutamine: inotropic without chronotropic
- ■ Norepinephrine/epinephrine: if not responding to dopamine/dobutamine
  b. Diuretics: Lasix 1–2 mg/kg q8h used to reduce preload
  c. Vasodilators: nitroprusside (rarely indicated in ED), hydralazine, captopril
- For some infants, systemic perfusion may be dependent on the patency of the ductus arteriosus such as interrupted aortic arch, hypoplastic left heart, and severe coarctation of the aorta. In such cases, infants present in shocklike syndrome when the ductus closes. These infants may benefit from infusion of PGE 0.05 µg/kg/min

► **Endocarditis (*see* Appendix 3)**
- **Pathophysiology:** nonbacterial thrombotic endocarditis → colonized with bacteria → multiply forming vegetation → embolize to other organs.
- **Etiology:**
  1. *Staphylococcus/Streptococcus* account for approximately 80% of cases
  2. Neonatal: *S. aureus* and *S. epidermidis* (umbilical venous catheter [UVC] contamination)
  3. *S. epidermidis*: < 60 days postoperative
  4. *Salmonella:* most common enterobacteria
  5. *Candida/Aspergillus*: most common fungal agent
- **Diagnostic**:
  1. Suspect in: congenital heart disease with fever, ill neonate with septicemia, immunocompromised with fever, fever postcardiac repair
  2. Classic presentation: fever, malaise, weight loss, murmur (85%), splenomegaly, chest pain, back pain, vomiting, arthralgias
  3. Rare findings: splinter hemorrhages, petechiae, Janeway lesions, Osler nodes
  4. Complications: myocardial abscess, emboli (kidney, spleen, CNS), mycotic aneurysm
  5. Ancillary data:
     a. Three blood cultures
     b. CBC: anemia (normochromic, normocytic) and thrombocytopenia

      c. Echocardiogram (negative study does not rule out)
- **Management:**
  1. ICU admission: if ill
  2. IV antibiotics: penicillin (unless prosthetic valve—methicillin-resistant *S. aureus*, therefore vancomycin), treat specific organism identified
  3. Prophylaxis: 1 hour before and 6 hours after procedure

▶ **Myocarditis**
- **Pathophysiology:**
  1. Inflammatory cells in the myocardium with damaged myocytes
  2. Cardiomyopathy:
     a. Dilated = congestive
     b. Hypertrophic
     c. Restrictive
- **Etiology:**
  1. Coxsackie B + other enteroviruses
  2. Tuberculosis
  3. Immunocompromised hosts: CMV, EBV, HBV, toxoplasmosis, candida, and cryptococcus
  4. Noninfectious:
     a. Collagen vascular disease
     b. Endocrine
     c. Radiation-induced
     d. Drug-induced (direct = cocaine, alcohol, etc.), (indirect = lithium, sulfonamides, phenytoin)
- **Diagnostic:**
  1. Suspect in: unexplained CHF or dysrhythmias
  2. ↑ WBC, ↑ ESR, ↑ LDH, ↑ CK, ↑ AST
  3. Throat, stool, urine, CSF for viral culture
  4. PPD if suspect TB
  5. ECG: nonspecific, atria/ventricular dysrhythmias, variable heart block
  6. Chest x-ray: cardiomegaly, pulmonary edema
  7. Endomyocardial biopsy: gold standard
- **Management:**
  1. ICU admit
  2. Cardiovascular surgery involved
  3. Treatment: CHF—pressors PRN (Digoxin with caution, avoid β-blockers)

4. Treatment: cardiogenic shock endotracheal intubation and inotropic support
5. IV antibiotics
6. IV IG and immunosuppressants: being studied

▶ **Pericardial Diseases**

- **Pathophysiology:**
  1. Pericarditis: inflammatory condition of pericardium (due to infectious and noninfectious)
  2. Can lead to pericardial effusion: tamponade

- **Etiology:**
  1. Virus: Coxsackie, mumps, EBV, CMV
  2. Bacteria: *Streptococcus pneumoniae*, *Staphylococcus aureus*, *Neisseria meningitidis*, *Haemophilus influenzae*
  3. Fungi: Histoplasma, cryptococcus, candida
  4. Parasites: toxoplasmosis, schistosomes
  5. Collagen vascular disease: systemic lupus erythematosus (SLE), rheumatoid arthritis, sarcoidosis, Kawasaki, inflammatory bowel disease (IBD)
  6. Uremia, myxedema, gout
  7. Neoplasm
  8. Trauma
  9. Anemia: sickle cell, thalassemia
  10. Drug-induced: isoniazid (INH), procainamide

- **Diagnostic:**
  1. Presents: upper respiratory infection (URI), fever, chest pain, respiratory distress; tamponade = jugular venous distention (JVD), hepatomegaly, pulsus paradoxus >10, ± rub
  2. Complications: associated with myocarditis, CHF, dysrhythmias
  3. Constrictive pericarditis: associated with TB
  4. ↑ WBC
  5. Blood culture, BUN, ABG
  6. For noninfectious causes: antinuclear antibodies (ANA), rheumatoid factor (RF), thyroid function, purified protein derivative (PPD)
  7. ECG: diffuse ST elevation with T inversions PR depression (particularly in lead II)
  8. Echo: evaluate effusion, perform pericardiocentesis

- **Management:**
  1. Pericardiocentesis
  2. IV antibiotics: nafcillin and cefotaxime
  3. Dialysis if uremic
  4. Indomethacin: older patient
  5. Steroids: do not use for viral cases. Useful for cases associated with SLE; however, steroids should not be given until an infectious etiology is ruled out

▶ **Rheumatic Fever**
- Pathophysiology:
  1. Inflammatory disease of connective tissue
  2. Associated with preceding group A streptococcal infection
- Diagnostic:
  1. 2–6 weeks after streptococcal pharyngitis
  2. Symptoms: fever, malaise, weight loss, joint pain
  3. Jones criteria:
     a. Major:
        - Carditis
        - Polyarthritis
        - Chorea
        - Erythema marginatum
        - Subcutaneous nodules
     b. Minor:
        - Arthralgia
        - Fever
        - ↑ ESR, ↑ CRP
        - Prolong PR
  4. ECG: first-degree AV block
  5. Echocardiogram: valvulitis
  6. Chest x-ray: cardiomegaly, pulmonary edema
- **Management:**
  1. Supportive care:
  2. ASA high dose: arthritis/carditis
  3. Haldol: chorea
  4. Penicillin treatment and prophylactic (erythromycin if penicillin-allergic)

▶ **Deep Vein Thrombosis (DVT)**
- DVT = 1.2/10,000 hospitalizations
- Pulmonary embolism = 7.8/10,000 hospitalization in children and adolescents

- **Etiology:**
  1. Indwelling catheter (21%)
  2. Surgery (13%)
  3. Trauma (9%)
  4. Systemic lupus erythematosus (SLE) (7%)
  5. Tumor (6%)
- **Predisposition:** AT3, protein C & S deficiency, pregnancy, oral contraceptive pills (OCP), SLE, nephritic syndrome, low flow states (polycythemia, CHF)
- **Diagnostic:**
  1. Classic DVT: red, warm, swollen, painful LE (Homans sign)
  2. Classic physical examination: shortness of breath, pleuritic pain, cough, hemoptysis, tachycardia, tachypnea
  3. ABG: A-a gradient
  4. ECG: S1Q3T3
  5. Chest x-ray: usually normal, Hampton hump, Westermark sign
  6. Ventilation-perfusion scan (VQ) scan or CT scan
  7. Angiogram: gold standard
- **Management:**
  1. Elevate extremity
  2. Heparin/low-molecular-weight heparin (titrate to keep PTT at about twice the control)
  3. Coumadin (INR = 2–3) for 3 months
  4. Vitamin K = antidote for coumadin (hemorrhagic complications) + fresh frozen plasma (FFP)
  5. Hemorrhage is the major side effect of heparin. Therefore, its use is contraindicated in:
     a. Bleeding disorders
     b. CNS bleeding
     c. Surgery of the eye, brain, or spinal cord

CHILD ABUSE AND NEGLECT

▶ Child abuse is defined as maltreatment of a child by parents, guardians, or other caregivers, and may take the form of physical, sexual, or emotional abuse.

▶ Child abuse is the most frequent cause of death in infants outside the neonatal period, and a leading cause of morbidity and
   mortality throughout childhood.

Physical Abuse

▶ Refers to infliction of physical injury, and does not require
   intent
▶ Children < 4 years of age are at ↑ risk for physical abuse due
   to:
   • Verbal or physical inability to resist
   • ↑ Time spent in direct contact with caregivers
   • Greater need for assistance in daily life activities
▶ Characteristics of the abused child:
   • Premature birth
   • Neonatal separation
   • Multiple birth
   • Congenital defect/mental retardation
   • Difficult temperament
   • Conditions interfering with parent-child bonding
▶ Characteristics of the abusive caregiver:
   • Aberrant childhood nurture or abuse
   • Previous loss of child to foster care or avoidable death
   • Fear of injuring child
   • Violent behaviors toward others
   • Substance abuser
   • Mental illness (particularly depression) or poor impulse
      control
   • Young mental age
   • Unrealistic expectations of child
▶ Characteristics of the abusive family:
   • Socially isolated with poor support system
   • Financial stress or unemployment
   • Marital problems (including spouse abuse)
   • Inadequate child spacing or unwanted pregnancy
   • Inadequate housing
   • Stressful life events
▶ **Historical Indicators of Physical Abuse:**
   • Child claims to have been injured
   • No history at all is offered

- History of inflicted injury
- History changes over time or different caretakers give different histories
- Serious injury blamed on another child
- Child developmentally incapable of acting as described
- History provided is inconsistent with injuries suffered
- Delay in seeking medical care

▶ **Physical Examination Indicators of Physical Abuse:**
- A lack of physical findings does not exclude abuse.
- Injury doesn't match history.
- Multiple injuries of various types and ages.
- Pathognomonic injuries: loop marks, cigarette burns, immersion burns (stocking glove distribution), fractures of posterior ribs, metaphyseal fractures, spinous process fractures, spiral femur fractures, "bucket handle" fractures = epiphyseal-metaphyseal junction fractures, retinal hemorrhages outside the neonatal period.
- Overall poor care.
- Spiral femur fractures in nonambulatory children.
- Multiple fractures of various ages.
- Shaken baby = retinal hemorrhage + subdural hematoma (predominantly para falcine).
- Tin ear syndrome = ecchymosis of an ear + retinal hemorrhage + ipsilateral subdural hematoma and possible ipsilateral vitreous hemorrhage.

▶ **Psychosocial Indicators of Physical Abuse:**
- Parents distant from both child and clinician
- Child withdrawn, passive, or depressed
- Child unusually friendly or pseudomature

▶ **Management of Suspected Physical Abuse:**
- Medical professionals are required to report all cases in which they suspect abuse to specific agencies. This responsibility cannot be delegated.
- Attend to the patient's medical needs first. If a medical emergency exists, treat the patient first and then make reports to the proper agencies.
- **Laboratory studies:** platelet count, PT, PTT, if contusions or hematomas are present. This prevents the accused or their lawyers from claiming that the patient had chronic bleeding disorders.

- **Radiographic studies:**
    1. Kempe (skeletal) series indicated for children < 2 years of age with evidence of abuse and for children < 1 year of age in the presence of neglect.
    2. Other x-rays as clinically indicated.
    3. Head CT should be obtained in suspected abuse in a child with head injury or abnormal neurologic findings and in the presence of injuries consistent with shaken baby syndrome (such as rib fractures) even in the face of normal neurologic examination.
- **Differential consideration:** Physician should be aware of other conditions that could mimic abuse such as: Mongolian spots, erythema multiforme, hemophilia, folk medicine practices including coin-rubbing (practiced mainly by Vietnamese immigrants causing linear ecchymoses), and cupping (practiced by Eastern European immigrants producing circular lesions as a result of placing heated hemispheric object on the skin). Cigarette burns should not be confused with impetigo since the latter has more variation in its sizes.

▶ **Neglect and Emotional Abuse:**
- Common physical findings in neglected infants are development delay, grossly poor hygiene, severe diaper dermatitis, alopecia or friction burns from prolonged contact with the crib sheets, and failure to thrive.

▶ **Disposition:**
- The child's safety must be considered at the time of disposition.
- Children requiring admission due to a medical or surgical condition obviously should be admitted.
- If the physician questions the home environment or is uncomfortable with discharge home, then the child should be admitted.
- Children may be sent home if there is no medical condition that warrants admission, the abuser will not have access to the child, and the parent(s) are comfortable with taking the child home.

Sexual Abuse

▶ **Historical Components Suggestive of Sexual Abuse:**
- Inappropriate knowledge of adult sexual behavior

- Compulsive masturbation
- Excessive sexual curiosity
- Sleep disturbances
- Aggressive behavior
- Running away
- Suicide attempt
- Abrupt behavioral change
- Diminished school performance
- Abdominal pain
- Sexually provocative behavior and promiscuity

▶ **Physical Exam Findings Suggestive of Sexual Abuse:**
- Genital injury
- Rectal injury
- Vaginal/urethral discharge
- Vaginal/rectal pain or bleeding
- Pregnancy
- Evidence of physical abuse
- Sexually transmitted diseases (gonorrhea, syphilis, chlamydia) are definitive of sexual abuse in children and infants.

▶ **Management of Suspected Sexual Abuse:**
- Attend to the patient's medical needs first. If there are signs of significant bleeding, acute abdominal signs, systemic signs of serious infection, or any other possible medical emergencies, treatment takes precedence over forensic issues.
- **Laboratory studies:**
  1. Cultures for *Neisseria gonorrhoeae* from the oropharynx, rectum, and vagina/cervix should be obtained for girls, and from the oropharynx, rectum, and urethra for boys as indicated. DNA probes are **not** acceptable. A new test, the urine nucleic acid amplification test, may be useful as a screening tool for GC and chlamydia.
  2. Chlamydia cultures should be obtained from the vagina/cervix or urethra. DNA probes are **not** acceptable.
  3. Urinalysis and pregnancy tests should be obtained as indicated.
  4. A vaginal wet mount for *Trichomonas* is indicated for vaginal discharge.

5.   Forensic evidence collection should include hair combings, clippings, cuttings of the patient's pubic hair, and any foreign material (indicate its location).

6.   In most cases, follow-up HIV testing will be necessary.

- Notify the family of your concerns without being accusatory. Clarify that you are concerned about the child's safety, and that you are required by law to report your concerns.

- Documentation should include:
  1.   Pertinent history including quotes from patient (if any)
  2.   Specific observations of behavior
  3.   Complete physical examination including detailed descriptions of all injuries; pictures are helpful.
  4.   Disposition and follow-up plans to include evaluation of siblings.

- If coitus has occurred during sexual abuse, postmenarchal girls with a negative pregnancy test should be offered pregnancy prophylaxis treatment, which consists of 2 tablets of Ovral (0.05 mg of ethinyl estradiol, 0.5 mg of norgestrel) within 72 hours of assault and 2 more tablets 12 hours later. Repeat pregnancy test 2 weeks later is recommended.

▶ **Disposition:**
- Similar to that of physical abuse

DERMATOLOGIC DISORDERS

▶ **Types of Skin Lesions**
- **Macule:** flat, not palpable, circumscribed: nevi, tinea versicolor, erythema marginatum
- **Papule:** raised above the skin, < 1 cm: acne, molluscum contagiosum, pityriasis
- **Vesicles/bullae:** elevated and contain clear fluid: miliaria, bullous impetigo, varicella
- **Nodules:** deep in the skin, epidermis can be moved over top—lymphadenitis, lipoma
- **Pustules:** localized accumulations of inflammatory cells—folliculitis

▶ **Acne**
- Caused by *propionibacterium acnes* and is not exacerbated by chocolate, caffeine, or other foods.
- **Treatment:** most widely used is topical benzoyl peroxide.

▶ **Atopic Dermatitis**
- Occurs on the cheeks, extensor surfaces of legs, and antecubital fossae. The appearance is that of dry skin to severe disruption of skin surface with open fissures. It is associated with cataract development in up to 13% of patients with severe atopic dermatitis.
- **Treatment:** includes moisturizers, topical steroids, diphenhydramine for itching, and antibiotics for superinfection.

▶ **Cellulitis**
- Most commonly caused by *S. aureus* but strep is also implicated. The rapidly progressing form is called erysipelas and is caused by group A beta-hemolytic streptococcus (GABHS). The involved area appears erythematous, tender, warm, indurated, and edematous.
- **Outpatient treatment** is with dicloxacillin or cephalexin.
- **Inpatient treatment** is indicated for facial cellulitis, children with immune compromise, outpatient failure, or signs of toxicity. Erysipelas usually requires parenteral treatment.
- Consider methacillin-resistant *staphyococcus* (MRSA) in patients with recurrent abcesses or failure to respond to antibiotics. Use clindamycin or trimettoprimsulfametto xazole (may see clindamycin induction however). Vancomycin for inpatients.

▶ **Periorbital Cellulitis**
- Caused by *S. aureus* or GABHS. Patients who are not immunized against *H. influenzae* can develop meningitis.
- The cellulitis is limited to the skin anterior to the orbital septum, with associated lid swelling and edema. Eye movements are normal and there is no proptosis.
- CT scan may be needed to differentiate from orbital cellulitis, the latter being associated with restricted eye movement, proptosis, and commonly toxicity.
- **Treatment:** older children with early infections can be treated as outpatients with Augmentin and close follow-up. However, children who are toxic and have high fevers should be admitted for IV antibiotics (cefotaxime). All patients with orbital cellulitis should be admitted.

▶ **Folliculitis**
- Superficial infection of the hair follicle, usually with *S. aureus*.
- **Treatment:** patients can be treated with oral antibiotics such as cephalexin or dicloxacillin. (Consider treatment with tri-

methoprim-sulfamethoxazole or clindamycin for methicillin-resistant *S. aureus*, MRSA.)

▶ **Impetigo**
- The most common skin infection in children and is caused by *S. aureus* or GABHS. It may appear as bullous lesions with thin blisters that rupture, or classically with pustules that rupture and develop golden crusting.
- Neonatal impetigo can lead to disseminated infection. Acute glomerulonephritis may follow impetigo due to GABHS.
- **Treatment** with 2% mupirocin has been shown to be as effective as systemic antibiotics for small isolated lesions. Oral dicloxacillin or cephalexin may be necessary for severe cases. (Consider trimethoprim-sulfamethoxazole or clindamycin for MRSA.)

▶ **Perianal *Streptococcus***
- Infection is due to GABHS involvement of the skin in the perianal area. It is a superficial process and not a cellulitis.
- The area appears well marginated around the anus and patients may present with perianal itching, or pain on defecation. The majority of cases occur in children < 10 years old, boys > girls.
- **Treatment** is with oral penicillin.

▶ **Staphylococcal Scalded Skin Syndrome**
- Usually seen in children < 5 years of age and is caused by *Staphylococcus*.
- Patients present with erythema rapidly followed by bullae and large areas of desquamation; the skin can be rubbed off in thin layers (Nikolsky sign). Crusting around the mouth and nose is characteristic.
- **Treatment:** fluid loss and electrolyte imbalance occur and therefore treatment focuses on fluid replacement; inpatient IV antibiotic treatment is with cefazolin or nafcillin.

▶ **Cold Panniculitis**
- Due to cold nodules that develop in the subcutaneous fat due to cold exposure. The lesion is hard, not warm, and the child does not appear ill. Cases usually occur in infants and toddlers.
- **Treatment** is benign neglect!

▶ **Contact Dermatitis**
- A lymphocyte-mediated reaction to particular allergen.

- The skin response is that of an abrupt, weepy, vesicular rash, or urticarial reaction. It is unusual in children < 8 years of age.
- **Treatment** includes topical steroids. Systemic steroids are indicated for severe reactions; antihistamines should be given for itching.

▶ **Diaper Dermatitis**
- Appears as reddened, dry skin in the diaper region, which may have vesicles and scaly lesions. If it is due to an irritant it usually spares intertriginous folds, whereas candidal diaper dermatitis usually involves intertriginous areas.
- **Treatment** involves keeping the skin dry by frequent diaper changes, applying cornstarch powder or zinc oxide emollients. Sparse use of hydrocortisone 1% cream may help severe cases. Candidal dermatitis can be treated with topical antifungal agents. Combination antifungal and steroid medications (such as Lotrisone) are not typically recommended.

▶ **Erythema Multiforme**
- A hypersensitivity reaction commonly associated with infections or drug exposure (sulfa-related antibiotics, penicillins, Dilantin). It appears as an urticarial rash, with classic target lesions that develop over days, not hours.
  1. **Erythema multiforme minor:** lesions found primarily on skin, benign disorder. **Treatment:** managed conservatively.
  2. **Erythema multiforme major:** prodromal symptoms of fever and malaise, and involvement of mucous membranes in addition to skin. **Treatment:** patients may require hospitalization if unable to eat or drink

▶ **Stevens-Johnson Syndrome/Toxic Epidermal Necrolysis (TEN)**
- A mucocutaneous eruption with associated prodrome of 1–14 days of fever, malaise, headache, vomiting, target lesions, and blistering of at least 2 mucous membranes: the eyes and mouth are most commonly involved. It is associated with antibiotic use, phenytoin, *Mycoplasma pneumoniae*, and various viral infections.
- Stevens-Johnson syndrome involves < 10% of the body surface area, Stevens-Johnson-TEN overlap syndrome involves 10–30% of the body surface area, and TEN involves > 30% of total body surface area.
- **Treatment:** patients should be admitted and treated using burn protocol.

▶ **Tinea Capitis**
- A fungal infection of the scalp, common in children between 2–10 years. It is caused by *Trichophyton tonsurans* (which does not fluoresce under Wood lamp) or *Microsporum audouinii* (which does fluoresce).
- There are four patterns of lesions: "black dot" appearance, kerion, discrete pustules, or flaky dandruff.
- **Treatment** is with oral griseofulvin 20 mg/kg/day for 6 weeks.

▶ **Tinea Corporis**
- A superficial fungal infection of the skin. Although the classic ringworm shape is the most recognizable form, patients may also have vesicles, papules, pustules, or eczematous patches. There is typically no regional lymph node involvement.
- Treatment is with topical antifungal agents.

▶ **Tinea Versicolor**
- Caused by *Malassezia furfur*. It is rare before puberty and commonly involves the upper trunk and arms with patients presenting with hypopigmentation of the skin. Cases are more prominent in the summer.
- **Treatment** involves using selenium sulfide shampoo and topical antifungal agents.

▶ **Henoch-Schönlein Purpura** (HSP)

Peaks in the winter and is usually seen in children 2–10 years of age. A useful mnemonic for the associated findings is: **ARENA**

A—Abdominal pain, with melena or heme-positive stools and possible intussusception

R—Rash, purpuric (palpable) and usually symmetrically distributed over the buttocks and lower extremities

E—Edema

N—Nephritis: patients may have hematuria and hypertension

A—Arthritis: present in two-thirds of patients, typically affecting the knees and ankles

Treatment: steroids have been used for patients with severe abdominal pain and also in patients with renal involvement.

▶ **Herpes Simplex**
- Infections are usually caused by HSV-1 or HSV-2. The primary infection occurs in an individual with no circulating

antibody against the virus.

- **HSV-1:** the most common presentation is gingivostomatitis, with most patients < 5 years of age. Patients present with high fever, irritability, and vesicles on the tongue, gingivae, and buccal mucosa. Regional lymphadenopathy may be present.
- **Herpetic whitlow:** grouped vesicles on one or more fingers. If this diagnosis is suspected do not perform an incision and drainage.
- **HSV-2:** occurs through sexual contact. The primary infection is asymptomatic in up to 75% of patients. **Treatment** of primary genital herpes is with oral acyclovir.

▶ **Varicella**
- Has an incubation period of 14–21 days. Patients present with a mild prodrome consisting of 1–2 days of respiratory symptoms, malaise, and low-grade fever.
- The rash starts on the trunk as small red macules or papules that progress to vesicles: "dew drop on a rose petal." It is characteristic to see lesions at all stages.
- The patient is no longer contagious when all of the lesions are crusted. Complications of varicella infection include cellulitis, encephalitis, and pneumonia.
- **Treatment:** high-risk patients should be treated with varicella-zoster immune globulin (IG) within 96 hours of exposure. A varicella vaccine is available.

▶ **Herpes Zoster**
- A late complication of chickenpox infections; the virus can persist in a latent form in spinal sensory nerve root ganglia and erupt several years later. Patients present with radicular pain with vesicles appearing along the distribution of a single dermatome; the thoracic and trigeminal nerve dermatomes are commonly involved.

▶ **Measles**
- Caused by an RNA virus of the *Paramyxovirus* group. Patients present with a prodrome of upper respiratory symptoms, brassy cough, coryza, and conjunctivitis. Children are usually sick and uncomfortable.
- Koplik spots present on the buccal mucosa (tiny white spots on erythematous buccal mucosa opposite the lower molars) are diagnostic of measles.

- The exanthem appears 14 days after exposure and starts behind the ears at the hairline and spreads from the head to the feet over 3 days. The rash is erythematous and maculopapular and progresses to become confluent.
- Otitis media is the most common complication and pneumonia is the most common reason for associated hospitalization.
- **Treatment:** measles vaccine given within 72 hours of exposure can be helpful. Immune serum globulin may prevent or ↓ the symptoms of measles if it is administered within 6 days of exposure.

▶ **Rubella**
- Patients present with a prodrome of upper respiratory symptoms with postoccipital and postauricular lymphadenopathy. A pink maculopapular rash is present and coalesces on the trunk on the 2nd day and subsequently fades on the 3rd day of illness.
- Patients are usually not very sick. Congenital rubella syndrome was a major problem.

▶ **Erythema Infectiosum (Fifth Disease)**
- Caused by parvovirus B19. The rash develops abruptly and is associated with bright red cheeks: "slapped cheek." Although the rash fades after a few days, it can reappear if the patient is exposed to warm water or sunlight.
- Patients who are pregnant and have been exposed to fifth disease should consult with their obstetrician. Patients with sickle cell disease are at risk for aplastic crisis if they are infected with parvovirus.

▶ **Roseola**
- Caused by human herpes virus 6. Age range is 6 months–3 years with an incubation period of 5–15 days. Patients present with the sudden onset of high fever lasting 3–4 days. When the patient becomes afebrile, a faint maculopapular rash develops over the trunk and resolves in 48 hours. Febrile seizures may occur.
- **Treatment** is symptomatic.

▶ **Hand-Foot-Mouth Disease**
- Caused by coxsackie A16 and is more common in the late summer and fall. Patients present with vesicles on the

CHAPTER 6 / SPECIFIC DISEASES

palms, soles, buttocks, and in the mouth. Herpangina produces small vesicles on the uvula, tonsillar pillars, and the soft palate.

- **Treatment** is symptomatic.

▶ **Pityriasis Rosea**
- Rare in children < 4 years of age and is more common in adolescents and young adults. The rash starts as a single oval scaly patch known as a herald patch; crops of oval scaly patches then develop on the trunk parallel to the skin cleavage lines and create the "Christmas tree" pattern. The face and extremities are usually spared. Secondary syphilis is the most important differential consideration.
- **Treatment:** exposure to sunlight may help with the itching.

▶ **Molluscum Contagiosum**
- Caused by the *pox virus* and is seen more commonly in children < 5 years of age. Papules can spread by autoinoculation or to others by direct contact. The lesions are soft, flesh-colored, round papules that have a dimple in the center.
- **Treatment:** spontaneous resolution can occur but curettage, cryotherapy, or application of vesicants may also be used.

▶ **Seborrheic Dermatitis**
- Scaly crusting eruption that occurs on the scalp, face, and intertriginous areas. It is common in infants < 6 months of age, but can also be seen in adolescents. Patients present with greasy, yellow scales on the scalp and eyebrows, diaper rash can also be present.
- **Treatment:** includes selenium shampoo and low-potency steroids for inflamed areas.

▶ **Pediculosis** (Head Lice)
- Caused by *Pediculus humanus capitis*. Patients present with an itchy scalp and nits that attach to the hair shaft and are very difficult to remove. Caucasians are more commonly affected than African Americans.
- **Treatment:** permethrin cream and hot water washing of clothes and linens. Lindane can cause neurologic toxicity in younger children.

▶ **Scabies**
- Caused by *Sarcoptes scabiei*. Patients present with severe

itching and erythematous papules that may become secondarily infected. In infants and young children, vesicles may be present on the palms and soles and also on the face and scalp. Older children and adults often have burrows between the web spaces of the fingers. Scabies is very contagious.

- **Treatment:** patients should be treated with permethrin; a second treatment in 1 week may be necessary. A variety of other agents are also available. All household contacts should be treated and all bedding and clothes should be washed in hot water.

► **Cutaneous Larva Migrans**
- Caused by the dog hookworm *Ancylostoma braziliensis*. The hookworm burrows into the skin of the human host and causes severe itching. The larva wanders through the epidermis. The larva eventually dies and the rash typically resolves within 1 month.
- **Treatment:** thiabendazole 10% suspension can be used for 7 days or oral thiabendazole can be given to eradicate the larva.

► **Pinworms**
- Most common human roundworm (*Enterobiasis vermicularis*). Patients present with perianal itching or vulvovaginitis. The worm migrates out of the rectum at night to lay her eggs.
- The Scotch tape test can be used to make the diagnosis: a piece of tape is applied to the perianal region and then placed on a microscope slide. This helps to identify the eggs.
- **Treatment:** mebendazole (100 mg tablet); may need to be repeated in 2 weeks.

► **Sunburn**
- Most common sun reaction; patients present with erythema, edema, and may have blister formation.
- **Treatment:** severe reactions may respond to oral prednisone for 5 days. Prevention is the key. PABA-containing sunscreen may cause photodermatitis.

DEVELOPMENTAL MILESTONES

► **Developmental milestones are presented in Table 6-4.**

TABLE 6-4
DEVELOPMENTAL MILESTONES

Age	Milestones
Newborn	Turns head from side to side
	Fixates to light
	Visual preference to human face
1 month	Smiles
	Tracks a moving object
4 months	Lifts head and chest
	Rolls and reaches for objects
	Coos
6 months	Sits unsupported
	Bears some weight
9 months	Cruises on furniture
	Crawls
	Says mama and dada
1 year	Walks
	Has a pincher response
	Says three words other than mama
2 years	Walks up and down stairs
	Uses at least three words together
	Uses a spoon
3 years	Rides a tricycle
	Stands on one foot
	Counts three objects
	Knows first and last name

EAR, NOSE, AND THROAT (ENT) DISORDERS

Signs And Symptoms

▶ **Drooling and Dysphonia**
  • Most babies do not have control of saliva until 1 year of age.
  • Hoarseness indicates a problem in the larynx or true vocal cords, and can be caused by inflammation (infections, allergy, chemical, or thermal), obstruction, trauma, or neurologic disease.
  • Dysphagia can result from anatomic obstruction or neurologic problems.
  • Consider retropharyngeal abscess, peritonsillar abscess, tracheitis, epiglottitis, caustic ingestion, foreign body, and oral lesions in the younger child who has difficulty controlling secretions (peritonsillar abscess more common > 12 years of age).
  • Systemic poisons that cause drooling include organophosphates, mercury, anticholinesterase eye drops, and iodides.
  • Evaluation is dependent on severity of symptoms and air-

way compromise, but may include soft-tissue films of the upper airway, chest x-ray, and barium swallow in the stable patient. In acute and equivocal cases, stabilization and endoscopy in the operating suite may be necessary.

▶ **Ear Discharge**
- Usually a manifestation of inner or middle ear problem and includes cerumen, CSF, pus, and blood.
- Differential includes:
  1. External ear canal problems: impaction, trauma, foreign body, otitis externa, and tumor.
  2. Middle ear problems: penetrating injury, bullous myringitis, acute otitis media, tumors, and trauma.
  3. Inner ear problems: round window trauma, and head trauma.
- Diagnosis may be apparent with history and examination.
- Raccoon eyes or Battle sign are suggestive of basilar skull fracture.
- CSF may be evaluated by checking a glucose level with glucose oxidase paper, and head CT with bone windows may be necessary.
- **Management:** is dependent on the cause.

▶ **Ear Pain**
- May be related to primary ear disease or referred pain from CN V, VII, IX, and X but most pain is related to middle or outer ear disease.
- Differential includes trauma, infection, foreign bodies, frostbite, perichondritis, and referred pain from the oral and pharyngeal areas.
- Ramsey-Hunt syndrome is inflammation of CN VII (facial nerve) from herpes zoster. It includes facial paralysis, vesicles on the pinna, or in the external canal, and associated pain, which could occur weeks after resolution of the vesicles.
- Topical anesthetic drops may help differentiate primary ear pathology from referred pain.
- Evaluation is dependent on the history and examination and if unrevealing may require plain films of the sinuses, mastoid bone, C-spine, and/or CT or MRI.

▶ **Epistaxis**
- Most children < 10 years of age have nosebleeds from anterior source (Little's area).

- Little's area contains Kiesselbach's plexus (an arterial and venous network on the anterior-inferior portion of the nasal septum), which is formed from the sphenopalatine branch (of the maxillary artery) and the septal branches of the superior labial artery (derived from the facial artery).
- Trauma is most common cause (mainly by the patient's own finger = epistaxis digitorum), but may also be caused by foreign body, idiopathic thrombocytopenia purpura (ITP), thrombotic thrombocytopenia purpura (TTP), leukemia, and hereditary bleeding disorder. Rendu-Osler-Weber syndrome (hereditary hemorrhagic telangiectasia) is an autosomal dominant disorder presenting after puberty with pathologically dilated small vessels.
- Nosebleeds of high-risk children have the following characteristic: frequency: > 25/year, >10 minutes, volume loss per episode > 30 cc, presence > 67% of their lifetime and bilaterally.
- May require silver nitrate sticks, topical vasoconstrictors/anesthetics nasal sponges, petroleum gauze packing, or nasal catheters. Cauterization will worsen bleeding if applied to angiofibroma, a gray mass in the nose.
- Evaluation is dependent on the history and concern of underlying cause.
- Recognize hypovolemia, hypotension, or bleeding disorder for factor replacement. May get CBC, PT, and PTT
- Usually self-resolving with more severe cases requiring ENT or hematology evaluation.

▶ **Halitosis** (Bad Smelling Breath)
- Usually associated with an oral infection or nasal foreign body, but may also be related to poor hygiene and diet.
- Paraoral causes of halitosis include sinusitis, retained foreign bodies, tonsillar infections, bronchiectasis, and lung abscess.
- Certain odors have systemic medical significance such as ammonia odor of uremia and the acetone odor of DKA. The breath odor of hepatic failure is musty like a mixture of rotten eggs and garlic.

▶ **Acute Hearing Loss and Tinnitus**
- The causes range from trivial (cerumen impaction) to life-threatening (head trauma or meningitis).

- Tinnitus is a perception of noise in the ear without an outside source.
- Vertigo is a hallucination consisting of an illusion of motion and sensation of disorientation with space (lesion along the CN VIII).
- Should be evaluated and characterized as conductive, sensorineural, or both. Vertigo suggests a lesion in the labyrinth or along CN VIII.
- More common causes include cerumen, foreign body, acute otitis media, cholesteatoma, trauma to ossicles. Should also consider temporal bone fracture, inner ear infection, and vasculitis. Isolated tinnitus may represent arterial venous malformation (AVM), hemangioma, or aneurysm, but usually is caused by middle or inner ear dysfunction.
- Usher syndrome: retinitis pigmentosa, mental retardation, vestibulocerebellar ataxia, and sensorineural hearing disorder.
- Jervell and Lange-Nielsen syndrome: prolonged QT, syncope, and sensorineural hearing loss.
- Examination should include the Weber test (lateralization of sound to one ear); with conductive loss, the diseased side will hear best; with sensorineural loss, the diseased side will have ↓ sensation. Rinne test (evaluation for air versus bone conduction, normally the sound is heard twice as long in the air). In the conductive hearing loss, bone conduction is better than air conduction. With sensorineural loss, vibration will be heard for a shorter time on the diseased side.
- The fistula test: to determine perilymphatic fistula. Application of positive or negative pressure to the external auditory canal via pneumatic otoscopy produces nystagmus, dizziness, or a sensation of motion.
- Evaluation may include a head CT, cerebral angiography, and tests confirming specific disease association.

▶ **Nasal Discharge and Rhinitis**
- More common causes are allergic, infectious, toxic exposure, and trauma.
- Unilateral purulent discharge more likely due to a foreign body.

- Nasal polyps are unusual, raising suspicion of cystic fibrosis or asthma.
- Bacterial rhinitis is usually a complication of viral rhinitis. *S. pneumoniae*, *H. influenza*, *Branhamella catarrhalis*, and staphylococcal species are the pathogens.
- Examination may reveal an allergic salute (a characteristic transverse crease at the junction of the nasal bone and cartilage occurs as a result of the child's repeated rubbing of the nose) or allergic shiners (dark infraorbital coloring from venous congestion). These signs are present in children with long-standing allergic rhinitis.
- Unrevealing examination may prompt allergic testing or evaluation for CSF.
- **Management** is dependent on the cause: antihistamines or inhaled steroids for allergic, antibiotics for infectious.

► **Neck Mass**
- < 2% of neck masses are malignant. More common causes include lymphadenitis, trauma, and developmental anomaly (congenital torticollis, branchial cleft cysts, cystic hygroma, lymphangiomas, and vascular abnormalities).
- Congenital muscular torticollis is usually seen during the first 2 weeks of life, presenting as a firm, nontender, nonenlarging mass in the sternocleidomastoid muscle (SCM).
- A fistula along the border of the SCM muscle is pathognomonic of a branchial cleft cyst, and thyroglossal duct cysts are usually midline.
- Pulsating mass is suggestive of vascular involvement.
- Evaluation includes a thorough history and examination, but may also include imaging if there is concern of airway compromise.
- A painless, firm neck mass should be considered malignant unless proved otherwise.
- Life-threatening masses require immediate interventions and airway stabilization.
- Inflammatory causes may have a trial of antibiotics and congenital or neoplastic causes require referral.

► **Neck Pain and Torticollis**
- Should consider muscular spasm, bony injury or mass, soft-tissue mass or infectious process, ocular or neurologic problems.

- Klippel-Feil syndrome is congenital fusion of the cervical vertebra.
- Plain films, soft-tissue films, and CT may demonstrate other abnormalities.
- Immobilize cervical spine if concern of trauma.
- **Management** includes analgesics and antiinflammatories.
- Intravenous diphenhydramine or benztropine mesylate should be administered if phenothiazine-induced dystonia is suspected.

▶ **Oral Mass**
- 90% are benign, but rhabdomyosarcomas are most common malignancy.
- Hemangiomas account for one third of all pediatric oral masses and are usually noted at birth.
- Obstruction of a salivary gland duct can cause formation of a retention cyst or ranula (blue pale translucent, covered with mucosa, having a "frog belly" appearance. These are located on one side of the floor of the mouth and can get quite large).
- Epstein pearls are epithelial inclusion cysts usually found in the midline of the hard palate in newborn infants (multiple, small pearly white lesions).
- Epulis results from a persistent inflammatory hyperplasia of the gingival.
- Pyogenic granuloma projects from the gingival surface on a pink or red stalk with a propensity for bleeding.
- Evaluate the patient's age, onset of mass, associated pain, bleeding, fever, malaise, and breathing pattern.
- Plain films of the airway are indicated if airway compromise is suspected.
- **Management** is specific for etiology.

▶ **Sore Throat**
- May be a result of inflammation or trauma. Viral causes are the most common (rhinovirus, coronavirus, and Epstein-Barr). Group A streptococcus is the most common bacterial cause. Consider other etiologies such as *Neisseria gonorrhea, Corynebacterium diphtheriae, Chlamydia trachomatis,* and *Mycoplasma pneumoniae* in adolescents with pharyngitis.
- Consider lymphoma, leukemia, histiocytosis X in ill patients with persistent pharyngeal inflammation. Other etiologies

include oral ulceration (syphilis, candida, autoimmune such as SLE, and Reiter syndrome, leukemia, or stress-related), gingivitis, and angioneurotic edema.

- Examination may reveal tonsillar erythema, exudates, sand paper rash, lymphadenopathy, hepatosplenomegaly, fever, dysphagia, stridor, and drooling.
- Evaluate for streptococcal infection with a rapid assay and obtain a culture only if the rapid assay is negative.
- Obtain CBC, EBV titers, monospot, rapid plasma reagin (RPR), gonococcal cultures as indicated clinically.

▶ **Toothache**
- Nearly 40% of these complaints are the result of dental caries and 30% are traumatic. Referred pain from the trigeminal nerve also possible.
- Infection may extend to involve deep fascial plains causing Ludwig angina, which is life-threatening. *Bacteroides, Peptostreptococcus, Actinomyces,* and *Streptococcus* species are common pathogens of orofacial infections arising from odontogenic sources.
- Dry socket is pain caused by either failure of clot formation or dislodgement of clot and is most common after pulling wisdom teeth.
- Imaging (panoramic x-rays of the dentition and mandible is the most useful) may be helpful if examination is non-revealing and a CBC and culture if the patient appears toxic.
- A CT scan of the orofacial area may be required if deep fascial space infection is suspected.
- Referral to dentist for caries, incision, and drainage when necessary, analgesia, and inpatient treatment for deep infections.

Diagnostic Entities

▶ **Foreign Body in the Ear and Nose**
- Self-insertion is the most common cause, then trauma, and animals (insects).
- Rhinolith is a nasal foreign body that has become mineralized. It will continue to ↑ in size as mineral salts are deposited onto its surface.
- At 9 months, the infant develops pincher grasp to pick up small objects.

- History may reveal the problem or the patient may present with purulent discharge and bleeding.
- Complications are related to insertion, examination, or removal.
- Plain films may be helpful if there is suspicion of foreign body but the object may not be radiopaque.
- Removal should be done with complete immobilization of the patient and may occasionally require sedation, a good light source, and a nasal speculum. May require topical vasoconstrictor to ↓ edema.
- Irrigation may be useful in removal of small aural foreign bodies close to the tympanic membrane (using a 30- to 60-mL syringe attached to a plastic infusion catheter or butterfly needle tubing). The presence of vegetable matter is a relative contraindication to this procedure because of the possibility of swelling of the foreign body causing further obstruction.
- After removal evaluate for trauma, if the ear canal is affected begin treatment for otitis externa.

▶ **Lymphadenitis**
- Lymphadenitis is the most common cause of neck mass in children.
- Normally, palpable head and neck nodes are detected in 25% of children and 34% of neonates, but a change in size or symmetry should be evaluated.
- The most common microbiologic causes of lymphadenitis are *S. aureus* and Group A streptococcus (look for local signs of infection of the mouth, throat, and scalp).
- Less common causes include tularemia, *Mycobacterium*, brucellosis, toxoplasmosis, EBV, Kawasaki disease, and Kikuchi disease (necrotizing lymphadenitis: affects Asian females as tender swelling of the cervical lymph nodes with fever and leukopenia mimicking lymphoma). Cat-scratch disease is frequently suspected on the basis of a cat scratch within 10 days of lymphadenitis. A specific antigen skin test (Hanger-Rose test) exists for this disorder.
- Complications include airway compromise and abscess formation. Systemic toxicity and sepsis can occur in neonates and children with altered immunity.
- Laboratory studies are not usually helpful but imaging may be helpful to determine any effect on the airway.

- In unusual cases, the laboratory may be of some assistance:
  1. Infectious mononucleosis: elevated number of atypical lymphocytes and a positive monospot test
  2. Leukemia: markedly ↑ or ↓ WBC with immature forms on peripheral blood smear
- Needle aspiration should be avoided in the ED particularly if suspecting mycobacteria to avoid chronic drainage.
- Most cases respond to oral antibiotics such as cephalexin (25–50 mg/kg) or amoxicillin-clavulanic (25–50 mg/kg).
- If advanced disease, toxic-appearing, young, immunocompromised, or unresponsive to outpatient therapy then the child should be admitted with possible ENT consultation.

▶ **Mastoiditis**
- Results as a complication of purulent otitis media (OM) with *Strep. pneumoniae, Staph. aureus, Strep. pyogenes, E. coli, Proteus*, and anaerobes.
- Symptoms include OM, fever, pain, erythema over the mastoid with unilateral outward and downward protrusion of the pinna.
- Complications include labyrinthitis, encephalitis, intracranial abscess, meningitis, and cranial nerve inflammation.
- Elevated erythrocyte sedimentation rate and leukocytosis are often noted but are not diagnostic. CT of the temporal bones should be performed to rule out complications of mastoiditis such as bone resorption, intracranial abscess, and facial nerve involvement.
- Differential diagnosis may include trauma, basilar skull fracture, cervical lymphadenopathy, and parotitis.
- Patient requires ENT consultation, intravenous antibiotics, and admission to the hospital.

▶ **Acute Otitis Externa**
- Inflammation of the ear canal that is dependent on a moist environment with the presence of microorganisms (swimmer's ear).
- Symptoms initially include pruritis then pain and occasionally discharge.
- *Pseudomonas* is the most common bacterium present in cultures but others include *Staphylococcus* species, *Streptococcus* species, diphtheroids, *Aspergillus*.
- Complications include extension to local cellulitis. Malig-

nant otitis externa is rare in children and sequelae are generally limited to facial nerve paresis, stenosis of the external canal, and hearing loss. Susceptible children include diabetic adolescents and the immunocompromised. More severe cases could invade the deeper tissue of the external acoustic meatus causing local thrombosis, vasculitis, and necrosis.

- Uncomplicated otitis externa requires no laboratory evaluation and is treated with appropriate cleaning and topical treatment. Acetic acid solutions (Otic-Domeboro or Vosol), the combination antibiotic-corticosteroid preparations (Cortisporin, Lidosporin), 4 drops instilled 4 times daily, or ofloxacin otic, 5 drops instilled 2 times daily, are effective. It is preferred to use suspensions (instead of solutions) in cases with known or suspected perforation. A wick is most helpful when edema of the canal is present, and should be removed 1–2 days after placement.
- Also consider foreign body, eczema, and furuncles.
- Hospitalization and ENT consultation are indicated if there is suspicion of malignant otitis externa.
- Treatment includes IV antibiotics and surgical debridement.

► **Otitis Media**
- It is a very common diagnosis in febrile children presenting to the ED with a peak age between 6 and 13 months of age.
- Supine position and shorter eustachian tube predisposes children to OM.
- Bacterial etiologies are similar for other upper respiratory infections (*S. pneumoniae*, *H. influenzae*, and *Moraxella catarrhalis*).
- In neonates may also include Group B streptococcus, *S. aureus*, and Gram-negative enteric pathogens.
- It is very important not to overdiagnose OM in the young febrile child. A febrile, crying child can have tympanic membranes that appear red, or lack a light reflex and bony landmarks. Presence of tympanic membrane mobility with insufflation will help differentiate this as a normal variant associated with crying.
- Whenever the diagnosis of OM is entertained, other coexisting bacterial illnesses must be carefully considered, such as meningitis.
- Trauma to the tympanic membrane or dysbaric injury (diving,

ascent to high altitudes, or slap to ear) can cause physical findings similar to OM. Careful history and assessment of tympanic membrane mobility can help differentiate these conditions.

- Canal should be cleaned for appropriate visualization.
- Complications include tympanic membrane perforation, cholesteatoma, mastoiditis, labyrinthitis, facial paralysis, and hearing loss (particularly with chronic serous OM with effusion). More serious complications include intracranial extension such as meningitis, encephalitis, brain abscess, or lateral sinus thrombosis. These complications should be considered in any child with known OM and associated irritability, intractable headache or vomiting, and lethargy. The presence of stiff neck, focal seizure, or other focal neurologic abnormality should further heighten one's level of suspicion.
- Tympanocentesis can relieve pain and provide fluid for culture in the toxic-appearing child, or immunologically compromised child (including neonates).
- CT of the head should be obtained if there is concern of intracranial complications.
- Usually respond to oral antibiotics as an outpatient unless ill-appearing or other concerns or complications.
- In a recent study, the American Academy of Pediatrics and American Academy of Family Physicians, Clinical Practice Guidelines included:
  1. If a decision is made to treat with an antibacterial agent, the clinician should prescribe amoxicillin for most children. (This recommendation is based on randomized, clinical trials with limitations and a preponderance of benefit over risk.) In addition, when amoxicillin is used, the dose should be 80–90 mg/kg/d.
  2. If initial treatment fails, the guidelines recommend limiting the use of broad-spectrum antimicrobials to those that are most likely to be efficacious—amoxicillin-clavulanate, ceftriaxone, or cefuroxime axetil.
  3. The option of observing a child without initial antibacterial therapy should be limited to:
     a. Healthy children 6 months–2 years of age with nonsevere illness (fever < 39° C and no or mild otalgia) at presentation and an uncertain diagnosis based on limited abnormal findings on otoscopic exam.

    b. Children 2 years of age and older without severe symptoms at presentation or with an uncertain diagnosis. In these situations, observation provides an opportunity for the patient to improve without antibacterial treatment. The association of age younger than 2 years with increased risk of failure of watchful waiting and the concern for serious infection among children younger than 6 months influence the decision for immediate antibacterial therapy.

▶ **Parotitis and Salivary Gland Infections**

- May result from ↓ in salivary flow, primary or secondary infection.
- Mumps is the most common viral cause of parotitis, but may also be due to EBV, herpes simplex, influenza, parainfluenza, and coxsackie and bacterial superinfection.
- Suppurative parotitis presents with swelling, pain, erythema, cervical adenitis, trismus, and purulent discharge from Stensen duct. It is caused by coagulase-positive *Staph. aureus,* and *Strep. viridans.*
- Viral parotitis may be similar with clear drainage from Stensen duct.
- Granulomatous parotitis is caused by mycobacteria, cat-scratch disease, *Treponema pallidum,* and *Francisella tularensis.*
- Paralysis or weakness of the facial nerve indicates malignancy.
- Ludwig angina is life-threatening with swelling of the submandibular region, which often has the "bull-neck" appearance. The tongue may enlarge 2–3 times its normal size.
- Complications of suppurative (bacterial) parotitis include necrosis, osteomyelitis, septicemia, and facial nerve palsy.
- WBC may be elevated with suppurative infection, plain films may reveal a stone in the duct, and CT if concern of deeper infection.
- Suppurative parotitis is treated with systemic antibiotics (followed by oral antibiotics in nontoxic and IV antibiotics in toxic patients).
- Viral parotitis is treated with heat and rest.
- Ludwig angina requires immediate airway stabilization, surgical drainage, and IV antibiotics.

▶ **Peritonsillar Abscess**
- Most common deep infection of the head and neck but is rare in children < 12 years of age.
- Usually polymicrobial.
- Symptoms include gradual ↑ in pharyngeal pain, otalgia, trismus, dysphagia, odynophagia, and drooling with a hot potato voice.
- Exam may include cellulitis, shift of the uvula, torticollis toward the opposite side.
- Complications include necrotizing fasciitis, airway obstruction, mediastinitis, lung abscess, sepsis, and thrombophlebitis.
- WBC may be elevated and throat culture will often document a streptococcal infection.
- May require needle aspiration and CT of the head and neck for extension of infection.
- Usually requires hospitalization, IV antibiotics, and surgical drainage. Penicillin (100,000 units/kg/d) is usually sufficient, but the results of the Gram stain and the cultures of the material from the infected tonsil will determine the final choice of therapy since *S. aureus* is occasionally recovered.

▶ **Retropharyngeal Abscess**
- 96% of cases in children < 6 years of age and 50% between the ages of 6–12 months.
- Results from suppuration of the retropharyngeal nodes most commonly caused by *S. aureus* and Group A streptococcus.
- Symptoms are usually characterized by prodromal nasopharyngitis or pharyngitis that progresses to an abrupt onset of high fever, dysphagia, severe throat pain, hyperextension of the head, stridor, meningismus (due to irritation of the paravertebral ligaments), and drooling.
- Complications include airway compromise, rupture of abscess into esophagus, lungs, or mediastinum. Blood vessels may be eroded and hemorrhage can occur.
- WBC may be elevated but not helpful for decision making. Soft tissue lateral of the neck may demonstrate retropharyngeal mass. Normal prevertebral space anterior to C2: ≤ 7 mm; anterior to C3 and C4: ≤ 5 mm or < 40% of the AP diameter of the C3 and C4 vertebral bodies. Adequate films are important for proper interpretation of these spaces.

- Differential includes epiglottitis, croup, peritonsillar abscess, cystic hygroma, hemangioma, neoplasm, trauma.
- **Management:** airway maintenance is vital because airway obstruction and aspiration can occur at any time. Patients will require hospitalization for IV antibiotics, hydration, analgesia, and surgical drainage. Antibiotic choices include clindamycin 30 mg/kg/d in 4 divided doses or combination of penicillin (10,000 units/kg/d) and cefazolin (100 mg/kg/d) both in 4 divided doses. If the patient is stable, consider obtaining a CT as the patient may have retropharyngeal cellulitis, which can be treated with antibiotics alone.

▶ **Sinusitis**

- Inflammation of the lining of the paranasal sinuses by infection or allergy.
- Maxillary and ethmoidal are aerated soon after birth, and frontal and sphenoid are visible radiographically by 7 and 9 years, respectively.
- Predisposing factors include allergies, rhinitis, choanal atresia, cleft palate, neoplasm, septal deviation, adenoid hyperplasia, Kartagener syndrome, and cystic fibrosis.
- Acute infection usually due to *H. influenzae*, *Strep. pneumoniae*, Group A streptococcus, *Staph. aureus*, *B. catarrhalis*.
- Chronic infection (> 30 days) is due to staphylococci and anaerobes.
- Symptoms to differentiate from URI include fever, purulent discharge, periorbital swelling, rhinorrhea > 10 days.
- Only 8% of patients will have tenderness over the frontal sinus, but 76% will have poor transillumination (limited in children before 8–10 years of age).
- Complications include sepsis, facial cellulitis, periorbital and orbital cellulitis, osteomyelitis, cavernous sinus thrombosis, epidural abscess, brain abscess, and meningitis.
- WBC may be helpful along with a culture.
- Radiographic imaging is recommended only if the diagnosis is unclear or patient appears ill, recurrent episodes, or chronic disease.
- X-rays include: (mucosal thickening > 4 mm is suggestive of infection):
  1. Water's (maxillary)
  2. Caldwell's (frontal and ethmoid)

3. Submentovertex (sphenoid)
4. Lateral (sphenoid)

- CT is recommended for the seriously ill child, chronic or recurrent disease, or suspected suppurative complications.
- Differential includes URI, allergy, foreign body, neoplasm, and polyp.
- **Treatment** with oral antibiotics for 2–3 weeks such as amoxicillin (40–50 mg/kg/d). Alternative drugs for penicillin-allergic children and those with recurrent disease are the same as for OM. Ill-appearing patients require inpatient management.

▶ **Streptococcal Tonsillopharyngitis**

- Usually Group A streptococcus in children > 3 years of age and purulent rhinitis is the predominant presentation of streptococcal URI in children < 3 years of age.
- Involves Waldeyer ring of lymph tissue.
- Symptoms include pain, dysphagia, fever, exudates, and cervical adenopathy in school-age children. Younger children may have headache, vomiting, abdominal pain, and a scarlatiniform rash (fine, erythematous, sandpaper-like). Infants commonly have excoriated nares.
- Complications include peritonsillar abscess (Quinsy), retropharyngeal abscess, OM, cervical adenitis, or sinusitis. Life-threatening complications include "postanginal sepsis" (bacteremia from septic thrombophlebitis of the tonsillar vein).
- Throat culture and rapid assay are helpful, WBC may be elevated but is nonspecific. Infants should have their nose cultured rather than their throats.
- Differential for exudative pharyngitis includes EBV, diphtheria, and adenovirus.
- **Management** with analgesia and antibiotics. Although a single dose of benzathine penicillin (25,000–50,000 international units/kg) obviates all problems with compliance, oral phenoxymethyl penicillin for 10 days provides an acceptable alternative. Amoxicillin (50 mg/kg/d with a maximum of 750 mg) can also be given once per day. Erythromycin is used for penicillin-allergic patients; the dosing of zithromax for strep pharyngitis is 12 mg/kg qd × 5 days, and represents a more expensive alternative (limited data on its effect on complication prevention). Limited data on the use of

steroids in the treatment of pharyngitis in children with available literature not supporting its use.

ENDOCRINE AND METABOLIC DISORDERS

▶ Endocrine and metabolic disorders are presented in Table 6-5.

EYE DISORDERS
General Information

The Eye Examination

▶ Include all of the following components in the eye examination:
  - Visual acuity: newborns are able to fixate and follow target by 6 weeks. "E" test by age 4 years, Snellen acuity chart by 5–6 years old
  - External structures of eye: lids and lashes include lid eversion particularly if a foreign body is suspected
  - Conjunctiva/cornea: includes use of fluorescein
  - Anterior chamber examination with slit lamp: look for hyphema (blood present) or hypopyon (pus)
  - Pupils: assess size, shape, symmetry, and reactivity
  - Extraocular movement
  - Direct ophthalmoscopy: look for papilledema, retinal hemorrhages, or other lesions
  - Visual field examination by confrontation
  - Tonometry: do not perform if there is suspected globe rupture or penetrating injury

▶ Penetrating ocular injury or ruptured globe by history or initial exam
  - Treatment mnemonic is "**SANTA**"
    S—Nonpressure eye **S**hield
    A—**A**nti-emetic
    N—**N**PO
    T—**T**etanus
    A—**A**ntibiotics
  - No further manipulation: consult ophthalmologist

Impaired Vision

General

▶ Trauma and infection are the most common causes of visual disturbance.

TABLE 6-5
ENDOCRINE AND METABOLIC DISORDERS

	Definition / Pathophysiology	Diagnosis	Management
FAILURE TO THRIVE (FTT)	Weight < 3rd/5th percentile or weight > 20% below ideal weight for height **or** slowing of growth velocity **or** fall off from previous growth curve. **Psychosocial:** developmental delay, chronic illness, family factors. Most common cause of FTT is social deprivation. **Congenital:** Turner syndrome, Noonan syndrome, Williams, inborn errors of metabolism. **GI:** cystic fibrosis, inflammatory bowel disease, pyloric stenosis, Hirschsprung disease. **Cardiopulmonary:** congenital heart disease, cystic fibrosis, bronchopulmonary dysplasia, asthma. **Renal:** anatomic, urinary tract infection, renal tubular acidosis; immunologic: DiGeorge, AIDS. **Endocrine:** hypopituitarism, thyroid, diabetes mellitus.	Growth charts, comparison with parents. Selected tests for specific diagnoses (dependent on suspected underlying diagnosis).	Therapeutic trial (including admission on adequate calories) may help in the diagnosis of psychosocial.

HYPOGLYCEMIA

Definition: glucose—< 40 mg/dL in child; < 30 mg/dL in neonate
Balanced by: intake gluconeogenesis glycogenolysis lipolysis
Regulated by insulin
Opposed by glucagon, cortisol, catecholamines, growth hormone

Infants: nonspecific symptoms (irritability, lethargy, vomiting, pallor, cyanosis, ↑HR, ↑RR).
Children: nervous, diaphoretic, tremor, altered level of consciousness, seizures, coma.
Differential: ↓ intake/absorption, inborn errors, hypopituitarism, hypothyroid, adrenal insufficiency, nesidioblastosis, Beckwith-Wiedemann, sepsis, Reye, salicylates, ethanol, propranolol.

Ancillary data (before giving glucose): serum glucose, plasma insulin and glucagon, serum lactate, toxin screen for ethanol; urine for ketones, glucose, and reducing substances.
Treatment: 0.25–0.5 g/kg dextrose = 5–10 cc/kg D_{10} (infant); 2–4 cc/kg D_{25} (child); 1–2 cc/kg D_{50} (adolescent); glucagon 0.1–0.2 mg/kg IM.

CONGENITAL ADRENAL HYPERPLASIA

90–95% due to deficiency in 21-hydroxylase (see chart below).
2 variants: simple virilizing ($1/3$) and salt wasting ($2/3$, develop at any age and to varying degrees).
3% due to 11-β-hydroxylase deficiency.

Classic virilizing: girls at birth; boys and classic salt wasters at risk for diagnosis in first few weeks of life.
Adrenal crisis: lethargy, vomiting, dehydration, cardiovascular instability.
Nonclassic: may present in late childhood with precocious pubic hair, accelerated growth, early fusion of epiphyses, hyperpigmentation.

Ancillary data: ↓Na, ↑K, ↓glucose, low cortisol; ECG, ABG, blood, and urine for cortisol precursors.
Management: fluid boluses, hydrocortisone 25 mg IV bolus (or 50 mg/m²).

continued

TABLE 6-5
ENDOCRINE AND METABOLIC DISORDERS (CONTINUED)

	Definition / Pathophysiology	Diagnosis	Management

CONGENITAL ADRENAL HYPERPLASIA	Cholesterol
	→
	Pregnenolone
	→
	Progesterone
	→
	  21-hydroxylase ↑
	11-desoxy-corticosterone → ↑
	  11-β-hydroxylase
	Aldosterone
		17-OH-pregnenolone
		→
		17-OH-progesterone
		→
		11-dexycortisol
		→
		Cortisol
			Dihydroepiandrosterone (DHEA)
			→
			Androstenedione
			→
			Testosterone
			→

ADRENAL INSUFFICIENCY	**Primary (Addison disease):** destruction of adrenal cortex **Secondary (pituitary)** and **tertiary (hypothalamus):** aldosterone controlled by RAS. **Etiology:** primary rare in childhood, 80% due to autoimmune destruction; secondary and tertiary more common, mostly due to CNS tumors or chronic exogenous steroid administration.	**Addisonian crisis:** fatigue, weakness, anorexia, abdominal pain, vomiting; fever, shock, coma; ↓glucose, ↓Na, ↑K, acidosis, decreased cortisol. **Waterhouse-Friderichsen syndrome:** adrenal hemorrhage with overwhelming sepsis esp. meningococcemia. May be insidious: weight loss, malaise, nausea/vomiting, hyperpigmentation, salt craving, dizziness.	**Ancillary data:** chemistries, ECG, cortisol, corticotrophin. **Management:** IM/IV hydrocortisone 50 mg/m^2.

SYNDROME OF INAPPROPRIATE SECRETION OF ANTIDIURETIC HORMONE (SIADH)

Osmoregulation occurs in anterior hypothalamus: produces ADH, secreted by posterior pituitary, in kidney increases resorption in collecting tubule.

Etiology:

CNS: meningitis/encephalitis, abscess, Gullain-Barré, trauma, tumor, hypoxia, Rocky mountain spotted fever, cerebral thrombus, cavernous sinus thrombosis, hydrocephalus, porphyria.

Intrathoracic: pneumonia, empyema, positive pressure ventilation, tumor, pneumothorax, asthma, CF.

Medications: chemotherapy, carbamazepine, morphine, phenothiazine; *misc.*: lymphadenitis, arthritis, sepsis, diabetic ketoacidosis.

Diagnosis: Na < 120 mg/dL causes lethargy, headache, disorientation, anorexia, nausea, vomiting, seizures.
Serum/urine sodium, serum/urine osmolarity.

Management: Fluid restrict to $1/2$–$2/3$ maintenance; if symptomatic give 3% saline (4 cc/kg) to correct give approximately 125 mg/dL, given over 15 min or as a bolus:

mEq Sodium (Na) needed = $0.6 \times$ weight $\times$ (125–actual Na)

continued

TABLE 6-5
ENDOCRINE AND METABOLIC DISORDERS (CONTINUED)

Definition / Pathophysiology	Diagnosis	Management
Defect in synthesis / secretion (central) or renal response (nephrogenic) to ADH. **Etiology:** **Central:** 50% idiopathic, also head injury, tumor, infection, septo-optic dysplasia, histiocytosis-X, sarcoid, sickle-cell disease, cerebral hemorrhage/thrombosis **Nephrogenic:** Idiopathic (rarely in infants, x-linked), more renal (polycystic kidneys, UPJ obstruction, pyelonephritis), K, Ca, toxins (alcohol, phenytoin, Lithium, demeclocycline, contrast dyes), histiocytosis-X, sarcoidosis, sickle cell.	**Diagnosis:** polyuria (sudden onset in central, less in nephrogenic), polydipsia with dehydration, change in mental status, coma.	**Ancillary data:** serum osm > 290 mOsm/L Serum Na > 145 mg/dL Urine osm < 150 mOsm/L. **Management:** boluses to restore intravascular volume; replace free water deficit over 24–48 hrs by: First calculate: Total body water (TBW) = weight (kg) × 0.60 Then free water deficit equals: (measured serum Na$^+$/140 × TBW) – TBW

DIABETES INSIPIDUS

DIABETIC KETOACIDOSIS (DKA)

Defined as: (1) **glucose > 250 mg/dL** and (2) **ketonemia** or **ketonuria** and (3) **acidemia (pH < 7.3 or bicarbonate < 15 mEq/L)**

Insulin deficiency and increase in counter-hormones (epinephrine, glucagons, cortisol, GH)

Etiology: toxic insult (infection, etc.) in genetically predisposed child → chronic autoimmune destruction of β-cells and decreased insulin production (anti-islet cell antibodies in 85%).

New onset: polyphagia, anorexia, polyuria, polydipsia, dehydration, ill-appearing but appropriate. If severe, **Kussmaul breathing** (deep, rapid), tachycardia, orthostatic changes, vomiting, abdominal pain.

Complications: dehydration (up to 100–150 cc/kg); lactic acidosis, ketones form β-hydroxybutyric acid and acetoacetic acid; **hyperosmolar nonketotic coma** *(glucose 800–1200) rare in children.*

Cerebral edema: usually 8–12 hrs after initiation of treatment, mortality 90%. Signs: headache, agitation, pupil changes, ophthalmoplegia, papilledema, abnormal vital signs, seizures, posturing. Treat with mannitol.

Ancillary data: chemistries, PO_4 (lost in urine), ABG; anti-islet cell and anti-insulin antibodies for new onset, HgA1C for prior diagnosed. corrected Na = measured Na + [1.6 × (glucose − 100)/100]

Management: (1) volume replacement (10–20 cc/kg NS); (2) replace fluids/electrolytes over 24–48 hrs with 1/2 NS + potassium (1/2 KCl and 1/2 KPhos; 40 mEq/L if K<3); (3) *Insulin ~0.1 units/kg/h (↓ glucose by no more than 100 mg/dL/h: risk of cerebral edema); add dextrose to fluids once glucose < 300 mg/dL.*

Bicarbonate is controversial only if pH < 7.0 or cardiovascular instability— consult with endocrinologist prior to administration (give 1–2 mEq/kg over 1–2 h), correct only to 7.1.

continued

TABLE 6-5
ENDOCRINE AND METABOLIC DISORDERS (CONTINUED)

	Definition / Pathophysiology	Diagnosis	Management
PHEOCHROMOCYTOMA	70% adrenal medulla chromaffin cells; 30% sympathetic chains (intra-abdominal); associated with neurofibromatosis, von Hippel-Lindau, Sturge-Weber, TS, MEN II. **Pathophysiology:** catecholamines synthesized from tyrosine, metabolized to normetanephrine, metanephrine then vanillylmandelic acid.	**Triad:** headache, palpitations, and diaphoresis. Also HTN (sustained) leading to CHF, retinopathy, hypertensive crisis. Associated with headache, visual blurring, tremors, flushing. Palpable mass in 10%.	**Ancillary data:** ECG, urinary catecholamines (increased in 95%), CT/MRI to localize tumor. **Management:** surgical excision, phentolamine (do not use β-blockers).
HYPERTHYROIDISM	Graves disease almost always cause, F > M, 60% in children >10 years old. Autoimmune, antithyroglobulin antibodies, antimicrosomal antibodies, TSH receptor antibodies stimulate follicular cells. **Etiology:** antibodies to *Yersinia enterocolitica* and other microorganisms may cross-react with TSH receptor.	Goiter (97–100%), nervousness (60–92%), tachycardia (65–91%), exophthalmos (55–78%), tremor, weight loss (50–67%), change in school performance/behavior, heat intolerance, diaphoresis, palpitations, **Thyroid storm:** precipitant (infection, trauma, etc.) leads to fever, marked tachycardia, progression to CHF or cardiogenic shock; CNS symptoms progress to confusion, psychosis, coma; GI symptoms common.	**Ancillary data:** serum T_3, T_4, TSH, T_3-resin uptake; ECG, chest x-ray if storm. **Management:** thyroidectomy, radioiodine, antithyroid drugs. **Thyroid storm:** antipyretics/cooling blankets, β-blockers (propranolol 0.1 mg/kg), PTU (5–10 mg/kg/24 h) inhibits thyroid hormone synthesis and decreases conversion of T_4 to T_3; can use methimazole (0.5–0.7 mg/kg), Lugol solution (5% iodine and 10% K iodide) 5 gtt/q8h PO 1 hour after PTU to inhibit release of thyroid hormone.

	Etiology	Clinical	Ancillary data / Management
THYROTOXICOSIS, NEONATAL	Maternal TSH-receptor-stimulating-antibody ($\frac{1}{2}$ life 10–14 d, up to 12 wks).	Heart rate > 160, microcephaly, craniosynostosis, restless, hyperthermic, respiratory distress, CHF.	**Ancillary data:** T_4, T_3, TSH, T_3-resin uptake, ECG, chest x-ray (CHF). **Management:** propranolol 1–2 mg/kg/24 h, PTU 5–10 mg/kg/24 h or methimazole 0.5–0.7 mg/kg/24 h, iodide 1 gtt PO q8h
HYPERTHYROIDISM, CONGENITAL	**Primary:** thyroid dysgenesis 80%; others: inborn errors of thyroid hormone synthesis. **Secondary:** hypopituitarism, septooptic dysplasia.	Classic is unusual (puffy facies, depressed nasal bridge, macroglossia, large fontanelles, umbilical hernia, abdominal distension, hypotonia), more often feeding difficulties, lethargy, constipation, jaundice.	**Ancillary data:** T_4, TSH, T_3-resin uptake, thyroid-binding globulin; consider sepsis evaluation and glucose level. **Management:** IVF for shock, levothyroxine 10–15 mg/kg/24 h.
HYPOTHYROIDISM, ACQUIRED	Autoimmune (lymphocytic thyroiditis) with antithyroid antibodies, antimicrosomal antibodies, thyroid-stimulating antiglobulin. **Etiology:** majority autoimmune, also decreased response to TSH, hypothalamic/pituitarism, iodine deficiency.	Insidious, failure to gain weight, decreased growth, lethargy, poor appetite, constipation, cold intolerance, precocious/delayed puberty, flattened affect, puffiness, goiter, bradycardia, slow deep tendon reflexes.	**Ancillary data:** low T_4, reduced T_3 resin-uptake, high TSH. **Management:** levothyroxine 10–15 mg/kg/24 h neonate, 2–3 mg/kg/24 h for adolescent.

HR, heart rate; RR, respiratory rate; ECG, electrocardiogram; ABG, arterial blood gas; RAS, reticular-activating system; CNS, central nervous system; ADH, antidiuretic hormone; CF, cystic fibrosis; UPJ, ureteropelvic junction; GH, growth hormone; NS, normal saline; MEN, multiple endocrine neoplasia; HTN, hypertension; CHF, congestive heart failure; TSH, thyroid-stimulating hormone; T_3, 3,5,5'-triiodothyronine; T_4, tetraiodothyronine (thyroxine); PTU, propyl thiouracil.

▶ **Normal Visual Acuity:**
  • 20/40 in 3-year-old
  • 20/30 in 4-year-old
  • 20/20 at 5 or 6 years of age
▶ Difference of more than one line between eyes on the eye chart is abnormal.

Differential

▶ Infectious disorders like conjunctivitis (secondary to excessive discharge), herpes simplex keratoconjunctivitis, *N. gonorrhoeae*, periorbital or orbital cellulitis
  • Recurrent herpes keratoconjunctivitis most common infectious cause of blindness in United States
▶ **Uveitis:** symptoms include: blurred vision, unilateral eye pain, photophobia, and headache
▶ **Endophthalmitis:** unilateral, painful, visually impaired eye with a hypopyon
▶ **Trauma:**
  • Blowout fracture: damage to medial wall and orbital floor, incarceration of the inferior rectus muscle causes restricted upward gaze and double vision.
  • Corneal abrasions: ↑ uptake with fluorescein staining.
    1. No longer treated with eye-patch.
    2. Use antipseudomonal agent in patients who wear contact lenses.
  • Hyphema: blood accumulation in the anterior chamber. Complications include: re-bleeding, elevated intraocular pressure with glaucoma, corneal bloodstaining.
    1. Elevate patient's head.
    2. Atropine 1% one drop TID.
    3. If eye pressure is > 30 mm Hg, a topical β-blocker should be given such as Timolol.
    4. If there is no response with topical medication, give mannitol or acetazolamide.
    5. Avoid acetazolamide in patients with sickle cell, as this medication can cause increased sickling and increased intraocular pressure.
  • Lens subluxation: diplopia and iridodonesis (trembling of iris).
  • Berlin edema or commotio retinae: contusion of the retina from blunt trauma. Patients present with decreased visual

acuity, "milky white haze" of the retina, and retinal hemor-rhages.

- Posterior segment trauma: vitreous hemorrhage and sudden visual loss.
- Retinal detachment: macular involvement suggested by "curtain" across visual field. Typically a result of trauma in children.
- Chemical burns: immediate copious eye irrigation and pH testing of eye.
- Ultraviolet light: corneal damage, red eye, photophobia, lacrimation, blepharospasm.

▶ Transient cortical blindness: secondary to blunt head trauma, no papillary or retinal findings on exam

▶ Retinal vein or artery occlusion: rare in pediatrics, sudden painless unilateral loss of vision

- Retinal artery: pale optic disk and cherry red spot of fovea on funduscopic exam
- Retinal vein: retinal hemorrhages, blurred optic disk, engorged tortuous veins known as the "blood and thunder" retina

Management

▶ All patients with acutely impaired vision must be seen by an ophthalmologist.

Paralysis and Movement Disorders

General

▶ **Strabismus:** muscle imbalance that causes improper eye alignment

▶ **Esotropia:** persistent inward deviation of the eyes

▶ **Exotropia:** divergent or outward eye deviation

▶ **Nystagmus:** involuntary rhythmic oscillation of the eyes

▶ **Motor Innervation of the Six Extraocular Muscles**

- Cranial nerve IV innervates superior oblique
- Cranial nerve VI innervates the lateral rectus
- Cranial nerve III innervates remaining extrinsic ocular muscles

Differential

▶ **Primary Muscle Disorder**

- Orbital floor fracture: inferior rectus entrapment, restricts upward gaze

- Thyroid ophthalmopathy: inflamed extraocular muscles, restricts eye movements
► **Cranial Nerves** (CN)
  - CN III: exotropia, downward eye deviation, ptosis, pupillary dilation, impaired adduction more frequently congenital, also due to ↑ ICP (tumor, trauma)
  - CN IV: head tilt to side opposite palsied superior oblique muscle, commonly congenital, acquired sources include trauma or midbrain tumor
  - CN VI: lose lateral eye movement, horizontal diplopia, most commonly acquired, tumor, hydrocephalus, meningitis, viral illness (benign), Gradenigo syndrome (painful 6th nerve palsy secondary to inflammation from otitis media or mastoiditis)
► **Conjugate Gaze Disorders**
  - Involve a defect in paired movement of eyes
  - Hydrocephalus, midbrain tumors, ventriculoperitoneal shunt malfunction, brain stem tumor
► **Diplopia** (double vision). Causes include: CNS tumors and bleeds, myasthenia gravis, head trauma, blowout orbital fractures, shunt malfunctions, and poisonings.
► **Nystagmus**
  - Vertical nystagmus is pathologic
  - Spasmus mutans: presents in first year of life, triad horizontal pendular nystagmus, head nodding, and torticollis
  - May be secondary to drugs like phenytoin and barbiturates

Diagnostic Evaluation
► Perform head CT in setting of: head trauma, focal neurologic findings, ↑ ICP, suspected orbital cellulitis
► Orbital CT scan for blunt trauma with suspected fracture and extraocular muscle entrapment
► Lumbar puncture for suspected meningitis or encephalitis

Red Eye

General
► **Conjunctival hyperemia:** reactive vascular tissue, responds to noxious stimuli with vasodilation and tear secretion
► Most commonly result of infection, allergy, or trauma

Differential
► **Infectious**
   • Conjunctivitis: bacterial (*S. pneumoniae, H. influenzae*), viral (adenovirus, herpes)
   • Herpes simplex: keratoconjunctivitis, dendritic pattern with fluorescein staining, never use steroids if herpes infection suspected
► **Allergic:** bilateral itchy, watery eyes, injected conjunctiva
► **Trauma:**
   • Foreign bodies and corneal abrasions are the most common causes.
   • Ultraviolet keratitis will show fine central corneal stippling with fluorescein exam.
   • Cyanoacrylate "super glue" instillation.
      1. Can cause the eyelids to adhere to the cornea.
      2. Glue should be moistened with erythromycin ointment to remove as many glue clumps as possible. The patient should then use the erythromycin ointment 5–6 times a day.
      3. An ophthalmology follow-up should be obtained in 1–2 days.
   • Chemical burns: alkalis are particularly serious as they cause a liquefactive necrosis. Acid burns cause a coagulation necrosis.
      1. Irrigate the eye with at least 1–2 liters of NS until a normal eye pH of between 6 and 8 is obtained.
      2. Any patient with corneal clouding or an epithelial defect should have an ophthalmology consultation.
► **Glaucoma:** uncommon in children, findings include photophobia, tearing, blepharospasm, corneal haziness. Requires immediate ophthalmology consult.
► **Iritis:** photophobia, hazy vision, miotic pupil, circumlimbal injection, punctate keratopathy, and "flare and cell" on slit lamp exam.
► Systemic diseases associated with red eyes include: Kawasaki disease, Stevens-Johnson syndrome, juvenile rheumatoid arthritis (JRA), scarlet fever, systemic lupus erythematosus (SLE).

Management
► **Corneal Abrasions:** broad-spectrum antibiotic ointment or drops

- • Never prescribe topical anesthetics or topical steroids for corneal abrasions.
- ▶ **Traumatic Iritis:** treat in consultation with an ophthalmologist
  - • Cycloplegics to reduce ciliary spasm
  - • Topical steroids to reduce inflammation

Chalazion and Hordeolum

General
- ▶ Eyelid infections are commonly associated with *S. aureus*, occasionally *S. epidermidis.*
- ▶ External hordeolum: acute infection of the glands of Zeis (sebaceous glands attached to hair follicles).
- ▶ Internal hordeolum: infection of meibomian glands, produces an abscess in the tarsal plate.
- ▶ Chalazion: localized painless swelling of the lid, chronic lipogranulomatous reaction, due to obstruction of meibomian glands.

Clinical Findings
- ▶ Hordeolum: eyelid edema, hyperemia, painful, points externally or internally
- ▶ Chalazion: typically painless

Management
- ▶ **Hordeolum**
  - • Warm compresses, gentle eyelash scrubs with baby shampoo, antibiotic ointment
- ▶ **Chalazion**
  - • Treat similarly to hordeolum
  - • May require incision and curettage by ophthalmologist

Conjunctivitis

- ▶ The most common cause of red eye in children.
- ▶ The conjunctiva is a transparent mucous membrane that covers the eye—palpebral conjunctiva covers the surface of the eyelids, bulbar conjunctiva covers the eyeball (except for the cornea).
- ▶ Conjunctiva responds to infection with vasodilation and inflammatory cell response.

Ophthalmia Neonatorum
▶ Defined as conjunctivitis in the first month of life
▶ **Etiology:**
  • Gonococcal: symptoms appear 2–4 days after delivery, hyperpurulent discharge, lid edema, chemosis, and most cases occur within first 2 weeks of life. Complications include corneal ulceration, perforation, and systemic toxicity. Diagnosis begins with a Gram stain showing intracellular Gram-negative diplococci and confirmed by culture.
  • Chlamydia (*C. trachomatis*): accounts for 20–40% of neonatal conjunctivitis, occurs at 5–14 days after delivery, complications include pneumonia. Diagnosis is by culture.
  • Herpes simplex: symptoms occur 2–14 days after delivery, fluorescein may show dendritic lesions, Tzanck preparation may show multinucleated giant cells or intranuclear inclusions. Confirm diagnosis with culture. It usually starts as unilateral conjunctivitis with clear ocular discharge.
  • Other organisms: other bacteria include *Staph. aureus, Strep. pneumoniae, Haemophilus* species, Gram-negative rods, and enterococci. Generally occur in the first 14 days of life.
▶ **Management:** in all cases, send discharge for Gram stain, Giemsa stain, and chlamydial/gonococcal culture
  • Gonococcal conjunctivitis: complete septic workup including lumbar puncture, admit for IV penicillin G (50,000 units/kg/24 h) or ceftriaxone sodium (50 mg/kg/24 h unless meningitis is suspected and then the dose is increased to 100 mg/kg/24 h), ophthalmology consult.
  • Chlamydia: outpatient treatment is acceptable, oral erythromycin (50 mg/kg/24 h) for 14 days, topical treatment alone is not acceptable for chlamydial pneumonia.
  • Herpes simplex: complete septic workup including lumbar puncture; admit for topical and IV viral therapy, ophthalmology consult.
  • Other bacteria: topical erythromycin or polymyxin B ophthalmic ointment.

Childhood Conjunctivitis
▶ **Etiology:**
  • Bacterial: nontypeable *H. influenzae, S. pneumoniae,* and *M. catarrhalis,* most common

- Viral: most commonly caused by adenovirus
- ▶ **Bacterial:** mucopurulent discharge, conjunctival injection, pain is uncommon, normal vision
    - Concurrent otitis media (OM) and conjunctivitis: usually secondary to nontypeable *H. influenzae*
    - Viral: discharge thin and watery
    - Herpes keratoconjunctivitis: unilateral, painful, fluorescein exam may show dendritic lesion (most common with recurrent disease)
    - Allergic conjunctivitis: itchy eyes with watery discharge, bilateral involvement
- ▶ **Management:**
    - Bacterial: topical ointments or drops including polymyxin B (Polysporin), sulfacetamide sodium (10%) (Sulamyd), erythromycin ointment, trimethoprim-polymyxin B (Polytrim)
    - Viral: supportive, cool compresses, artificial tears
    - Concurrent OM and conjunctivitis: systemic antibiotics

Periorbital Cellulitis

- ▶ **Definition:** an infection in the tissues around the eye anterior to the orbital septum
- ▶ Peak incidence between 2–4 years
- ▶ **Etiology:**
    - *Staph. aureus, Strep. pyogenes,* or anaerobes, following local skin or lid infection, or trauma
    - *Strep. pneumoniae* or *H. influenzae* (much less common due to *H. influenzae* immunization) following sinusitis, OM, upper respiratory tract infections
- ▶ **Diagnostic Findings:**
    - Unilateral lid swelling, erythema, tenderness, and warmth
    - Fever present in majority of cases, but can present without fever
    - Proptosis, or pain with eye movement should not be present and suggests an orbital cellulitis
- ▶ **Evaluation:**
    - CT scan of orbit is indicated to differentiate from orbital cellulitis if any question exists
- ▶ **Management:**
    - If *H. influenzae* or *S. pneumoniae* are possible sources, then IV

antibiotic combination such as nafcillin 150 mg/kg/24 h, and ceftriaxone 100 mg/kg/24 h or cefuroxime 75–100 mg/kg/24 h should be administered.

- If *S. aureus* periorbital cellulitis is suspected (particularly if infection is following insect bite), consider antibiotic coverage of MRSA such as Septra or clindamycin.
- For an afebrile patient with cellulitis secondary to trauma, who has a normal CBC, IM ceftriaxone (50–75 mg/kg) and oral cephalexin (50 mg/kg/24 h divided QID) may be attempted; however, only attempt if 24-hour follow-up is assured.

Orbital Cellulitis

▶ **Definition:** infection of the orbital tissues posterior to the orbital septum

▶ Occurs secondary to sinus infection approximately 75% of the time

▶ **Etiology:**
- *Staph. aureus* following trauma or surgery
- *Strep. pneumoniae*, nontypeable *H. influenzae*, GABHS secondary to sinus infection

▶ **Clinical Findings:**
- Acute-onset unilateral lid edema and erythema, commonly associated with fever, conjunctival injection, proptosis, pain with extraocular movements, ↓ ocular mobility

▶ **Complications:**
- Meningitis, intracranial abscesses, septicemia, orbital abscesses, cavernous sinus thrombosis, visual loss

▶ **Evaluation:**
- Lab studies: CBC, blood culture, lumbar puncture in neonates
- CT scan of the head is the radiologic study of choice

▶ **Management:**
- Ceftriaxone (100 mg/kg/24 h divided q12h IV) and clindamycin (15–40 mg/kg/24 h divided q6–8h IV)
- Ophthalmology and ENT consultation
- In newborns with orbital cellulitis, strongly consider performing a lumbar puncture, as bacterial seeding is the most common mechanism of infection in this age group
- Admit

FOREIGN BODIES OF GI TRACT AND AIRWAY
Gastrointestinal Foreign Bodies

▶ Majority occur between 6 months–6 years.

▶ Equal in males and females.

▶ Less than 50% have witnessed event.

▶ Coins are most popular nonfood item.

▶ Most common sites of obstruction:
  • Objects lodge at one of three sites:
    1. Inferior edge of the cricopharyngeus muscle (most common)
    2. Level of the aortic arch crossing
    3. Gastroesophageal junction

▶ **Complications of Impaction in Esophagus Include:**
  • Intramural ulceration
  • Perforation
  • Hemorrhage
  • Tendency to lodge at areas of acute angulation

Esophageal Foreign Bodies

▶ Many are asymptomatic.

▶ Symptoms and signs include: gagging, choking, coughing, stridor, refusal to feed, drooling, dysphagia, neck or throat pain, vomiting, foreign body sensation.

▶ Less than 1% result in perforation.

▶ Perforation can result in mediastinitis, pneumothorax, retropharyngeal abscess, sepsis.

▶ **Radiologic Studies:**
  • AP and lateral soft-tissue neck and chest x-rays identify radiopaque objects.
  • Coins in the esophagus lodge in the coronal plain.
  • Coins in the trachea lodge in the sagittal plane.
  • Contrast studies or endoscopy identify objects not seen on plain films.

▶ **Management:**
  • All esophageal bodies must be removed. (In what time frame? If they do not pass into the stomach within 24 hours)
  • Endoscopy is the procedure of choice.

- IV glucagon (0.03–0.1 mg/kg/dose) for bodies lodged in distal third esophagus. Success rate of 30–50% is limited to adult studies and rarely applicable to pediatric patients.
- Esophageal bougienage: use of a dilator to push it down, high risk of perforation.
- Balloon catheter: safe and effective, only use if lodged < 48–72 hours.

Gastric and Intestinal Foreign Bodies

▶ 80–90% will pass uneventfully.
▶ Intestinal perforation is rare.
▶ **Management:**
  - Conservative approach is appropriate for asymptomatic patients.
  - Sewing needles, toothpicks, or other long slender objects (> 5 cm) should be removed from stomach or proximal duodenum endoscopically.
  - Surgical consultation for children with abdominal pain, fever, vomiting, bleeding.
▶ **Button Batteries**
  - If battery in esophagus, immediate endoscopic removal is mandated.
  - If past the lower esophageal sphincter, asymptomatic patients can be observed.
  - Symptomatic patients require surgical consultation.
  - Larger batteries in the stomach (> 15 mm) need follow-up films in 48 hours; those that persist need endoscopic removal.

Airway Foreign Bodies

▶ Greater than 75% occur in children < 3 years of age.
▶ Organic debris most frequently retrieved, peanuts most common.
▶ Objects rarely radiopaque.
▶ Most lodge in a main stem bronchus (right more common than left).
▶ **Diagnostic Findings:**
  - Classic triad includes: acute-onset wheezing, coughing, absent or diminished breath sounds.

- 50–90% of patients have suggestive history.
- Other signs/symptoms include cyanosis, dyspnea, and choking.
- One fourth of children present asymptomatically.
- Delay in presentation may be misdiagnosed as croup, asthma, and pneumonia.

▶ **Radiologic Studies:**
- AP and lateral views of the chest and neck.
- Differential inflation of affected lung most common abnormality identified (lateral decubitus films).
- Fluoroscopy may help in localizing the foreign body.

▶ **Management:**
- Initial management includes adequate oxygenation and ventilation.
- Partial obstruction: no blind finger sweeps, abdominal thrusts, or back blows—may cause complete obstruction.
- Complete obstruction (apneic, unconscious) series of 5 back blows and chest thrusts for kids < 1 year of age. Abdominal thrusts for older children.
  1. If this fails, perform laryngoscopy and try to remove the foreign body with Magill forceps.
  2. If foreign body is in subglottic area, orotracheal intubation and pushing it into main stem bronchus may be lifesaving.
  3. If unable to intubate then needle cricothyrotomy may bypass the obstruction.

GASTROINTESTINAL DISORDERS
Differential Diagnosis of Abdominal Pain

▶ **Infancy**
- Intussusception: most common between 5 and 12 months, visceral pain
- Volvulus: intestinal obstruction and vascular compromise, visceral
- Incarcerated hernias: inguinal, femoral, umbilical, visceral
- Hirschsprung disease: most common cause of obstruction in neonates
- Necrotizing enterocolitis (NEC): primarily in neonates
- Colic: usually < 3 months of age, unknown etiology

- Perforation: NEC, ulcers, abuse, trauma
▶ **Childhood**
    - Gastroenteritis: most common cause of abdominal pain in children
    - Appendicitis: peak incidence is 9–12 years
    - Pancreatitis: most cases occur > 10 years of age
    - Henoch-Schönlein purpura (HSP): abdominal pain occurs in two thirds of children
    - Hemolytic uremic syndrome (HUS): usually preceded by gastroenteritis or URI
    - Ulcer disease: less common in children than adults
    - Constipation: common cause of abdominal pain
    - Urinary tract infection (UTI): bacteriuria indicates UTI
    - Functional causes: somatization, hypochondriasis, factitious
▶ **Adolescence**
    - Ectopic pregnancy: most occur at 6–12 weeks of gestation
    - Pelvic inflammatory disease (PID): gonorrheae, chlamydia, *Mycoplasma hominis*
    - Testicular torsion: abrupt-onset scrotal or lower abdominal pain
    - Inflammatory bowel disease (IBD): usually includes multiple other symptoms
    - Biliary tract disorders: associated with thalassemia, sickle cell
▶ **Extra-Abdominal Causes:**
    - Sickle cell anemia
    - Pneumonia
    - Diabetic ketoacidosis (DKA)
    - Lead intoxication
    - Porphyria
    - Poisonings
▶ **Normal Stool Patterns:**
    - In first 2–3 months, 1 bowel movement per feeding to 1 every other day
    - 2 months–1 year, 2–3 bowel movements per day
    - 1–5 years, 1–2 bowel movements per day
▶ **Jaundice**
    - **Definition:** syndrome characterized by hyperbilirubinemia and yellow appearance of the patient
    - **Conjugated versus unconjugated:**

1. Conjugated: direct component of the serum bilirubin > 30%
2. Unconjugated: direct component is < 15% of serum bilirubin

- **Unconjugated hyperbilirubinemia:**
    1. Physiologic jaundice
        a. Occurs in 60% of newborns
        b. Does not occur on 1st day
        c. Peaks about 3rd day of life
        d. Declines to normal over first 10–14 days of life
    2. Breast milk jaundice
        a. Etiology unknown
        b. Peaks at 10–27 days, and persists for 3–10 weeks
        c. May treat by substituting formula
    3. Jaundice in first 24 hours (or that rises faster than 0.5 mg/dL/h)
        a. Always considered abnormal
        b. Consider hemolytic disease, TORCHS infections, and sepsis
    4. Persistent or occurs after 1st week of life
        a. Considered pathologic
        b. Consider hemolytic anemia, Crigler-Najjar and Gilbert syndrome, sepsis, UTI, GI tract obstruction, congenital hypothyroidism
    5. Treatment: consider phototherapy if total bilirubin is > 20 mg/dL, exchange transfusion if phototherapy fails or child looks sick and total bilirubin is > 25 mg/dL

- **Conjugated hyperbilirubinemia**
    1. Is always pathologic
    2. Differential includes obstructive causes, infectious causes, drugs/toxins, metabolic causes

▶ **Anal Fissure**
- The most frequent cause of rectal bleeding in 1st year of life
- Associated with constipation: hypothyroidism, diabetes insipidus (DI), bowel obstruction

▶ **Perianal Abscess**
- Infections of perianal glands and ducts, originating from crypts of morgagnii
- Healthy boys < 3 years of age

- 25–30% have associated anal fistula
- Condyloma acuminatum: human papillomavirus (HPV), maternal transmission in first 2 years of life; suspect abuse in older children
- Treatment includes: incision and drainage, Augmentin or Keflex, sitz bath

► **Juvenile Polyps**
- Common cause of lower GI bleeding in school-age children and account for 90% of all GI polyps in children
- Always benign, more common in males
- Peak incidence: 3–4 years
- Bright red blood on surface of stool
- Can be lead point for intussusception
- 70% found in rectum and palpable on digital exam
- Autoamputation possible, or polypectomy via colonoscopy

► **Hemorrhoids**
- Usually external (varicosities of inferior rectal veins)
- Associated with constipation or anorectal disease in Crohn disease
- Internal hemorrhoids associated with portal hypertension
- Conservative treatment: sitz bath, stool softener

► **Rectal Prolapse**
- Painless protrusion of rectum through anus
- Partial prolapse most common in < 3 years of age
- Predisposing factors: prune belly, meningomyelocele, exstrophy of bladder, cystic fibrosis, rectal polyps
- Spontaneously resolve, use stool softeners, manual reduction
- Phenol and glycerin or 30% saline injections around rectal wall cause fibrosis

► **Acalculous Cholecystitis Predisposing Factors:**
- Acute systemic disturbance such as burns, sepsis, dehydration; infection with *Salmonella/Shigella/Ascaris*
- Ultrasound: signs of inflammation without calculi

► **Hydrops of Gallbladder**
- Acute noncalculous distension of gallbladder without inflammation
- Predisposing illness: upper respiratory tract infection, Kawasaki syndrome, leptospirosis
- 40% have jaundice and 75–100% have a right upper quadrant (RUQ) mass

▶ **Gastroenteritis**
- **Rotavirus** accounts for 30–60% of all diarrhea in infants 3–15 months of age.
- **Norwalk virus** accounts for 40% of GI outbreaks in older children in schools, camps.
    1. Lasts 12–60 hours, infective for 2 days, malabsorption of lactose and fat for up to 2 weeks.
- **Adenovirus** is the second most common cause of diarrhea in children with an incubation period of 3–10 days and a duration of 5–12 days.
- *Campylobacter* is the leading cause of bacterial gastroenteritis in the United States.
    1. Person to person, pet-person transmission with an incubation period of 2–5 days
    2. Fever, abdominal cramping, bloody diarrhea with leukocytes in stool
- *Salmonella* more common in children < 5 years of age
    1. Fecal-oral and person-person
    2. Fever, watery diarrhea, stools with streaks of blood
    3. If < 3 months, hospitalize for IV antibiotics due to the risk of associated bacteremia and sepsis (including meningitis)
    4. After infancy, antibiotics may prolong carrier state
    5. *Salmonella typhi*: fever, malaise, headache, hepatosplenomegaly, rose spots, and a relative bradycardia
- *Shigella*: as few as 100 organisms cause disease
    1. Bloody diarrhea with 10–25 stools/day
    2. Nonfocal seizures
    3. White blood count (WBC) < 10,000 with left shift
    4. Treatment: Bactrim or ampicillin for 5 days
- *Yersinia*
    1. Fever, vomiting, bloody diarrhea, toxicity
    2. Pseudoappendicitis
    3. Treat with aminoglycosides, cefotaxime, Bactrim, or tetracycline
- *E. coli* O157:H7 associated with HUS
- **Food poisoning** presents with vomiting/prostration within 12–16 hours of eating
    1. *Clostridium perfringens*: resolves in 24–48 hours.
    2. *Clostridium botulinum* typically found in home preservatives, and honey:

      a. ptosis, mydriasis, nystagmus, paresis of extraocular muscles.
3. ***Clostridium difficile*:** pseudomembranous colitis attack rate is 32% in day care centers.
    a. Clindamycin, cephalosporins, and amoxicillin/ampicillin are the most common causative antibiotics, although almost any antibiotic may be responsible.
    b. Typical onset is 7–10 days after the initiation of antibiotics, but may present up to 8 weeks after the antibiotic is discontinued.
    c. Patients present with frequent, mucoid watery stools. Fecal leukocytes may be present.
    d. Treat with oral vancomycin or Flagyl.
4. **Cholera** presents with rice water stools. Treatment is with Bactrim or tetracycline.
- **Parasitic agents**
1. Cryptosporidium
    a. Acid fast stain
    b. AIDS, day care attendees
    c. Chlorine kills it
2. *Giardia lamblia* is the most common parasitic pathogen in the United States
    a. Lasts a long time: up to 4 weeks
    b. Cysts seen microscopically, enzyme-linked immunosorbent assay (ELISA) tests
    c. Treat with quinacrine hydrochloride, furazolidone, or Flagyl

▶ **Viral Hepatitis**
- **Hepatitis A virus** (HAV): RNA virus
1. 20–25% of clinical hepatitis in developed countries
2. Fecal oral spread, uncooked shellfish
3. Highest contagiousness in preicteric phase
4. Fever, vomiting/diarrhea, anorexia, dark urine, light stools
5. High aminotransferase, detection of antibody to HAV
6. Anti-HAV IgM: recent infection, anti-HAV IgG peaks at 1–2 months
7. Treatment is supportive
8. Passive immunization of all household and day care contacts with IG

- **Hepatitis B:** DNA virus
  1. Blood-borne, sexual contact
  2. 60–70% of cases are subclinical
  3. Treatment
     a. Vaccine available
     b. Hepatitis-B immune globulin (HBIG) exposed infants < 12 months, all persons whose sexual partners have acute hepatitis B, infants of mothers with hepatis B surface antigen (HBsAg) within 12 hours of delivery
- **Hepatitis D:** RNA virus can only infect patients positive for HBsAg
  1. Mortality 2–20%
  2. Treatment is supportive, α-interferon, liver transplant
- **Hepatitis C:** non-A non-B, RNA virus, parenteral transmission with 10–20% developing cirrhosis

▶ **Inflammatory Bowel Disease** (IBD)
  - **Ulcerative colitis**
    1. Confined to mucosa and submucosa; begins in rectum, spreads proximally
    2. Bloody diarrhea, dramatic onset
    3. Severe colitis
       a. Toxic megacolon
       b. Five or more grossly bloody stools a day
       c. Oral temperature > 100° F
       d. Tachycardia > 90
       e. Hematocrit < 30%
       f. Serum albumin < 3
       g. 3–20% risk of carcinoma
       h. Thumb printing on x-ray
       i. Barium study: mucosal irregularity, effaced haustrations
  - **Crohn disease**
    1. Involves one or all layers of bowel
    2. Associated with fistulas and abscesses
    3. Insidious onset
    4. Extraintestinal signs: growth failure, polyarthritis, ankylosing spondylitis, skin manifestations, uveitis, hepatobiliary dysfunction

5. X-rays with incomplete small bowel obstruction (SBO), distended bowel loops, air-fluid levels
6. Barium: cobblestoning, segmental lesions
- **Treatment options for IBD:**
    1. Steroids
    2. Cyclosporine A in fulminant colitis
    3. Surgery
        a. Profuse hemorrhage
        b. Perforation
        c. Toxic megacolon and obstruction
        d. Failed medical management
        e. Immunosuppressives (6 MP [6 mercaptopurine], azathioprine) for Crohn disease
        f. Flagyl

▶ **Acute Pancreatitis**
- Cullen sign: bluish periumbilical area
- Grey Turner sign: bluish flanks
- Most common causes: posttrauma and viral etiology

▶ **Reye Syndrome**
- An acute noninflammatory encephalopathy with cerebrospinal fluid (CSF) < 8 leukocytes, or histology of brain showing cerebral edema; hepatopathy by biopsy or autopsy or by threefold rise in aspartate aminotransferase (AST) or alanine aminotransferase (ALT) or ammonia and no more reasonable explanation for cerebral or hepatic abnormalities.
- Linked to aspirin use and varicella infection.

▶ **Appendicitis**
- Rovsing sign: pain in right lower quadrant (RLQ) upon palpation to left lower quadrant (LLQ)
- Obturator sign
- Psoas sign
- 30% of cases are ruptured at surgery
- Classic x-ray findings
    1. Loss of psoas shadow on right
    2. Localized air-fluid levels in cecum and terminal ileum
    3. Scoliosis of lumbar spine
    4. Fecalith (up to 10% of the time), gas in appendix
    5. Obliteration of right properitoneal fat line and free air

- Management includes:
  1. Fluid resuscitation
  2. Initiate antibiotic therapy (triple coverage—ampicillin, clindamycin, and gentamicin) if signs of peritonitis
  3. Rapid surgical consultation

▶ **Hirschsprung Disease**
  - The absence of ganglion cells from rectum to sigmoid
    1. Cone-shaped transition zone and dilated proximal colon on lateral film.
    2. Newborns present with failure to pass a meconium stool. Older children present with chronic constipation.
    3. Treatment: decompressing colostomy followed by definitive repair and colostomy closure at 1 year of age, although some centers are performing primary repairs.
    4. Complications of surgery: stenosis and anastomotic leak with perineal abscess formation (Hirschsprung enterocolitis).

▶ **Inguinal Hernias**
  - In females, it is due to failure of the canal of Nuck to close. In males, it is due to failure of processus vaginalis to obliterate.

▶ **Intussusception**
  - More common in male infants 3–12 months with peaks in the spring and autumn.
  - Dance's sign: elongated mass in right upper quadrant (RUQ) with absent bowel in right lower quadrant (RLQ).
  - Ultrasound and CT scan are the best modalities of diagnosis unless classic signs and symptoms of intussusception are present then air not barium is diagnostic and therapeutic tool.
  - Signs and symptoms include colicky abdominal pain, heme-positive stools (currant jelly stools are a late finding), and vomiting.
  - Surgery consult should be obtained prior to performed enema in case of reduction failure or complications.

▶ **Meckel Diverticulum**
  - The most frequent congenital abnormality of small intestine
  - Painless, massive GI bleeding
  - Vestige of omphalomesenteric duct

- Rule of 2's:
  1. 2% of the population
  2. 2 feet (40–100 cm proximal to ileocecal valve)
  3. Children < 2 years of age
- Meckel scan test of choice: 95% accurate if gastric mucosa is present

▶ **Pyloric Stenosis**
- Usually present between 2 and 6 weeks of life.
- Nonbilious vomiting is the first complaint, which eventually becomes projectile.
- Hypokalemic, hypochloremic metabolic alkalosis may be present.

▶ **Malrotation and Midgut Volvulus**
- A complete twisting of loop of bowel about the mesenteric base of attachment.
- Sudden onset acute abdomen and shock in newborn. Bilious emesis is common. Usually abdominal distension is absent (upper and not lower GI obstruction).
- 75% of cases within first month of life.
- Double-bubble sign on film, upper GI helpful. However, immediate management involves obtaining an emergent surgical consultation, placing an NG tube, starting antibiotics if perforation is suspected and aggressive IV hydration.

GYNECOLOGIC AND OBSTETRIC DISORDERS
Examination

▶ **Prepubertal**
- Position: frog leg (knee-chest more threatening), consider in mom's lap. If uncooperative, never force move to exam under anesthesia by gynecology.
- Normal hymenal shape may be fimbriated, circumferential, or posterior rim; diameter ~ 1 mm per year of age.
- Equipment: moistened Q-tip for specimen B culture lateral vaginal wall for *C. trachomatis*; chocolate agar for *N. gonorrhoeae*. Inject 2–3 cc saline and aspirate for seminal washings.

▶ **Pubertal**
- Ask about sexual activity with parent out of the room.

- Position: lithotomy, speculum and bimanual, consider Huffman speculum if virginal.
- Equipment: wet preps from posterior vagina, endocervical swabs for *C. trachomatis* and *N. gonorrhoeae.*

Vaginal Bleeding

▶ **Prepubertal**
- **Neonatal:** physiologic withdrawal of maternal estrogen, no treatment, reassurance only.
- **Vulvovaginitis:** bleeding due to pruritis/scratching from pinworm, enteric infections (*Shigella,* GAS). Treat with sitz baths, treat pinworm/enteritis (see vaginal discharge section).
- **Trauma:** straddle injuries commonly cause bruising, **rarely** cause hymenal tears. Difficult exam, consider 2% lidocaine jelly or under anesthesia; if bleeding Gelfoam or gynecology to suture. If penetrating (broom handle, etc.) then rule out injury to bowel, bladder, rectum.
- **Foreign body:** usually **not** foul-smelling discharge, knee-chest position best for visualization, consider gentle irrigation with 25 cc syringe of NS and urethral catheter, consider rectal exam for large objects.
- **Lichen sclerosus: rare**, affects vulvovaginal/perianal skin, white papule, atrophic plaques, ecchymoses, and excoriations.
- **Genital tumors: rare**, sarcoma botryoides or embryonal rhabdomyosarcoma, bleeding, vaginal discharge, abdominal mass, grapelike lesions; clear-cell adenocarcinoma in DES exposure (0.2%).
- **Urethral prolapse:** doughnut-shaped friable red-blue mass; sitz baths/emollients, surgery if necrotic.
- **Precocious puberty:** cyclic vaginal bleeding, with breast development/pubic hair < 8 years old. Differential includes idiopathic (most common), tumor (ovary/CNS), McCune-Albright syndrome.

▶ **Postpubertal**
- Dysfunctional uterine bleeding: irregular, due to immaturity of pituitary/ovarian axis causing anovulatory cycles and withdrawal bleeding.
  1. History: duration and amount (> 6 pads/day), oral contraceptive pills, pregnancy

2. Physical examination: hemodynamic stability, pelvic exam
3. Laboratory studies: CBC, UCG (urine pregnancy test)
4. Management: **Hgb > 11 mg/dL** reassure, follow-up in 2 months; **Hgb 9–11 mg/dL** oral contraceptive pill (4 per day for 4 days, 3 per day for 3 days, 2 per day for 2 days, 1 per day for 1 day) and iron, continue for 4 months; **Hgb < 9 mg/dL** fluids/transfusion if required (get coagulation profile first), estrogen 25 mg IV q4h
5. Dysmenorrhea
6. Primary (no pathology, usually starts 6–18 months after menarche)
7. Secondary (PID, endometriosis, congenital malformations, psychosocial factors)
8. Treatment primary: NSAIDs on days 1–3 ± low-dose oral contraceptive pills

- Pregnancy complication:
  1. Spontaneous abortion: 25% of pregnancies result in spontaneous abortion
  2. Septic abortion: fever
  3. Ectopic pregnancy: may present with shock, stabilize hemodynamically, then emergent obstetric consult for definitive management
  4. Molar pregnancy
  5. Abruptio placenta or placenta previa: in second or third trimester, **avoid pelvic exam**, stabilize with IV, monitor fetal heart rate, obtain CBC, PT/PTT/INR, and obstetric consult
- Contraceptive complication: oral contraceptives with breakthrough bleeding
- PID: always consider and culture for *C. trachomatis* and *N. gonorrhoeae*
- Endometriosis: pain, vaginal discharge, dyspareunia, spotting prior to menses
- Coagulation disorders: heavy first menstrual period, consider von Willebrand, factor VIII/IX
- Trauma: assault, accidental, foreign body (retained tampon)
- Systemic illness: renal dialysis, immune thrombocytopenic purpura (ITP), viral induced thrombocytopenia

- Endocrine disorders: hypo/hyperthyroidism, polycystic ovary syndrome, prolactinomas, Cushing disease, Addison disease; consider checking prolactin, luteinizing hormone (LH), follicle-stimulating hormone (FSH)
- Tumors: cervical polyps, hemangiomas (**rare**), cervical cancer

Vaginal Discharge

▶ **Prepubertal**
- Vulvovaginitis:
    1. Nonspecific: mixed bacteria, due to poor hygiene. Avoid irritants, 1% hydrocortisone if severe, if recurrent consider amoxicillin 10–14 days or topical estrogen cream.
    2. Post-URI infection: with GAS, *S. pneumoniae*, *H. influenzae*, *N. meningitides*.
    3. Shigella: bloody discharge in 50%, may persist weeks after diarrhea.
    4. Chlamydia: consider abuse, look for gonorrhea, and treat with erythromycin.
    5. Gonorrhea: purulent discharge, consider abuse; treat with ceftriaxone ± tetracycline/doxycycline for 7 days.
    6. *Trichomonas:* may occur in first few months of life, can be vertical.
    7. Skin organisms: staphylococcus, β-hemolytic *Streptococcus*, *Proteus*, *Candida*.
- Foreign body.
- Systemic illness: varicella, measles, scarlet fever, and diphtheria can cause vaginal manifestations.
- Structural: prolapsed urethra, labial adhesions, ectopic ureter, congenital fistula (rectum/posterior vagina).
- Skin diseases: seborrhea, psoriasis, atopic dermatitis, lichen sclerosus.

▶ **Postpubertal**
- Infection
    1. *Candida:* white, treat with nystatin topical or oral single-dose fluconazole 150 mg PO
    2. *Gardnerella vaginalis* (bacterial vaginosis): fishy odor with KOH, clue cells, pH > 5. **Treatment:** metronidazole (clindamycin cream if pregnant in 1st trimester)
    3. *Trichomonas vaginalis*: pruritis, frothy discharge, trichomonas on wet mount, pH 5–7. **Treatment:** metronidazole.

4. Gonorrhea: 7–10% adolescents; vaginitis, cervicitis, sal-pingitis. Symptoms 3–8 days after exposure. **Treatment:** cefixime 400 mg PO or ceftriaxone 250 mg IM/IV or erythromycin 500 mg QID for 7 days.

5. Chlamydia: often asymptomatic but **is the most common** sexually transmitted disease (STD) (10–30% teens). Syn-dromes: (1) mucopurulent cervicitis; (2) PID; (3) asymp-tomatic. Treat with azithromycin 1 g PO, or doxycycline for 7 days.

- Foreign body: tampon, diaphragm, condom; consider rectal exam to try and dislodge.

Breast Disorders

▶ **Prepubertal**
- Neonatal: physiologic engorgement 2–3 weeks after birth ± milk. If mastitis, needs sepsis workup, cover with penicilli-nase-resistant antibiotic (nafcillin).
- Premature thelarche: breasts prior to 8 years old, uni/bilat-eral, no further evaluation unless genital changes also present.

▶ **Postpubertal**
- Normal: tenderness of breast bud, asymmetry
- Gynecomastia: breast development in boys during adoles-cence, < 3 cm is normal, counseling and surgery referral if larger
- Nipple irritation: sports (jogging, biking), lubricate and use sports bra, avoid nipple hair removal
- Breast infection
  1. Lactational mastitis postpartum: fever, tenderness, mass; treat with ampicillin or erythromycin, warm com-presses
  2. Nonlactational: trauma (foreplay, sports, epidermal cysts), treat the same
- Breast masses—history: tenderness, timing, size change, menstrual relation, and drainage from nipple
  1. Fibroadenoma: 95% of breast masses, firm/rubbery, smooth, mobile, 3–15 cm, multiple or bilateral, slow growth usual, if rapid then biopsy.
  2. Trauma: sports injuries with contusion, hematoma, fat necrosis causing mass; pre-existing lump noticed after

trauma. Acute injuries: prescribe cool compresses, analgesics.

3. Other: cystosarcoma phyllodes, intraductal breast papilloma, breast carcinoma. Firm, nonmovable, indiscreet from breast tissue, rapidly enlarging: refer for biopsy.

External Genitalia

▶ Bartholin gland abscess: often gonorrhea and chlamydia; erythematous, unilateral, fluctuant mass in posterior vulva. Incision and drainage, consider drainage catheter if large, antibiotics to cover gonorrhea/chlamydia.

▶ Imperforate hymen/hematocolpos: asymptomatic until menarche, blue/purple bulging hymen.

▶ Labial adhesions, trauma/dermatitis/infection denudes epithelium, connective tissue bridge forms. 1–6 years old: may present with UTI. Consider abuse if thick raphe. Estrogen cream nightly (QHS), when separated continue to apply Vaseline jelly to prevent recurrence.

▶ Lichen sclerosus: burning, pruritis, nocturia, dysuria, bleeding, perianal involvement may occur. Treat with steroid or antifungal creams.

▶ Urethral prolapse: usually 2–12 years old, 95% in black girls. Doughnut-shaped friable red-blue mass. Treat with sitz baths/emollients, consider estrogen cream or zinc oxide cream; surgery if necrotic.

Sexually Transmitted Diseases (STD)

Chlamydial Infection

▶ **General:** most common STD in adolescence, caused by *C. trachomatis*, commonly asymptomatic

▶ **Diagnostic Findings:**
  • Vaginal discharge, pelvic pain, dysuria, cervical erythema/friability, diagnosis confirmed with ELISA, cell culture, or monoclonal antibodies
  • Complications include PID, perihepatitis (Fitz-Hugh-Curtis syndrome)

▶ **Management:** azithromycin 1 g PO once, or doxycycline 100 mg PO BID for 7 days, or erythromycin 500 mg QID PO for 7 days

Pelvic Inflammatory Disease (PID)

▶ **Diagnostic Criteria:**
- Lower abdominal pain
- Cervical motion tenderness
- Adnexal tenderness
- One or more of:
  1. Fever > 38° C
  2. WBC > 10,500 mm^3
  3. Pelvic abscess
  4. Purulent material
  5. Erythrocyte sedimentation rate (ESR) > 15
  6. Chlamydia monoclonal antibody
  7. Gram-negative diplococci
  8. WBC on oil immersion Gram stain

▶ **Treatment:**
- Cefoxitin (2 g q6h IV) or cefotetan (2 g q12h IV) + doxycycline (100 mg q12h IV) then doxycycline PO;
- Clindamycin (900 mg q8h IV) + gentamicin IV, then doxycycline (100 mg BID PO for 14 days) or clindamycin (450 mg QID PO for 14 days); or
- If nontoxic, compliant, cefoxitin 2 g IM or ceftriaxone 250 mg IM + doxycycline 100 mg PO for 14 days. Hospitalize if no improvement.

Herpes Genitalis

▶ **General:** HSV-1 commonly in oral lesions, HSV-2 more common with sexual transmission and in adolescence.

▶ **Diagnostic Findings:** Painful urination, ± fever, papules progress to vesicles on erythematous base. Stain shows multinucleated giant cells, if prepubertal do viral cultures.

▶ **Management:** If primary, treat with oral acyclovir 400 mg PO TID × 7–10 days (not if pregnant). Recurrent episodes acyclovir 400 mg PO TID × 5 days.

Syphilis

▶ **General:** *Treponema pallidum*, congenital or sexual transmission.

▶ **Diagnostic Findings:** open nontender lesions, then adenopathy, secondary is 6–20 weeks after with maculopapular rash palms/

soles, fever, splenomegaly, lymphadenopathy, condyloma lata. Rapid plasma reagin (RPR), dark field microscopy.

▶ **Management:** benzathine penicillin G 2.4 million U IM, recheck serology at 3–6 weeks.

Condylomata Acuminata

▶ **General:** human papillomavirus (venereal warts) can be vertically transmitted, transmitted via close contact/bath towel/bath with infected person.

▶ **Diagnostic Findings:** soft, nontender, nonulcerative, cauliflower-like, lesions or warts.

▶ **Management:** dermatologist or gynecologist with cryotherapy, podophyllin.

Gonococcal Infection

▶ **General:** Gram-negative intracellular diplococcus

▶ **Diagnostic Findings:** asymptomatic, vaginal discharge, pelvic pain secondary to PID, friable cervix, dysuria, urinary frequency

  • Complications: tuboovarian abscess, PID, Bartholin gland abscess, disseminated gonococcal arthritis

▶ **Management:** uncomplicated gonorrhea ceftriaxone (250 mg IM) plus azithromycin (1 g PO)—may substitute doxycycline (100 mg PO BID × 7 days) for azithromycin.

Menstrual Problems

Dysfunctional Uterine Bleeding

▶ **General:** irregular and sometimes excessive menstrual bleeding due to anovulatory cycles

▶ **Diagnostic Findings:**

  • History should include duration, amount, suggestion of bleeding diathesis, aspirin use

  • Physical: assess hemodynamic stability, pelvic exam to evaluate extent of bleeding

  • Laboratory studies: CBC, pregnancy test, ± coagulation studies

▶ **Management:**

  • Mild bleeding/no anemia: reassurance and follow-up

  • Moderate bleeding/anemia (hematocrit: 25–35%)/hemodynamically stable: combination estrogen and progestin in

tapering dose, iron supplements, close follow-up
- Severe bleeding/hemodynamic compromise: two large-bore IVs, type and crossmatch for blood, coagulation studies, isotonic fluid resuscitation, Premarin 25 mg q4–6h IV

Dysmenorrhea

▶ **Primary:** no pathology, usually starts 6–18 months after menarche
▶ **Secondary:** PID, endometriosis, congenital malformations such as bicornuate uterus causing obstruction, psychosocial factors
▶ **Management:** primary: NSAIDs on days 1–3 ± low-dose oral contraceptive pills

Pregnancy Complications

Miscarriage

▶ 20–25% have bleeding in the first 20 weeks, 50% of those miscarry.
▶ Landmarks: 10 weeks—Doppler heart tones; 12 weeks—palpable at symphysis pubis, 20 weeks—palpable at umbilicus; gestational age = symphysis to fundus height in cm. B-HCG 750–1000 IU/mL = detectable by transvaginal ultrasound; 1800 = detectable by conventional ultrasound.
▶ Spontaneous abortion: 25% of pregnancies result in spontaneous abortion, incomplete, complete, or threatened—present with bleeding, cramps.
▶ Missed abortion: fetus dies but remains in uterus, frequently occurs in 2nd trimester, sonography confirms diagnosis, requires curettage.
▶ Septic abortion: nonsterile attempt to perform therapeutic abortion, appear toxic, fever, treat with IV antibiotics.

Ectopic Pregnancy

▶ **General:** PID, intrauterine device (IUD), prior pelvic surgery, all predispose to ectopic.
▶ **Diagnostic Findings:** triad of abdominal pain, abnormal vaginal bleeding, and mass are present in only 45% of cases, may present with shock.
▶ **Management:** fluid resuscitation to stabilize hemodynamically, then obstetric consultation for definitive management (generally surgical).

Abruptio Placenta or Placenta Previa
- ▶ Occurs in 2nd or 3rd trimester
- ▶ Avoid pelvic examination
- ▶ **Abruptio placentae:** presents with vaginal bleeding and abdominal pain
- ▶ **Placenta previa:** due to implantation of placenta over cervical os, presents with painless vaginal bleeding
- ▶ **Management:**
  - • Stabilize with IV
  - • Monitor fetal heart rate
  - • Obtain CBC, PT/PTT/INR
  - • Obstetric consultation

HEMATOLOGY AND ONCOLOGY DISORDERS
Anemia
- ▶ Hgb < 11 mg/dL (varies with age—relative anemia—newborn/premature = 8 mg/dL, at 2 months = 10.5 mg/dL, at 3 months = 11 mg/dL)
- ▶ Erythropoietin → stimulates RBC production (life span 100–120 days)
- ▶ Most common cause from 9 months–2 years of age = nutritional iron deficiency
- ▶ Most common cause in women of childbearing age = menstruation
- ▶ Mentzer index > 13.5 = iron deficiency; < 11.5 = thalassemia minor
- ▶ Normochromic, normocytic → recent blood loss, transient erythroblastopenia of childhood (TEC), chronic anemia, renal disease, osteomyelitis, autoimmune disease
- ▶ Hemolytic anemia → hereditary spherocytosis (Coombs negative, aplastic crisis from parvovirus, splenectomy is curative), hereditary elliptocytosis, G6PD, Epstein-Barr virus, drugs, malignancy
- ▶ Hypochromic, microcytic, basophilic stippling → lead toxicity
- ▶ Transfusion → 3–5 mL/kg pRBC (cautious for volume overload/CHF)

G6PD Deficiency
- ▶ Inherited
- ▶ Enzyme deficiency ↑ RBC susceptibility to oxidative stress

▶ Hemolysis after exposure to infection, drugs, fava beans
▶ **Avoid:** ciprofloxacin, naphthalene, nitrofurantoin, sulfa components
▶ **Clinical Manifestations:** pallor, jaundice, hemoglobinuria
▶ **Peripheral Smear:** reticulocytosis, bite cells, Heinz bodies
▶ **Treatment:** remove inciting agent, transfuse packed RBC, folate

Sickle Cell

▶ Single amino acid substitution (valine for glutamate)
▶ **Peripheral Smear:** Howell-Jolly bodies
▶ **Heterozygote Variant:** β-thalassemia, Hgb SC
▶ **Death:** infection leading cause from 1–3 years old, cerebrovascular accident (CVA) and trauma from 10–20 years
▶ **Asplenia ↑ Risk:** *S. pneumoniae* (30–100× higher than healthy children < 5 years, requires penicillin prophylaxis), *H. influenzae*, *N. meningitides*, *Salmonella*, *E. coli*, *Mycoplasma*, *Staph. aureus*
▶ Fever is common chief complaint
  • ↑ Risk of bacterial infection (*Strep. pneumoniae*, *H influenzae*, *N. meningitides*, *Salmonella*, *E. coli*, *Mycoplasma pneumoniae*, *Staph. aureus*)
  • Laboratory studies: CBC, reticulocyte count, urinalysis, blood/urine/throat culture and chest x-ray and lumbar puncture (LP) (if mental status change or signs suggestive of meningitis)
  • Treatment: (immediate) cefotaxime or ceftriaxone ± vancomycin (for resistant pneumococcus in meningitis or overwhelming sepsis)
▶ **Complications**
  • Osteomyelitis: typical organisms include *Salmonella* and *S. aureus.*
  • Splenic sequestration: rapid pooling of blood volume in spleen, common symptom is syncope, profound anemia, children 5 months–2 years at highest risk, uncommon over 6 years of age, death within hours, treat with immediate transfusion.
  • Pain crisis: most common complication, precipitants include: infection, dehydration, hypoxia, cold, fatigue. **Treatment:** analgesics (morphine 0.15 mg/kg bolus, then 0.07 mg/kg/h IV infusion)/hydration (1½× maintenance), supplemental oxygen.

- Acute chest syndrome: chest pain, dyspnea, fever, pulmonary infiltrates/effusions, treat with antibiotics (cover atypical organisms), supplemental oxygen, may need exchange transfusion.
- Thrombotic and hemorrhagic strokes: headache, seizures, aphasia, focal motor deficits, coma, require CT scan of head, treatment varies with clinical scenario—anticonvulsants PRN, exchange transfusion if hemorrhagic infarct.
- Aplastic crisis: dyspnea, ↑ fatigue, may have high output CHF, marked anemia with ↓ or no reticulocytes, associated with infection (parvovirus B19), transfusion may be necessary.
- Other complications include: cholecystitis/cholelithiasis, priapism, retinopathy.

Thalassemia

▶ **Microcytic Hemolytic Anemia**
▶ **Defective Synthesis of Globin Chains**
▶ **Major** (Cooley or Mediterranean anemia): homozygous with severe anemia, hepatosplenomegaly, jaundice, growth retardation, abnormal development
  - Treatment: regular transfusion, iron chelation, splenectomy (risk for sepsis, require vaccinations and aggressive fever evaluation)
▶ **Heterozygous β-Thalassemia:** thalassemia minor or thalassemia trait → microcytosis, mild anemia, target cells
▶ **Thalassemia Intermedia:** homozygous variant, produce enough hemoglobin to survive without chronic transfusions, still susceptible to aplastic crises
▶ **α-Thalassemia:** deletion of genes: 1 = silent; 2 = asymptomatic; 3 = hemoglobin H disease; 4 = hydrops fetalis (fatal)
  - Hgb H: anemia, reticulocytopenia, splenomegaly, worse with infection

Neutropenia

▶ **Leukopenia:** WBC < 5000/mm^3
▶ **Neutropenia:** absolute neutrophil count (ANC) < 1500/mm^3; mild 1000–1500/mm^3; moderate 500–1000/mm^3; severe < 500/mm^3

▶ **Cause:** congenital (Schwachman-Diamond syndrome), infection (Epstein-Barr virus, influenza, measles, varicella, hepatitis A and B), neonatal alloimmune, drugs (phenytoin, antiinflammatories, antibiotics)

▶ **Management:**
- Afebrile: CBC, outpatient close observation, no antibiotics
- Febrile (previously healthy, well-appearing): more problematic

Thrombocytopenia

▶ **Causes:**
- ↑ Destruction of platelets: ITP, HIV-associated, SLE, sepsis, DIC, necrotizing enterocolitis, giant hemangiomas, drugs (heparin, valproic acid, quinidine), HUS, thrombotic thrombocytopenia purpura (TTP)
- ↓ Platelet production: leukemia, lymphoma, granulomas, storage disease, myelofibrosis, Wiskott-Aldrich syndrome, congenital giant platelet syndrome, viral infections, drugs (chemotherapeutic agents, sulfa, rifampin, chloramphenicol), idiopathic, toxin-induced, Fanconi syndrome
- Sequestration: splenomegaly

Bleeding Disorders

▶ History of excessive bleeding after procedures (e.g., tooth extraction), menorrhagia, epistaxis, recent aspirin use

▶ Consider checking: CBC, peripheral smear, bleeding time, PT/PTT/INR, fibrinogen, fibrin split products, D-dimer, factor and co-factor levels

Disseminated Intravascular Coagulation

▶ Activation of coagulation and fibrinolytic systems microthrombi formation, also consumption of clotting factors bleeding

▶ **Cause:** Gram-negative sepsis (meningococcemia), Gram-positive sepsis (*Strep. pneumoniae, Staph. aureus*), viral (herpes simplex virus, cytomegalovirus, influenza, measles, hepatitis B, varicella), rickettsia (Rocky Mountain spotted fever), chlamydial, fungal, *Mycobacteria, Protozoa* (malaria), trauma, pregnancy, malignancy, snake bites, anaphylaxis, hypothermia, hyperthermia

TABLE 6-6
HEMOPHILIA FACTOR REPLACEMENT

Factor	Degree of Hemorrhage	Factor Replacement (units/kg)
VIII	Moderate hemorrhage	25 units/kg
	Head injury (no CNS hemorrhage)	25 units/kg
	Life- or limb-threatening hemor-rhage	50 units/kg
IX	Moderate hemorrhage	50 units/kg
	Head injury (no CNS hemorrhage)	50 units/kg
	Life- or limb-threatening hemor-rhage	100 units/kg

- ▸ Peripheral smear: microangiopathic hemolytic anemia, schisto-cytes, thrombocytopenia
- ▸ PT/PTT prolonged, ↓ fibrinogen levels, ↑ fibrin split/degrada-tion products
- ▸ **Treatment:** treat underlying cause, transfuse clotting factors and platelets as needed
  - FFP: first-line therapy, dose of 10–15 mL/kg
  - Cryoprecipitate: primarily factor VIII and fibrinogen, dose of 1 unit/5 kg
  - Platelets: transfuse if severe thrombocytopenia ($< 20,000/mL^3$) and bleeding, dose of 1 pack/5–6 kg (max of 6 units)
  - Heparin therapy is controversial

Hemophilia

- ▸ PTT is increased
- ▸ **Treatment:**
  - Fluid replacement of spontaneous bleeding in deep muscles and joints: pain is presenting sign
  - Hemophilia A → X-linked, factor 8 deficiency
  - Hemophilia B → Christmas disease, factor 9 deficiency
  - Bleeding time and PT → normal
    1. PTT and thrombin major hemorrhage
    2. Factor replacement:
       a. Factor 8: 1 unit/kg → raises measured level 2%; $t\frac{1}{2} = 12$ h ($0.5 \times$ kg $\times$ desired increment % of fac-tor 8 level)

b.   Factor 9: 1 unit/kg → raises level 1.5%; t½ = 24 h
     (1 × kg × desired increment % of factor 9 level)
     ■ Oral aminocaproic acid: for oral mucosa bleeding,
       dose of 100 mg/kg/dose
     ■ Corticosteroids: recurrent joint bleeding
     ■ DDAVP (IV form of desmopressin): used in mild
       classic hemophilia (< 4 years old—risk of
       hyponatremia and seizure), dose of 0.3 µg/kg
       over 15–30 minutes

Immune Thrombocytopenic Purpura (ITP)

▶ Destruction of platelets on an autoimmune basis
▶ Occurs 2–3 weeks postvaccination, or after viral illness
▶ Most cases self-limited, 90% spontaneously resolve within 6 months
▶ Can be first manifestation of HIV
▶ **Diagnostic Findings:**
  • 2–10 years old
  • Sudden-onset bruising, petechiae, mucosal bleeding (epistaxis, menorrhagia), GI bleed
  • No associated weight loss, fatigue, fever, bone pain, adenopathy, or hepatosplenomegaly
  • Rare death: intracranial hemorrhage (< 1%)
▶ **Ancillary Data:**
  • Hemoglobin, hematocrit, white count and differential are normal
  • Platelets: usually < 50,000/mm^3 (if < 20,000/mm^3 risk of life-threatening hemorrhage)
  • Peripheral smear: normal (microangiopathic: consider TTP, HUS, DIC)
▶ **Management/Disposition:**
  • Controversial
  • CT scan if concern for intracranial hemorrhage
  • Restrict contact sports in all patients with ITP
  • No aspirin
  • Expectant waiting, IVIG, steroids
  • If platelet count < 20,000/mm^3: must raise count with IVIG, steroids, admit
  • Check bone marrow before starting steroids to rule out leukemia (bone marrow → normal or ↑ megakaryocytes)
  • "Chronic": > 6 months, evaluate for autoimmune disease

von Willebrand Disease (vWD)

▶ Quantitative or qualitative congenital abnormality of von Willebrand factor (VWF)

▶ **Pathophysiology:**
  • Inherited autosomal dominant
  • vWF protein facilitates adherence of platelets to damaged endothelium

▶ **Diagnostic Findings:**
  • Type I—most common (70–80%): ↓ vWF antigen and ↓ vWF activity on ristocetin co-factor assay
  • Type IIB—rare (3–5%): hyperresponsiveness to vWF therefore DDAVP contraindicated
  • Hemorrhage out of proportion to severity of injury
  • Ecchymosis, epistaxis, menorrhagia

▶ **Management:**
  • Type I: IV DDAVP (or intranasal)
  • Type IIA: DDAVP + vWF replacement
  • Type IIB: factor VIII and vWF replacement
  • Type III: trial of DDAVP, or vWF replacement
  • Platelet type vWD: platelet transfusion
  • Cryoprecipitate not recommended
  • Acute hemorrhage with type unknown: type and cross, treat with vWF, avoid DDAVP (if type unknown)

Complications of Common Malignancies

Fever and Neutropenia

▶ Temperature > 38.3° C

▶ **Differential Diagnoses:** infections, pyrogenic medications (includes: cytotoxic agents), blood products, malignant process

▶ **Neutropenia:** absolute neutrophil count (ANC) < 500/mm^3 (or < 1000/mm^3 and falling due to antineoplastic therapy)

▶ Careful/rapid evaluation for overwhelming sepsis

▶ Evaluation of common infection sites
  • IV/portacath sites
  • Lungs: chest x-ray
  • Perioral
  • Perirectal
  • Urinalysis and urine culture: avoid catheterization
  • Stool: including *C. difficile*

- **Management:** controversial
  - Prompt broad-spectrum antibiotics (vancomycin and ceftazidime) as the Gram-positive organisms are most common (staphylococci and streptococci), Gram-negative include (*E. coli, Klebsiella pneumoniae, Pseudomonas, Enterobacter*)
  - Continue antibiotics until the ANC > $1500/mm^3$
- Varicella: if seronegative or bone marrow transplant patient, then administer varicella zoster immune globulin (IG) within 96 hours of exposure (dose of 1 vial/10 kg)

Genitourinary Emergencies

- **Hemorrhagic Cystitis**
  - Dysuria, hematuria, leukocytes, 2-degree to inflammation/bleeding of bladder
  - Cyclophosphamide and ifosfamide are most common cause
  - Treatment: hydration, transfusion, correction of coagulopathy, IV or oral Mesna
- **Urinary Flow Obstruction**
  - Retention 2-degree lesions of spinal cord/bulky pelvic tumors (retroperitoneal sarcomas, lymphomas, ovarian/bladder wall tumor, "drop" metastases from brain)
  - Treatment: catheterization or nephrostomy

Hyperleukocytosis

- Peripheral leukocyte count > $100,000/mm^3$
- Death from CNS hemorrhage or thrombosis, pulmonary leukostasis, tumor lysis
- Occur in lymphoblastic leukemia (T-cell), acute myelogenous leukemia (AML)
- **Symptoms:** none, hypoxia, acidosis, blurred vision, mental status change
- **Treatment:**
  - Supportive: hydration, alkalinization, allopurinol
  - Controversial: exchange transfusion, leukophoresis, cranial radiation
  - Definitive: chemotherapy to ablate abnormal bone marrow cells

Metabolic Emergencies

▶ **Tumor Lysis Syndrome**
  • Direct result of degeneration of malignant cells
  • Triad: ($\uparrow$ uric acid) hyperuricemia, ($\uparrow$ K+) hyperkalemia, ($\uparrow$ PO_4) hyperphosphatemia
  • Complications: hypocalcemia, seizures, acute renal failure, ventricular arrhythmias, and death
  • Occurs before therapy or 1–5 days after specific chemotherapy
  • Most commonly seen with Burkitt and T-cell leukemia/lymphoma
  • Prevention: hydration (2–4 × maintenance fluid volume without K+), alkalinization (urine pH 7–7.5), allopurinol (inhibits xanthine oxidase)
  • $\uparrow$ K+ causes arrhythmias/death: treat with insulin/glucose, calcium gluconate, Kayexalate, dialysis

▶ **Hypercalcemia**
  • $Ca^+ > 10.5$
  • Associated with acute lymphocytic leukemia (ALL), non-Hodgkin lymphoma, neuroblastoma, Ewing sarcoma
  • Usually secondary to $\uparrow$ bone resorption
  • Includes GI, renal, neuromuscular, cardiovascular symptoms
  • Other exacerbating factors: thiazide diuretics, oral contraceptives, antacids, $\uparrow$ vitamin A or D, adrenal insufficiency, fractures, immobilization
  • Treatment: saline fluids, furosemide

Neurologic Emergencies

▶ **Acute Mental Status Change**
  • Lethargy, stupor, coma due to intracranial hemorrhage, CVA, metastases, 1-degree disease, CNS bacterial/fungal infection, sepsis, DIC, encephalitis, leukoencephalopathy
  • Evaluation: ABC, rule out herniation
  • Laboratory studies: CBC, serum glucose, electrolytes, LFTs, coagulation profile, toxin screen
  • If $\uparrow$ intracranial pressure $\rightarrow$ hyperventilate (PCO_2 30–35), dexamethasone, mannitol

▶ **Spinal Cord Compression**
  • 4% tumor-related compression

- 50% sarcoma metastases (remainder neuroblastoma, lymphoma, leukemia)
- Epidural compression most common
- Evaluation: strength, reflex, anal tone, sensory level
- MRI
- Rapidly progressive: immediate dexamethasone (1–2 mg/kg q6h)
- Treatment options include: surgery, radiation, chemotherapy

► **SIADH**
- Release ADH without relation to plasma osmolality: ↓ Na$^+$ and water intoxication
- Symptoms: fatigue, weight gain, lethargy, confusion, seizure, coma, death
- Diagnosis: urine osmolality
- Treatment: If Na$^+$ > 120 and asymptomatic → fluid restriction. If seizures → 3% NS (rate of correction of 2 mEq/dL/h)

Thoracic Emergencies

► Superior vena cava (SVC) syndrome
- Compression/infiltration/thrombosis of SVC
- Associated with T-cell leukemia, non-Hodgkin lymphoma
- Symptoms: tracheal compression, respiratory distress, stridor, wheezing, face/neck/upper extremity swelling, plethora, cyanosis, engorged chest wall veins
- Progresses rapidly
- Chest x-ray: anterior-superior mediastinal mass ± pleural/pericardial effusion
- Treatment: radiation is traditional therapy, steroids (consult oncologist), chemotherapy

► **Pleural/Pericardial Effusion**
- Transudate: sympathetic response to tumor in chest or abdomen, fluid overload, heart failure, ↓ protein, ↓ specific gravity, ↓ cell counts
- Exudates: protein > 2.5, specific gravity > 1.015, high cell count
- Thoracentesis indicated for fluid evaluation, rule out infection, relieve respiratory distress, eliminate reservoir for drugs (i.e., methotrexate)

▶ **Cardiac Tamponade**
- Compression with pericardial fluid, constrictive fibrosis after radiation, 1-degree cardiac tumor
- Symptoms: (like heart failure) cough, chest pain, shortness of breath, hiccups, nonspecific abdominal pain
- Signs: cyanosis, pulsus paradoxus > 10 mm Hg, friction rubs, diastolic murmur, atrial dysrhythmia
- Chest x-ray: "water bag" cardiac shadow
- ECG: low voltage, flat or inverted T wave, electrical alternans
- Differential diagnosis: CHF, myocarditis (infection versus therapy-induced)
- Treatment: hydration, oxygen, ultrasound-guided pericardiocentesis (diuretics contraindicated)

INFECTIOUS DISEASE

▶ Treatment for infectious diseases are outlined in Figures 6-1 to 6-3.

Fever

Strategies for Management

▶ *In febrile infants < 2 months of age, antibiotic administration as early as possible is optimal and a "Febrile Infant Protocol" has been proposed. This includes identification of febrile infants in triage, provision of acetaminophen by the triage nurse, and provision of information sheet about fever and the need for evaluation for the parents (see Table 6-7). If the parents consent to proceed with treatment, there is immediate transfer of the patient to a patient care room with nursing initiation of bladder catheterization, IV line placement (if patient is ≤28 days of age), and blood sampling for a CBC and blood culture prior to evaluation by a doctor. The doctor then evaluates the infant, performs an LP and antibiotics are administered, with the goal of antibiotic administration within 1–2 hours of arrival to the ED. If IV access is unsuccessful within 2 hours, antibiotics are administered IM. This approach significantly reduces overall time to antibiotic administration in this age group.*

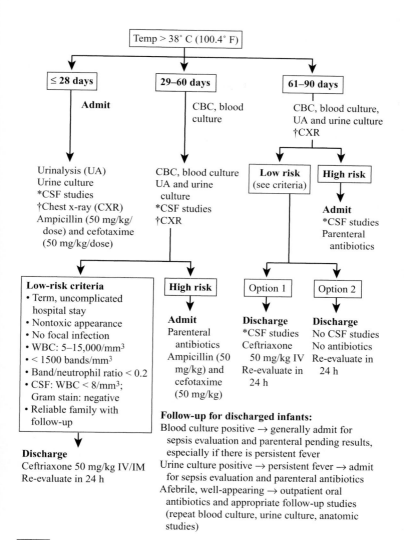

FIGURE 6-1

Recommended management of an infant 0–90 days of age with temperature > 38° C (rectally). *CSF studies include cell count, Gram stain, protein, glucose, and culture. †Chest x-ray if tachypnea, respiratory distress, abnormal breath sounds or pulse oximetry < 95% (room air, sea level).

Source: American College of Emergency Physicians Clinical Policies Committee; American College of Emergency Physicians Clinical Policies Subcommittee on Pediatric Fever. Clinical policy for children younger than three years presenting to the emergency department with fever. *Ann Emerg Med* 2003 Oct;42(4):530–545.

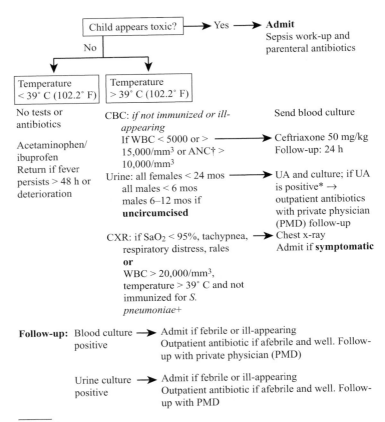

FIGURE 6-2

Recommended management of a child 3–36 months of age with fever without a source.
[+]Those immunized against *S. pneumoniae* should have a prevalence of bacteremia that is reduced by 90% compared with the general population. Similarly, the vaccine reduces clinical pneumonia by 10%, radiographic pneumonia by 32%, and pneumonia with definite consolidation by 73%. ***Urine screen positive:** Either positive leukocyte esterase (LE) **and** nitrites, **or** positive Gram stain for bacteria on urinalysis are most predictive of urinary tract infection (UTI). The presence of > 10 WBC/hpf has been used, but has much lower sensitivity for predicting bacteriuria with a reported 10% incidence of bacteriuria without pyuria. [+]ANC: absolute neutrophil count

Age	Temperature	Labs	Disposition	Treatment
0–1 month	≥ 38° C (≥ 100.4° F)	CBC/blood culture UA/urine culture CSF studies ± CXR	ADMIT	Ampicillin + cefotaxime
1–2 months	≥ 38° C (≥ 100.4° F)	CBC/blood culture UA/urine culture CSF studies ± CXR	ADMIT high risk DISCHARGE low risk with 24-hour follow-up	Ampicillin + cefotaxime Ceftriaxone

CBC, complete blood count; UA, urinalysis; CSF, cerebrospinal fluid; CXR, chest x-ray.

FIGURE 6-3

Management summary—0–2 months.

TABLE 6-7
DESCRIPTION OF WORKUP FOR THE PARENTS

Children's Hospital and Health Center San Diego Emergency Department

Febrile Young Infant

We want to make your visit as short as possible and care for your child's needs in a timely manner. Your infant has a high fever (over 104° F) and this could be a sign of serious illness. Due to your child's very young age, it is possible that this illness may be a bacterial infection. Young children do not have good defenses to fight these infections well, so it is important to find out if this is what is causing your child's high fever. We will need to collect a blood and a urine sample to check for possible bacterial infection.

The doctor will come in to examine your child as soon as possible, but with your permission, we would like to have the nurse collect the blood and urine sample now to avoid further delay. The doctor may feel more tests are needed after examining your child (such as a chest x-ray or a spinal fluid exam) to find out what is causing your child's fever. Collecting the blood and the urine now may make your visit to the emergency department shorter.

The blood sample is taken from a vein (usually on the arm). Sometimes an IV (intravenous line) is placed at the same time as drawing the blood.

The urine sample from a baby is best obtained with a catheter. The nurse will place a small tube into the opening to the bladder (the urethra) and collect the urine through this tube into a sterile cup. Before inserting the catheter, the nurse puts on sterile gloves and cleans the area with a special soap. Some children may experience discomfort during the procedure, but it does not take long.

The urine and blood samples are then sent to the lab. If a lumbar puncture is performed, the fluid will also be sent to the lab.

Please let the nurse know if you would like us to start these tests now or if you'd rather wait until the doctor has examined your child.

Meningococcemia

▶ Caused by a Gram-negative diplococcus with most cases occurring in children 6–12 months of age.

▶ The mortality of meningococcemia is higher than that of meningococcal meningitis.

▶ Patients present with a prodrome of an upper respiratory tract infection, headache, myalgia, nausea, and vomiting. The classic skin lesions are petechiae progressing to purpura.

▶ Contact prophylaxis should be given for close school and household contacts: rifampin can be used in children.

▶ Complications include disseminated intravascular disease (DIC), hypotension, cervicitis, and pericarditis.

Mononucleosis

▶ Caused by Epstein-Barr virus (EBV) and is most frequently diagnosed in adolescence.

▶ Diagnostic findings of EBV include a prodromal phase of anorexia, headaches, fatigue which lasts up to a week. This is followed by the acute phase—classic triad of fever, exudative tonsillitis, lymphadenopathy, splenomegaly, palatal petechiae, and conjunctival injection. A throat culture to exclude GABHS—group A beta-hemolytic streptococcus—should be performed.

▶ The most common complication of EBV is splenic enlargement and rupture with the greatest risk between 14–28 days. No athletic activity/sports for 1 month. Laboratory studies may show absolute lymphocytosis, with > 20% atypical lymphocytes. 40% of patients will have a positive heterophil antibody test in the first week of illness and 80% will be positive in the first 3 weeks. The heterophil antibody test may not be accurate in children < 4 years of age and therefore an IgM antibody test to EBV may be necessary.

Mumps

▶ Caused by a paramyxovirus with swelling of the parotid gland being the hallmark finding.

▶ Patients present with fever, malaise, and headache in addition to parotid swelling.

▶ Complications of mumps include: meningoencephalitis (males predominate), transverse myelitis, Guillain-Barré, deafness, orchitis.

Pertussis (Whooping Cough)

▶ Caused by *Bordetella pertussis* (Gram-negative bacterium)
▶ Diagnostic Findings:
- Incubation period is 6–20 days.
- First stage (catarrhal stage): 1–2 weeks, rhinorrhea, lacrimation, mild cough.
- Second stage (paroxysmal stage): 2–4 weeks, paroxysmal cough, inspiratory "whoop."
- Third stage (convalescent stage): gradual improvement in symptoms, lasts 1–4 weeks.
- Infants < 6 months of age with pertussis are at risk of apnea (the classic presentation is continuous cough until they turn "red in the face" instead of classic whooping cough).
- It should be considered in the differential diagnosis of Acute Life-Threatening Event (ALTE).
- Laboratory studies: show WBC > 15,000/mm^3, lymphocytosis, chest x-ray shows atelectasis or pneumonia. It should be considered in the differential diagnosis of leukemia due to the extreme elevated WBC and lymphocytosis.
▶ Management:
- Erythromycin estolate for 14 days (50 mg/kg/24 h).
- Bactrim is an alternative.
- Household and close contacts should be treated with erythromycin for 14 days.
- Contacts < 7 years should receive immunizations.
- Patients < 6 months should be hospitalized.
- Isolation for 5 days after starting erythromycin treatment.

Rabies

▶ An acute viral infection from an RNA virus.
▶ The highest incidence is in wild carnivores (skunks, raccoons, foxes). Uncommon in rodents and lagomorphs.
▶ Wounds from domestic animals that appear healthy should be managed by observing the animal for 10 days.
▶ Wounds from high-risk carnivores should be treated with human rabies immune globulin 20 IU/kg with half infiltrated at the site of the wound, and half given IM in gluteus, and human rabies vaccine (1 mL) in the deltoid on days 0, 3, 7, 14, and 28.

Tuberculosis

▶ Caused by *Mycobacterium tuberculosis*.
▶ The incubation period is 2–10 weeks.
▶ A positive TB skin test is: > 15 mm in healthy individuals > 4 years; > 10 mm in individuals < 4 years or with risk factors; > 5 mm in patients with HIV.
▶ **Management:**
  - Preventive therapy in asymptomatic patients is isoniazid (INH) (10 mg/kg/24 h) daily for 9 months.
  - Uncomplicated pulmonary TB requires INH, rifampin, pyrazinamide, for 2 months, then INH and rifampin for 4 months.
  - Other infections (meningitis, miliary disease, etc.) are treated with INH, rifampin, pyrazinamide, streptomycin for 2 months, then INH and rifampin for 10 months.

Tularemia

▶ Caused by *Francisella tularensis* with Dermacentor being the tick vector.
▶ The incubation period is 1–14 days, with patients presenting with headache, fever, malaise, anorexia, lymphadenopathy, and conjunctivitis.
▶ **Treatment** is with gentamicin.

Relapsing Fever

▶ Caused by *Borrelia recurrentis* with Ornithodoros being the tick vector.
▶ The incubation period is 5–9 days with patients presenting with relapsing fever, headache, malaise, myalgias, cough, meningismus, lymphadenopathy, and leukocytosis.
▶ **Treatment** is with tetracycline or chloramphenicol.

Rocky Mountain Spotted Fever

▶ Caused by *Rickettsia rickettsii* with Dermacentor being the tick vector.
▶ The incubation period is 2–14 days with patients presenting with resistant fevers, headache, malaise, arthralgias, petechiae, rash (including palms and soles), thrombocytopenia, hyponatremia.

▶ **Treatment** is with tetracycline or chloramphenicol.

Colorado Tick Fever

▶ Also transmitted by Dermacentor.

▶ The incubation period is 3–6 days with patients presenting with the sudden onset of fever, retro-orbital headache, myalgia, anorexia, meningismus, rash, conjunctivitis, and leukopenia.

▶ **Treatment** is supportive.

Ehrlichiosis

▶ Caused by *Ehrlichia chaffeensis* with Dermacentor being the tick vectors.

▶ The incubation period is 7–21 days with patients presenting with fever, headache, malaise, arthralgias, myalgias, nausea, vomiting, rash, and leukopenia.

▶ **Treatment** is tetracycline or chloramphenicol.

Lyme Disease

▶ Caused by *Borrelia burgdorferi* with Ixodes being the tick vector.

▶ The incubation period is 3–32 days with patients presenting with several stages:

- **Stage I:** erythema chronicum migrans, fever, flulike symptoms, rash present in about 60–80%
- **Stage II:** neurologic and cardiac manifestations, aseptic meningitis is most common neurologic finding, and AV block is most common cardiac finding
- **Stage III:** chronic arthritis, chronic neurologic complaints, acrodermatitis chronica atrophicans

▶ **Treatment** is with doxycycline.

Erythema Infectiosum (Fifth Disease)

▶ Transmitted by parvovirus B-19.

▶ The incubation period is 1 week with patient presenting with fever, malaise, headache, and erythematous erysipeloid rash on cheeks that spreads to arms, legs and trunk, and fades into a reticular "lace-like" pattern.

▶ Care is supportive. Patients who are pregnant or have sickle cell disease should be protected from exposure. Those with sickle cell are at risk for aplastic crisis and pregnant patients are at risk for fetal demise.

Hand-Foot-and-Mouth Disease

▶ Caused by coxsackievirus. Patients present with low-grade fever, malaise, and a rash involving the palms, feet, and mouth.

▶ **Treatment** is supportive with antipyretics and analgesics.

Roseola

▶ Caused by herpesvirus 6 with 95% of cases occurring in children between 6 months and 3 years.

▶ Patients present with the sudden onset of a high fever that lasts approximately 3 days. After defervescence, the patient develops a macular rose-pink rash that begins on the trunk and spreads to the proximal extremities.

▶ Supportive care is all that is necessary.

Rubella

▶ Transmitted by the togavirus and typically occurs in adolescents and young adults.

▶ Patients present with a prodrome of malaise, fever, and tender post-auricular nodes. Within 24 hours of fever, they develop a macular rash on the face and scalp that moves down the body, coalesces, and then fades. Forchheimer sign is petechiae on the soft palate.

Rubeola (Measles)

▶ Caused by *Paramyxovirus* and is more common in preschool children.

▶ Patients present with a prodrome of fever, malaise, cough, coryza, and conjunctivitis. Koplik spots are the earliest findings. The rash begins on the face, scalp, and neck, and spreads downward to affect most of body, and coalesces.

▶ Complications of the measles are otitis media, pneumonia, and meningitis.

▶ **Treatment** is supportive.

Human Immunodeficiency Virus (HIV)

▶ 90% of pediatric HIV is the result of vertical transmission from mother to infant. The risk of HIV infection following percutaneous exposure to known HIV-infected blood is 0.4%.

▶ Patients with acquired immunodeficiency syndrome (AIDS)/ HIV may present with recurrent fever, generalized lymphadenopathy, failure to thrive, recurrent oral candidiasis, chronic diarrhea, hepatomegaly, splenomegaly, encephalopathy, or severe or recurrent bacterial infections.

▶ The incidence of *Pneumocystis carinii* is highest in children < 12 months of age with a peak between 3–6 months of age. Chest x-ray may reveal diffuse bilateral alveolar infiltrates. The diagnosis can be confirmed by bronchoalveolar lavage.

▶ In children > 18 months of age, the diagnosis of HIV is made by enzyme immunoassay (EIA); if this test is positive, repeat and confirm by Western blot.

▶ In patients < 18 months of age, an HIV viral culture or polymerase chain reaction (PCR) and detection of p24 antigen. The HIV culture and PCR are very sensitive and specific by 6 months of age.

Infant Botulism

▶ Most common form of botulism in the United States.

▶ Caused by *Clostridium botulinum*, an anaerobic Gram-positive bacillus.

▶ Honey or corn syrup may be a source of bacillus in children < 12 months of age.

▶ Clinical features of botulism develop 12–72 hours after the ingestion of toxin and include:
- Blurred vision
- Dilated or fixed pupils
- Diplopia
- Constipation
- Irritability
- Respiratory distress
- Seizures
- Poor suck
- Poor cry
- "Floppy baby"

▶ The diagnosis can be confirmed by finding the toxin or organisms in the stool. Electromyogram (EMG) may also help to establish the diagnosis.

▶ Supportive care is necessary, as many infants require intubation. Patients with classic botulism should be treated with trivalent antitoxin. However, infants do not benefit from antitoxin.

Diphtheria

▶ Caused by *Corynebacterium diphtheriae*, a Gram-positive bacillus.

▶ The incubation period is 2–5 days.

▶ Patients with pharyngeal diphtheria present with fever, sore throat, cervical lymphadenopathy, a thick gray-white membrane, and tachycardia.

▶ The treatment is IV equine antitoxin and erythromycin or penicillin G for 2 weeks. Close contacts should be cultured and treated with oral erythromycin or IM penicillin G and booster immunizations should be administered.

▶ Patients with laryngeal diphtheria present with hoarseness or loss of their voice.

Malaria

▶ Caused by *Plasmodium falciparum, P. vivax, P. ovale*, and *P. malariae*.

▶ Symptoms include malaise, headache, vomiting, anorexia, and abdominal pain.

▶ *P. falciparum* may cause cerebral malaria, seizures, and a prolonged postictal period.

  • The diagnosis is confirmed by the presence of parasites in the peripheral blood smear, thick or thin preparations.

  • *P. falciparum* has the highest rate of chloroquine resistance and these patients should be treated with quinidine hydrochloride.

Perinatal Herpes Simplex (HSV)

▶ Transmitted via intrapartum exposure to genital HSV infection with HSV type 2 accounting for 70–80% of cases. Patients present with skin lesions, keratoconjunctivitis, buccal ulcers, jaundice, hepatomegaly, encephalitis, or seizures.

▶ **Treatment** is with IV acyclovir.

Herpes Simplex Encephalitis

▶ Present with fever, headache, altered level of consciousness, seizures, and focal neurologic findings.

▶ The spinal fluid reveals an elevated protein and WBC that ranges from 5–2000 cells/mm^3. CSF should be sent for either herpes culture or PCR.

▶ IV acyclovir should be initiated if the diagnosis is suspected.

Herpetic Gingivostomatitis

▶ Present with fever, irritability, inflammation of the gingiva and mucous membranes of the mouth, and may be dehydrated.

▶ Supportive care is indicated.

Herpetic Whitlow

▶ Present as an erythematous, painful distal phalanx that ultimately develops a vesicle. These may be confused with a felon. However, herpetic whitlow should not be incised and drained.

▶ **Treatment** is with analgesics.

Influenza

▶ Children at risk for infection include asthmatics, patients with chronic lung disease, or patients with sickle cell disease.

Tetanus

▶ Caused by *Clostridium tetani*, an anaerobic, spore-forming, Gram-positive bacillus organism that produces a neurotoxin-tetanospasmin.
  - **Generalized tetanus:** severe muscle spasms—jaw, face neck, back—trismus and opisthotonus.
  - **Localized tetanus** typically involves the muscle group closest to the contamination site and involves associated muscle spasms.
  - **Cephalic tetanus** involves the head and neck musculature.

▶ **Treatment** includes the administration of tetanus immune globulin (TIG), surgical debridement, penicillin, and the use of benzodiazepines to control the muscle spasms.

Kawasaki Disease

▶ May result in serious cardiac disease in up to 20% of untreated children.

▶ The peak incidence is 18–24 months of age with 80% of cases occurring in children < 4 years of age.

- ▶ The male to female ratio is 1.5:1, with the Asian population being at greatest risk.
- ▶ The diagnostic findings of Kawasaki disease include:
  - Fever for at least 5 days, and at least four of the following five:
    1. Bilateral bulbar nonexudative conjunctivitis
    2. Polymorphous rash
    3. Changes in lip and oral cavity: erythema, and cracking lips, strawberry tongue, diffuse injection of oral and pharyngeal mucosa
    4. Cervical adenopathy (nodes > 1.5 cm): unilateral
    5. Changes in peripheral extremities: erythema and induration of hands and feet, desquamation from fingers or toes
  - Findings are unexplained by another disease.
  - A high index of suspicion is required to diagnose Kawasaki disease in infants (may not have all signs and symptoms).
- ▶ **Complications of Kawasaki Disease:**
  - Coronary aneurysms
  - Valvular insufficiency
  - Congestive heart failure
  - Myocardial infarction
  - Dysrhythmias
  - Ruptured aneurysm
  - Pericardial effusion
  - Hydrops of the gallbladder
- ▶ **Treatment** includes the administration of IV gamma globulin (IVGG): 2 g/kg; aspirin: 100 mg/kg/24 h until the platelet count has normalized followed by 3–5 mg/kg/24 h × 2–3 months, and cardiac evaluation. IVIG may be repeated if fever persists. New therapies exist for refractory disease.

Toxic Shock Syndrome (TSS)

- ▶ Occurs most commonly in menstruating females who use tampons.
- ▶ Caused by a toxin from certain strains of *Staphylococcus*: TSST-1.
- ▶ **Diagnostic Findings:**
  - Fever > 39.2° C
  - Rash: diffuse macular erythroderma
  - Desquamation, 1–2 weeks after onset of illness: palms and soles

TABLE 6-8
TICK TRANSMITTED DISEASES

	Tularemia	Relapsing Fever	Rocky Mountain Spotted Fever	Colorado Tick Fever	Ehrlichiosis	Lyme Disease
Etiology	*Francisella tularemia*	*Borrelia recurrentis*	*Rickettsia rickettsii*	Colorado Tick Fever Virus	*Ehrlichia chaffeensis*	*Borrelia burgdorferi*
Tick vector	Dermacentor	Ornithodoros	Dermacentor	Dermacentor	N/A	Ixodes scapularis
Incubation	1–14 days	5–9 days	2–14 days	3–6 days	7–21 days	3–32 days
Diagnosis	Headache (HA), fever malaise, LAD, anorexia, conjunctivitis	Fever, HA, LAD, leukocytosis, meningismus	Fever, HA, periorbital edema, coma, centrifugal hemorrhagic rash, petechiae	Sudden onset of fever, leukopenia, orbital HA, conjunctivitis	Fever, HA, nausea, vomiting, rash	Erythema chronicum migrans, HA, chills, anorexia, encephalopathy, peripheral radiculopathy
Antibiotics	Gentamicin	Tetracycline PCN, or chloramphenicol	Tetracycline	None	Tetracycline or chloramphenicol	Doxycycline, amoxicillin

Source: Felter R, Bower J. Infectious disorders. In: Barkin R, ed. *Pediatric Emergency Medicine Concepts and Clinical Practice*, 2nd ed. St Louis: Mosby, 1997. p 955.

- Hypotension
- Involvement of three or more organ systems with negative blood, throat, CSF, Rocky Mountain spotted fever, measles, or leptospirosis studies:
  1. GI: vomiting and diarrhea
  2. Muscular (CK elevation)
  3. Renal: > 5 WBC per hpf or BUN or creatinine levels $\geq 2\times$ normal
  4. Hepatic: AST or ALT $\geq 2\times$ normal
  5. Hematologic: thrombocytopenia
  6. CNS: altered sensorium

▶ **Treatment** includes nafcillin or cefazolin. Steroid and IVIG may also be administered. Electrolyte and fluid monitoring are essential.

Tick-Transmitted Diseases

▶ Tick-transmitted diseases are listed in Table 6-8.

NEUROLOGIC DISORDERS
Ataxia

▶ **Differential Diagnosis**
- **Acute:**
  1. **Postinfectious causes** (varicella, influenza, coxsackievirus, echovirus, HSV, EBV, poliovirus, mycoplasma). Patients may have dysarthria and nystagmus. Head CT is negative and the CSF has mild pleocytosis. Mild symptoms may persist for up to 6 years of age.
  2. **Drug ingestion:** *very common*—phenytoin toxicity, alcohol, tricyclic antidepressants (TCAs), hypnotics, sedatives, benzodiazepines, lead, insecticides, phencyclidine (PCP).
  3. **Posterior fossa tumors:** medulloblastoma, astrocytoma, ependymoma, brain stem glioma. Patients present with headaches, vomiting, ataxia, and papilledema.
  4. **Head trauma**
  5. **Neuroblastoma:** Triad of ataxia, myoclonus, opsoclonus, also known as dancing eyes, dancing feet syndrome.

6. **Infections:** meningitis, encephalitis, labyrinthitis, Guillain-Barré, transverse myelitis, tick paralysis
7. **Metabolic:** Hartnup disease, maple sugar urine disease (MSUD), hypothyroidism
8. **Stroke/Vasculitis**

- **Chronic:**
  1. Tumor
  2. Hydrocephalus
  3. Friedrich ataxia
  4. Congenital (Dandy-Walker, Arnold-Chiari)
  5. Ataxia-telangiectasia
  6. Wilson disease
  7. Multiple sclerosis
  8. Vitamin B_{12}/E/folate deficiency

▶ **Diagnostic Workup**
- Toxicology screen
- Computed tomography (CT) versus magnetic resonance imaging (MRI)
- Lumbar puncture (LP)
- Electrolytes
- Ammonia level
- 24-hour urine for VMA (vanillylmandelic acid) and HVA (homovanillic acid) for occult neuroblastoma
- Also need abdominal films and chest radiograph
- Electroencephalogram (EEG)
- Electromyogram (EMG)

Coma/Altered Mental Status

▶ **Definitions:** lethargy = ↓ wakefulness; confusion = ↓ awareness; delirium = disorientation, fear, irritable, misrepresentation of stimuli; obtundation = slow response to stimuli, ↑ time asleep; stupor = deep sleep, aroused by repeated vigorous stimuli.

▶ **Breathing Patterns:** Cheyne-Stokes breathing = apnea/hyperpnea; apneustic breathing = inspiratory pauses with alternating expiratory pauses = pontine dysfunction/encephalopathy.

▶ **Pupil Size:** midbrain lesion = fixed to light but spontaneous fluctuation in size, constriction but reactive = metabolic or pontine; uncal herniation = unilateral fixed/dilated; Horner syndrome = hypothalamic damage → ipsilateral constriction, ptosis, anhidrosis; doll's eye tests for vestibular function; ocu-

TABLE 6-9
SHOCK/ALOC (ALTERED LEVEL OF CONSCIOUSNESS) IN THE NEWBORN: (THE MISFITS)

T—Trauma/NAT (nonaccidental trauma)
H—Heart disease: congenital
E—Electrolyte disturbances

M—Metabolic disturbances (congenital adrenal hyperplasia)
I—Inborn errors of metabolism
S—Sepsis
F—Formula dilution or overconcentration
I—Intestinal catastrophes
T—Toxins (home remedies)
S—Seizures/CNS abnormalities

lovestibular = flex to 30 degrees, inject 50 cc ice water. If the brain stem is intact, the eyes move toward the cold stimulus.

▶ **Posturing:** decorticate = flexion, cerebral cortex dysfunction; decerebrate = rigid extension, brain stem dysfunction; flaccid = deep brain stem dysfunction.

▶ **Glasgow Coma Scale:** also useful in nontrauma situations.

▶ Differential diagnosis of altered level of consciousness: **"THE MISFITS"** and **"Tips from the vowels"** (see **Tables 6-9** and **6-10**).

TABLE 6-10
"TIPS FROM THE VOWELS"

T—Trauma: *abuse* (look for bruising)
I—Insulin **(hypoglycemia)**: *ketotic* after prolonged fast (i.e., in morning), 18 months–5 years, often history of low birth weight
   Intussusception (change in mental status can present *before* abdominal changes)
P—Poisoning (ingestion): **ask if there are any** medications in the household
   Psychogenic
S—Shock, Seizure
A—Alcohol
E—Epilepsy
   Encephalopathy: Lead from paint chips fatigue, emesis, abdominal pain. Diagnosis: labs (lead level, free erythrocyte protoporphyrin, CBC), x-ray may show lead chips. **Treatment:** chelation.
I—Infection: with secondary *Reye's syndrome* (vomiting → change is mental status, recent illness or aspirin)
   Inborn Errors (*acidosis, emesis, seizures*; check serum amino acids and urine organic acids)
O—Opiates
U—Uremia

▶ **Management/Diagnosis**
- **ABCs** (immobilize C-spine)
- **D**—Dextrostix: give glucose 1 g/kg
- Disability: pupils—size, brief neurologic examination
- **E**—(full exam and history)

▶ **Prognosis:** poor if Glasgow Coma Score (GCS) < 9, age < 2, skull fracture, CT → bilateral edema, → intracranial pressure > 2 days, coma > 2 weeks, no improvement at 6 months. **Brain death** requires 24 hours observation if < 12 months old, 12 hours if > 12 months.

Headache

▶ **Pathophysiology**
- Pain-sensitive structures include the large arteries/veins, dura at skull base, cranial nerves V, VII, X, upper cervical nerves; pain insensitive structures include the brain, skull, dura, ependyma; intracranial sources refer pain to front of head; posterior fossa sources refer pain to the back of the head and neck.

▶ **Differential Diagnosis**
- **Inflammatory:**
  1. **Meningitis/encephalitis** (fever, altered mental status, nuchal rigidity); fever (frontal/bitemporal, throbbing)
  2. **Sinusitis** (sphenoid = occipital pain, ethmoid = eyeball pain); teeth
- **Vascular:** pulsatile, throbbing
  1. **Migraine** (common migraine) has no aura, bilateral pain with nausea/vomiting; (classic) is uncommon, has aura, neurologic symptoms, unilateral, nausea/vomiting, positive family history
  2. **Hypertension; hypoxia, cluster headaches** (retro/peri-orbital, unilateral autonomic symptoms, lasting 30–120 minutes)
- **Traction:** daily, progressive, morning, exacerbated by Valsalva, caused by mass lesions (neoplasm, hematoma, AV malformation, abscess), hydrocephalus, pseudotumor
- **Tension:** scalp/neck muscles, constant, squeezing
- **Trauma**
- **Toxins:** carbon monoxide, lead, alcohol, nitrites (meat)
- **Miscellaneous:** eye strain (infrequent cause, check refrac-

tive error), epilepsy, temporal arteritis, trigeminal neuralgia, altitude sickness, temporomandibular joint (TMJ) disease

Movement Disorders

▶ **Definitions**
- **Chorea:** quick jerks, seen with drugs (antiepileptic drugs [AEDs], oral contraceptive pill [OCP], psychotropics, stimulants, antiemetics), thyroid disease, and rheumatic fever.
- **Athetosis:** writhing movements, associated with perinatal injury; choreoathetosis is infectious/metabolic.
- **Ballismus:** irregular violent flailing, often viral encephalitis/subthalamic stroke.
- **Dystonia:** basal ganglia, ± grimace, simultaneous agonist/antagonist contraction, exacerbated by stress.
- **Torticollis:** tilt of head/neck, if fixed investigate C-spine, can occur in familial paroxysmal choreoathetosis, paroxysmal infantile-torticollis is intermittent.
- **Myoclonus:** involuntary rapid jerks.
- **Tics:** stereotyped purposeless movements/utterances, more with stress/excitement, in 10% of children; complex if mixed vocal/motor, tend to be chronic, **Tourette syndrome** is an inherited complex tic.
- **Tremors:** involuntary rhythmic oscillations of hands.
- **Spasmus mutans:** episodic abnormal head posturing/nodding and nystagmus. Affects infants 4–12 months and resolves spontaneously.
- **Parkinsonism:** tremor, rigidity, bradykinesia, abnormal posture.

▶ **Treatment:** based on specific diagnosis (i.e., treat phenothiazine dystonias with diphenhydramine 1 mg/kg PO/IV/IM or benztropine 1–2 mg IM).

Paralysis/Hemiplegia

▶ **Definitions**
- **Paralysis:** loss of function
- **Paresis:** partial/complete weakness
- **Paraplegia:** lower half of body
- **Hemiplegia:** one side of body
- **Quadriplegia:** all 4 limbs

▶ **Paraplegia Diagnosis**
- **Acute:**
  1. **Trauma** (compression, may be slowly progressive epidural hematoma; atlantoaxial dislocation in Down syndrome, mucopolysaccharidoses, Klippel-Feil syndrome)
  2. **Vascular** (anterior spinal artery occlusion)
- **Subacute:**
  1. **Tumor/infection/myelitis:** patients present with clumsiness and back pain that may be due to a tumor (astrocytoma/ependymoma/neuroblastoma) or abscess (hematogenous spread of *S. aureus*, also consider *Salmonella* and TB).
  2. **Polio:** anterior horn cells with asymmetric motor weakness.
  3. **Guillain-Barré:** ascending weakness with loss of deep tendon reflexes (oculomotor involvement = **Fisher syndrome**), similar presentation to tick paralysis (toxin-mediated).
  4. **Botulism:** flaccid paralysis, consider *toxins* (organophosphates, chemotherapeutic agents, lead, arsenic, mercury).
  5. **Myasthenia gravis** (usually starts bulbar).
  6. **Dyskalemic paralysis** (familial periodic or acquired 2-degree diuretics, amphotericin-B, albuterol, laxatives, licorice).
- **Congenital:** tethered cord in spina bifida; meningomyelocele, cerebral palsy.
- **Workup:** CBC; ESR, electrolytes; x-rays; LP (may cause decompensation if mass lesion), consider CT first (head/spine); MRI evaluates spinal cord.

▶ **Hemiplegia Diagnosis**
- **Acute:**
  1. **Vascular** (cerebral infarction ± hemorrhage)
     a. **Neonatal** 2-degree polycythemia, DIC, carotid birth trauma
     b. **Sickle cell disease** with vasoocclusive crisis (VOC)
     c. **Congenital heart disease** with polycythemia/dehydration
     d. **Vasculopathies:** i.e., SLE, Takayasu arteritis, polyarteritis nodosa

   e. **Coagulation disorders** such as protein C, S or anti-thrombin III deficiencies
   f. **Insulin-dependent diabetes mellitus (IDDM)** can have acute transient hemiparesis associated with headache (HA) during URIs
   g. **Neurofibromatosis** and **Sturge-Weber syndrome** more at risk of CVA
   h. **Focal intractable seizures** (*epilepsia partialis continua*)
   i. **Trauma** (cerebral artery injury thrombosis)
   j. **Todd paralysis** after seizure (minutes–days)
   k. **Familial hemiplegic migraines** (hemiplegia often followed by headache, nausea/vomiting)
- **Subacute:**
   1. **Moyamoya:** stenosis/occlusion of carotid with collaterals transient ischemic attacks (TIAs) and headaches
   2. **AV malformations:** cerebral aneurysm, infections (cavernous sinus thrombosis, vasculitis, thrombophlebitis, cat scratch disease, and mycoplasma pneumoniae) can unilateral cerebral infarction (carotid inflammation)
- **Workup:** CBC, ESR, consider sickle prep with reticulocyte count; coagulation and DIC panels. ECG/echo to evaluate for dysrhythmias, heart disease; head CT/ MRI.

Syncope

▶ **Pathophysiology**
- **↓ Peripheral vascular resistance/abnormalities of circulatory control**
   1. Orthostatic hypotension (hypovolemia, phenothiazines/antihypertensives, nitrates)
- **Vasovagal**
   1. Stress, anxiety, fear, pain with ↓ PVR
   2. Cough (after paroxysms)
- **Micturition** (? reflex, ↓ PVR)
- **Autonomic dysfunction** (primary dysautonomia)
   1. Riley-Day
   2. Shy-Drager syndrome
   3. Spinal cord injury
   4. Diabetes mellitus

- **Carotid sinus syndrome** (rare, exaggerated response to carotid massage)
- **Cardiovascular** (↓ cardiac output which decreases cerebral perfusion)
  1. Acquired heart disease (myocarditis)
  2. Tumor
  3. Dysrhythmias (Wolff-Parkinson-White)
  4. Prolonged QT syndromes (Romano-Ward, Jervell Lange-Nielsen with deafness)
  5. Drug-induced dysrhythmias: procainamide, quinidine, TCAs, phenothiazines, nonsedating histamines
  6. Metabolic especially hypoglycemia
  7. Neurologic (epilepsy, vertigo)
  8. Psychologic (hypocapnia, hysterical)
  9. Drugs
- Metabolic: especially hypoglycemia
- Neurologic (epilepsy, vertigo)
- Psychologic (hypocapnia, hysterical)
- Drugs

▶ **Workup**
- Accurate **history** most important.
- **Examination** → orthostatics (positive if ↑ HR of 20 bpm, bradycardia, ↓ SBP by 20 mm Hg when going from supine to any other position).
- **Laboratory studies:** CBC, electrolytes, consider pregnancy test, drug screen, ABG if necessary; ECG (normal QTc < 0.44 seconds); consider echocardiogram. Holter monitor, stress test. If the syncope is exercise-induced consider electrophysiology studies or catheterization.

Vertigo

▶ **Definitions**
- **Vertigo:** sensation of motion (spinning, rotation) ± nystagmus
- **Dizziness:** balance disturbed/lightheaded

▶ **Differential Diagnosis**
- **Infectious:** otitis media (OM), meningitis. Acute suppurative labyrinthitis 2-degree OM, cholesteatoma with labyrinth damage; vestibular neuritis (viral infection of laby-

rinth/vestibular nerve with vertigo, vomiting, ataxia 2-degree mumps, measles, EBV).

- **Epilepsy:** aura preceding or as only component of a complex partial seizure.
- **Migraine:** basilar artery, ± scotoma, blurred vision, paresthesias, loss of consciousness (LOC), and drop attacks.
- **Benign paroxysmal vertigo:** occurs in children aged 1–4 years with multiple brief episodes of disequilibrium, nystagmus, pallor, sweating, vomiting, no LOC, normal EEG, abnormal caloric response.
- **Drugs/toxins:** aminoglycosides, anticonvulsants.
- **Ménière disease:** uncommon in children; rupture of labyrinth with hearing impairment, tinnitus, vertigo, lasts 1–3 hours.
- **Motion sickness:** pallor, nausea/vomiting.
- **Hyperventilation:** psychogenic—if complains of vertigo without nystagmus, not true vertigo.
- **Trauma:** head injury, vestibular/labyrinthine concussion, tympanic membrane (TM) perforation, whiplash (basilar artery spasm).
- **Tumor:** posterior fossa.

Breath-Holding Spells

▶ **Two Types:**
  - **Cyanotic:** cries, exhales, holds breath, becomes cyanotic, limp and loses consciousness; may have posturing and tonic-clonic movements; autonomic respiratory mechanism resumes, arousal occurs, may be postictal.
  - **Pallid:** unexpected painful episode leads to crying or gasping, patient then drops to the floor due to vagally mediated syncope or asystole. The body may stiffen or the child may have tonic-clonic movements.

▶ **Diagnosis:** < 5 years old, try provocative test (apply compression over both eyeballs for 10 seconds, either bradycardia at a rate of < 50% of resting heart rate, asystole for > 2 seconds or precipitation of a spell; positive in > 60% of children with pallid, 30% of children with cyanotic).

Bacterial Meningitis

▶ Males > females, young > old, immunocompromised (sickle cell disease, malnutrition, diabetes mellitus, renal/adrenal insufficiency etc.), recent surgery/fracture of skull, newborns (vertical transmission from maternal genital/GI tract)

▶ **Etiology:**
- *S. pneumoniae* is the most common organism, followed by *N. meningitides* in patients >2 months of age. *H. influenzae* ↓ due to universal vaccination
- Newborns: half are due to Group B streptococcus and one fourth are due to *E. coli. Listeria, N. meningitides,* and *S. pneumonia* also occur.

▶ **Clinical Presentation:**
- Fever/hypothermia
- ALOC
- Vomiting
- Headache
- Stiff neck
- Petechial rash may be present
- Apnea
- Seizures
- Bulging fontanelle
- **Laboratory studies:** LP (delay only if unstable), electrolytes, blood culture, UA, CT if suspicion of raised ICP. If bloody tap, 1000 RBCs usually contribute 1–2 WBCs and raise the protein by 1.5 mg/dL. # of WBCs introduced = (peripheral WBC × RBCs in CSF)/peripheral RBCs.

▶ **Management:**
- Stabilize, LP, parenteral antibiotics (before LP only if unstable, third-generation cephalosporin and vancomycin), watch fluid administration as SIADH may develop, steroids if positive CSF Gram's stain or grossly purulent CSF (dexamethasone 0.15 mg/kg); admit.

Migraines

▶ **Pathophysiology:** neuronal event triggers biochemical and vascular changes, serotonin involved, also prostaglandins, prolactin, gamma-aminobutyric acid (GABA), dopamine, substance P, neuropeptide 7, vasoactive intestinal peptide (VIP).

▶ **Diagnosis:**
- Periodic headaches separated by symptom-free intervals, associated with at least three of the following:
  1. Abdominal pain with nausea/vomiting

2. Unilateral headache
3. Pulsing, throbbing quality
4. Aura: visual, sensory, motor
5. Family history
6. Relief by sleep

- **Five phases:**
  1. Prodrome
  2. Aura
  3. Headache
  4. Termination
  5. Postdrome

▶ **Classification:**

- **Common migraine:**
  1. At least five episodes
  2. Headache lasts 4–72 hours
  3. Headache has at least two of the following qualities:
     a. Unilateral
     b. Pulsating/throbbing
     c. Moderate-severe intensity
     d. Aggravated by physical activity
  4. At least one of the following occurs during the attack:
     a. Nausea or vomiting
     b. Photophobia and phonophobia
  5. At least one of the following is present:
     a. History and physical examination excludes an organic disorder
     b. Investigation rules out organic disorder
     c. Organic disorder present but migraine does not occur in temporal relation to disorder

- **Classic migraine:**
  1. At least two attacks
  2. At least three of the following are present:
     a. One or more completely reversible aura symptom occurs
     b. At least one aura symptom develops gradually over 4 minutes or 2 or more develop in succession
     c. No single aura is present for over 1 hour
     d. The headache follows the aura with a headache-free interval of < 60 minutes, or may accompany the aura
  3. History and physical examination exclude an organic disorder

- **Complicated:** associated with neurologic disturbances
- **Hemiplegic/hemisensory:** aphasia, paresthesias, hemiparesis, contralateral headache
- **Ophthalmoplegic:** third nerve palsy, usually < 10 years old, males > females
- **Basilar artery:** visual symptoms, vertigo, ataxia, decreased level of consciousness
- **Acute confusional state:** restless, combative, hyperactive
- **Migraine variants:** abdominal migraine, cyclic vomiting, benign paroxysmal vertigo
- **Posttraumatic:** after mild head injury, strong family history of migraine

▶ **Diagnosis:**
  - History (triggers, family history, pattern, psychosocial history), physical (funduscopy)
  - **Laboratory studies:** CT, consider EEG, LP

▶ **Differential:**
  - Intracranial pathology

▶ **Management:**
  - Reassurance, education, nonpharmacologic treatment (remove triggers, avoid oral contraceptives, reduce stresses, sleep well)
  - Pharmacologic
    1. **Acute:** APAP, NSAIDs, Excedrin, Reglan, Ergotamine, sumatriptan, opiates if severe symptoms are present
    2. **Prophylaxis:** propranolol, low-dose phenobarbital or Dilantin, Periactin
  - Follow up with neurology and primary care physician

Pseudotumor Cerebri

▶ **Pathophysiology:**
  - Increased volume of brain-free water with ↑ ventricular CSF pressure and ↓ absorption of CSF via villi

▶ **Etiology:**
  - Associated with various conditions (otitis media [OM], roseola, sinusitis, steroid use, hyperthyroidism, obesity, menstrual irregularities, OCP use, Addison disease, hypoparathyroidism, pregnancy, tetracycline, vitamin A, nitrofurantoin, allergy, minor head trauma, anemia, immune disorders, sarcoidosis)

▶ **Diagnosis:**
- As young as 4 months old, no sex predilection in children
- Headache (50–75%, worse in morning), visual changes, tinnitus, nausea/vomiting, dizziness, papilledema, retinal hemorrhages, rectus muscle palsy, ataxia
- **Complications:** usually self-limited, visual loss can occur with papilledema
- **Laboratory studies:** head CT, LP to exclude infection— opening pressure > 20 cm H_2O confirms the diagnosis

▶ **Management:**
- Serial LPs (pressure < 20 cm H_2O), Diamox 5 mg/kg/dose every 24–48 hours, address obesity, consider steroids; surgery if refractory (lumbar-peritoneal shunt, optic nerve sheath fenestration)

Seizures

▶ **Epileptic Syndromes**
- **Benign rolandic (childhood) epilepsy:** between 3–13 years, facial movements, grimacing, vocalizations, often wake from sleep; centrotemporal spikes on EEG, remission by age 20.
- **West syndrome (infantile spasms):** sudden tonic contractions of extremities, head, trunk in clusters; EEG shows hypsarrhythmia, associated with mental retardation, onset 4–18 months. **Treatment:** ACTH.
- **Lennox-Gastaut:** onset at 1–8 years of generalized seizures (atonic, atypical absence, myoclonic, tonic), EEG with spikes and slow waves, mental retardation.
- **Juvenile myoclonic epilepsy of Janz:** idiopathic, onset 12–18 years, myoclonic seizures on awakening, may also have tonic, tonic-clonic, absence. Precipitated by stress, lack of sleep, alcohol excess. EEG with fast spike-wave discharges. **Treatment:** valproic acid for life.
- **Neonatal seizures:** (1) subtle: eye deviation/flutter, sucking, respiration changes, apnea (2) focal clonic, (3) multifocal clonic, (4) tonic, (5) myoclonic.
- **Status epilepticus:** prolonged or frequently repeated (longer than 30 minutes or series of seizures between which consciousness is not regained).

▶ **Benign Familial Neonatal Convulsions (BFNC):** begin in first 3 days of life, strong family history

▶ **Benign Idiopathic Neonatal Convulsions (BINC, "fifth day fits"):** occur on day of life 5

▶ **Causes of Seizures in Children:**
- Idiopathic
- Birth-related injuries
- Infections: meningitis, encephalitis
- Tumors
- Head injury
- Metabolic disorders
- Electrolyte imbalances: hypo/hyperglycemia, hypocalcemia, hypomagnesemia
- Inborn errors of metabolism
- Cerebral degenerative disorders
- Eclampsia
- Noncompliance with antiepileptic drug regimen
- Drug interactions reducing efficacy of antiepileptic agent
- Cysticercosis
- Drug ingestions/toxins
- Ventriculoperitoneal shunt malfunction or infection
- Vascular-ischemic, hemorrhagic, or thrombotic (sickle cell) stroke
- Hypertensive encephalopathy

▶ **Toxins That Can Cause Seizures (PLASTIC):**
　　P—Pesticides, phenothiazines, phencyclidine
　　L—Lidocaine, lindane, lithium
　　A—Alcohol, amphetamines, antihistamines, antidepressants, anticholinergics
　　S—Salicylates
　　T—Theophylline
　　I—Insulin, Isoniazid, Inderal
　　C—Camphor, caffeine, carbon monoxide, cocaine

▶ **Types of Epileptic Seizures in Childhood:**
- **Partial seizures:**
  1. **Simple partial** (consciousness intact and no postictal state)
     a. Motor
     b. Sensory
     c. Autonomic
     d. Psychic

TABLE 6-11
DIFFERENTIAL DIAGNOSIS OF SEIZURES IN CHILDREN

Benign paroxysmal vertigo
Benign myoclonus of infancy
Benign sleep myoclonus
Breath-holding spells
Gastroesophageal reflux
   Sandifer syndrome
Migraine headaches
Night terrors, sleepwalking, somniloquy, narcolepsy
Shuddering attacks
Sleepwalking
Syncope
Toxins
Psychological/behavioral
   Attention deficit disorder
   Hyperventilation
   Hysteria and rage attacks
   Pseudoseizures
   Panic attacks
   Tics, Tourette syndrome

   2. **Complex partial** (consciousness impaired):
      a. Simple partial followed by impaired consciousness
      b. Consciousness impaired at onset of seizure
   3. **Partial seizures with secondary generalization:**
- **Generalized seizures**
   1. Atonic
   2. Infantile spasms
   3. Absence
      a. Typical
      b. Atypical
   4. Generalized tonic-clonic
   5. Tonic
   6. Clonic
   7. Myoclonic

▶ **Complications:** recurrence 27–61% after first seizure; higher if partial seizure, family history or prior febrile seizure. If second seizure, risk of recurrence is 50–75% within 6–12 months of first.

▶ **Ancillary Data:** Accu-Chek, electrolytes, toxicology, urine for amino/organic acids if suspicious. Head CT for focal seizures or focal neurologic findings, or if there is suspicion of child abuse. EEG as an outpatient (sleeping and awake).

TABLE 6-12
COMMON ANTICONVULSANT AGENTS

Drug	Type of Seizure	Side Effects	Maintenance
Carbam- azepine (Tegretol)	Generalized tonic-clonic, partial, benign rolan- dic seizures	Rash, liver disease, diplopia, aplastic anemia, leu- kopenia	10–40 mg/ kg divided BID or TID
Clon- azepam (Rivotril, Klonopin)	Myoclonic, aki- netic, infan- tile spasms, partial, Len- nox-Gastaut	Fatigue, behavioral issues, sali- vation	0.05–0.3 mg/kg/ d divid- ed BID or TID
Ethosuxim- ide (Zarontin)	Absence	GI upset, weight gain, lethar- gy, systemic lupus erythemato- sus, rash	20–40 mg/ kg/d divided qd or BID
Gabapentin (Neuron- tin)	Partial and sec- ondarily gen- eralized sei- zures	Fatigue, dizzi- ness, diar- rhea, ataxia	20–70 mg/ kg/d
Lamotrigi- ne (Lam- ictal)	Complex partial (atypical absence) Len- nox-Gastaut, myoclonic, absence, tonic-clonic	Headache, nausea, rash, Stevens- Johnson syndrome, lymphade- nopathy, diplopia, GI upset	
Phenobar- bital (Luminol)	Generalized tonic-clonic, partial	Sedation, behavioral issues	2–6 mg/ kg/d divided qd or BID
Phenytoin (Dilantin)	Generalized tonic-clonic, partial	Gingival hyperpla- sia, hirsut- ism, rash, Stevens- Johnson syndrome, lymphoma	4–8 mg/ kg/d divided BID, TID, or QHS

continued

TABLE 6-12
COMMON ANTICONVULSANT AGENTS (CONTINUED)

Drug	Type of Seizure	Side Effects	Maintenance
Primidone (Mysoline)	Generalized tonic-clonic, partial	Rash, ataxia, behavioral issues, sedation, anemia	10–25 mg/kg/d divided BID, TID, or QID
Topiramate (Topamax)	Refractory complex partial seizures, infantile spasms, adjunctive therapy for temporal lobe epilepsy	Fatigue, nephrolithiasis, ataxia, headache, tremor, GI upset	1–9 mg/kg/d
Tiagabine (Gabitril)	Adjunctive therapy for refractory complex partial (focal) seizures	Decreased attention span, tremor, dizziness, anorexia	Average dose 6 mg/d
Valproic acid (Depakote)	Generalized tonic-clonic, absence, myoclonic, partial, akinetic, juvenile myoclonic epilepsy of Janz, infantile spasms	GI upset, liver involvement, alopecia, sedation	10–60 mg/kg/d divided TID or QID
Vigabatrin (Sabril)	Infantile spasms, adjunctive therapy for refractory seizures	Weight gain, agitation, depression, behavioral changes, visual field constriction, optic neuritis	30–100 mg/kg/d divided qd or BID

▶ **Management:**
  • **Acute tonic-clonic status epilepticus:**
    1. ABCs
    2. Laboratory studies including drug levels if on anticonvulsants

TABLE 6-13
ETIOLOGY OF NEWBORN SEIZURES

Day 1 of Life	Days 2 and 3 of Life	Day 4 of Life to 6 Months of Age
Anoxia	Sepsis	Hypocalcemia
Hypoxia	Inborn errors of	Hyponatremia/
Trauma	metabolism	hypernatremia
Intracranial hem-	Trauma	Infection
orrhage	Hypocalcemia	Drug withdrawal
Drugs	Hypoglycemia	Inborn errors of
Infection	Hypomagnesemia	metabolism
Hypoglycemia/	Hyperphosphatemia	Hyperphosphatemia
hyperglycemia	Hyponatremia/	Hypertension
Pyridoxine defi-	hypernatremia	Congenital anomalies
ciency	Drug withdrawal	Developmental brain
	Congenital anomalies	disorders
	Developmental brain	Benign idiopathic
	disorders	neonatal seizures
	Benign familial neo-	
	natal seizures	
	Hypertension	

3. NS bolus (consider IO if status epilepticus and unable to obtain access)

4. Consider **Narcan** if pupils constricted or **thiamine** if malnourished, **3% NS** 4 cc/kg IV if suspect hyponatremia, 0.5–1 mL/kg 10% **Ca gluconate** if hypocalcemic; **magnesium sulfate** 25–50 g/kg IV if hypomagnesemic

5. **Anticonvulsants: lorazepam** 0.05–0.1 mg/kg or **diazepam** (shorter half-life) 0.2–0.3 mg/kg IV or 0.5 mg/kg rectal; **phenytoin** (to prevent recurrence) 15–20 mg/kg IV (side effects: bradycardia, dysrhythmias, hypotension);

TABLE 6-14
DRUGS USED IN THE MANAGEMENT OF NEONATAL SEIZURES

Diazepam	0.2–0.3 mg/kg IV or 0.5 mg/kg rectal
Lorazepam	0.05–0.1 mg/kg IV
Midazolam	0.1 mg/kg IV–0.2 mg/kg IM
Phenytoin	15–20 mg/kg IV (no faster than 1 mg/kg/min)
Fosphenytoin	15–20 mg/kg IV or IM (can be given 3 mg/kg/min IV)
Phenobarbital	18–20 mg/kg IV, then 5–10 mg q10 min (1 mg/kg/ min) (maximum 50–60 mg/kg)
Pyridoxine	50–100 mg IV
Lidocaine	1–2 mg/kg IV, then 4–6 mg/kg/h for refractory seizures

> **phenobarbital** 20 mg/kg IV/IM if continues (side effects: respiratory depression, hypotension; drug of choice in neonates); if refractory **pentobarbital** 20 mg/kg load followed by 1–2 mg/kg/h

- **Acute nonconvulsive status epilepticus:**
  1. Absence present with mental confusion, give lorazepam/diazepam; if with myoclonic/atonic seizures valproic acid is drug of choice
  2. Simple partial status treat same as tonic-clonic; complex partial—same management

Febrile Seizures

▶ Age range is 6 months–5 years. Overall incidence is 2.5%, this ↑ to 10–20% if there is a first-degree relative with a history of febrile seizures.

▶ **Definition of Simple Febrile Seizures:** age 6 months–5 years, generalized tonic-clonic seizure, only one in a 24-hour period, no evidence of meningitis, duration < 15 minutes. Complex febrile seizures fall outside of this definition.

▶ **Risk Factors for Recurrence:**
- Age < 12 months with first febrile seizure
- Temperature < 39° C with first seizure, or complex seizures
- Approximately 30% of patients will have recurrence, 50% occur within 6 months of initial seizure, 75% in 1 year, 90% have a recurrence within 2 years

▶ **Risk of Epilepsy:** ↑ if there is an abnormal neurodevelopmental examination prior to the febrile seizure or if the seizure was atypical/complex. If both risk factors present, the risk of epilepsy is ~10%, if one risk factor is present then there is 2–3% chance of epilepsy, and if no risk factors are present there is 0.9% incidence of epilepsy.

▶ **Ancillary Data:** LP if history and physical are suspicious for meningitis; no need for routine electrolytes/BUN/creatinine, magnesium, and calcium tests. CT not necessary for simple febrile seizures. CBC and urine with cultures if there is fever without source (same risk of bacteremia as those without fever).

▶ **Management:** seizure control as per status epilepticus; long-term management does not require seizure prophylaxis, antipyretic therapy does not prevent seizures.

ORTHOPEDIC INJURIES AND DISORDERS
Management Principles of Fractures in Children

▶ The physis (epiphyseal plate, growth plate) is commonly injured in children; 30–60% of physeal injuries occur in the distal radius and 80% of all physeal injuries occur in children between 10 and 16 years of age (median age: 13 years).

▶ The ligaments in children are very strong and therefore sprains are not common, as the physis will fracture before injury occurs to the flexible ligament. Salter-Harris III-V are at most risk for growth disturbances.

▶ **Fracture Types:**
  • **Salter-Harris I**
    1. **Incidence:** approximately 5% of injuries.
    2. **Location:** the epiphysis separates from the metaphysis through the physis with maintenance of the nutrient blood supply. May be occult on radiograph or there may be widening of the physis.
    3. **Treatment:** immobilization (splint), elevation, ice, and orthopedic follow-up.
    4. **Prognosis:** excellent with very infrequent growth disturbance.
  • **Salter-Harris II**
    1. **Incidence:** the most common type of fracture accounting for 75% of physeal injuries.
    2. **Location:** fracture is through the metaphysis and physis.
    3. **Treatment:** closed reduction if there is angulation or displacement, splinting/casting and orthopedic follow-up.
    4. **Prognosis:** good with infrequent growth disturbance.
  • **Salter-Harris III**
    1. **Incidence:** accounts for 10% of physeal injuries.
    2. **Location:** fracture is through the epiphysis and physis.
    3. **Treatment:** orthopedic consultation in the ED is typically required as "near perfect" alignment of the articular surfaces is imperative. Open reduction may be required.
    4. **Prognosis:** generally good but depends on the extent of displacement and blood supply disruption.
  • **Salter-Harris IV**
    1. **Incidence:** accounts for approximately 10% of physeal injuries.

2. **Location:** fracture is through the metaphysis, physis, and epiphysis. Most commonly involves the distal humerus.

3. **Treatment:** higher requirements for operative intervention in order to achieve anatomic reduction.

4. **Prognosis:** significant risk of growth disturbance.

- **Salter-Harris V**
  1. **Incidence:** < 1% of physeal injuries.
  2. **Location:** crush through the physis with minimal or no displacement of the epiphysis. May be radiographically occult. Most commonly diagnosed retrospectively when bone growth abnormalities are detected on serial radiographs.
  3. **Treatment:** orthopedic consult in the ED if diagnosis is suspected with casting followed by limited use of the affected region.
  4. **Prognosis:** worst prognosis with likely focal bone growth arrest.

▶ The types of Salter-Harris fractures are always in reference to the physis:

    S—Same as the physis = > Salter-Harris I

    A—Above and including the physis (metaphysis) = > Salter-Harris II

    L—Below and including the physis (epiphysis) = > Salter-Harris III

    T—Together: metaphysis and epiphysis = > Salter-Harris IV

    ER—Everything **R**uined! = > Salter-Harris V (see **Figure 6-4** on facing page)

Upper Extremity Injuries

▶ Clavicle
- **Clavicular fractures**
  1. Most commonly fractured bone in childhood
  2. The most common site of fracture is between the middle and lateral thirds
  3. **Diagnostic findings:** pain with movements of the upper arm and neck; local tenderness, swelling, and crepitation at the fracture site; older children; downward and inward placement of the patient's shoulder. Keep the injured arm close to the body and support it with the other hand.

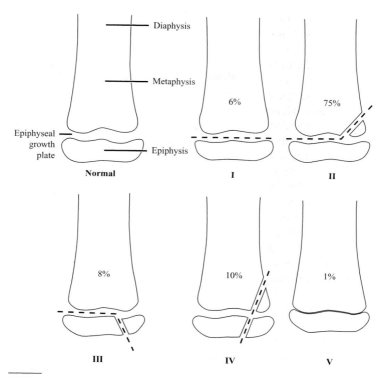

FIGURE 6-4

ER = Everything ruined! = > Salter Harris V.

   4. **Treatment:**
      a. Immobilization with a figure of eight splint for a total of 3–4 weeks (day and night for the first 2 weeks and during the day only for the remainder), sling, or sling and swathe are appropriate.
      b. Displaced clavicle fractures in children over 6 years should be referred to orthopedics and may need reduction.
   • **Acromioclavicular sprain/separation**
      1. Rare in children
      2. **Diagnostic findings:**
         a. Pain with movement of the upper extremity (UE) and the lateral portion of the clavicle may be displaced upward with ligamentous rupture

  b. If x-rays are unrevealing then they should be repeated with the child holding a 30 g weight or 1 oz/kg to widen the space:
- No displacement: first-degree sprain
- < 1 cm displacement: second-degree sprain
- > 1 cm: third-degree sprain

 3. **Treatment:** first- and second-degree sprain—treat with sling and swathe; third-degree may require surgical repair and orthopedic consultation

▶ **Scapular Fractures**
- Fractures are usually related to crush or high-energy trauma
- Often associated with other injuries
- **Diagnostic findings:** tenderness and swelling with inability to move the arm upward
- **Treatment:** immobilization with a sling and swathe but other injuries should be addressed

▶ **Shoulder**
- **Shoulder dislocation**
  1. Anterior dislocation is more common (95%)
     a. Usually from a fall on an outstretched arm
     b. Before the physis closes, the mechanism usually causes a humeral fracture
  2. **Diagnostic findings:**
     a. Flattened deltoid and prominent acromion with limitation of abduction or external rotation (posterior dislocation presents with the shoulder flattened anteriorly).
     b. Radiographs should be done before and after reduction.
  3. **Treatment:**
     a. Reduction may be done by several methods:
        - Longitudinal traction with external rotation or prone patient on the stretcher with the arm hanging off the side holding a 10 lb weight
        - Traction-counter traction
        - Scapular manipulation
     b. The axillary nerve, which innervates the deltoid muscle, is particularly vulnerable, and should be assessed before and after reduction.
     c. Immobilization with a sling and swathe for 4 weeks.
     d. Referral to orthopedic after the second dislocation.

- **Brachial plexus injury**
  1. May be seen as complication from delivery that was not diagnosed in the nursery or from direct trauma.
  2. Patient will have a decreased range of active motion with normal passive motion. Moro may be asymmetric.
  3. Evaluate with x-ray and evaluation by a neurologist for follow-up and therapy (80% return to normal function by 1 year).
- **Pulled shoulder**
  1. Forceful traction on a child's arm occasionally causes a partial tear in the joint capsule of the shoulder without dislocation.
  2. Patient will have pain but normal x-rays.
  3. Treat with sling; repeat films may reveal a Salter-Harris I fracture.
- **Rotator cuff injury**
  1. Includes the supraspinatus, infraspinatus, and teres minor muscles
  2. Mechanism often strenuous movement such as throwing
  3. **Diagnostic findings:** pain with abduction or external rotation, with point tenderness over the point of insertion of the rotator cuff into the tuberosities
  4. **Treatment:**
     a. Minor injuries may be treated with immobilization in sling, passive range of motion exercises, and pain management.
     b. Avulsion fractures of the tuberosity may require surgical repair.

▶ **Humerus**
- **Proximal humeral epiphyseal fractures**
  1. Salter-Harris II fractures are most common in children over 11 years.
  2. Diagnostic findings:
     a. Swelling and pain with any motion.
     b. Assessment should include a test of the deltoid function for evidence of axillary nerve injury.
     c. AP and lateral films are needed for the diagnosis.
  3. Longitudinal growth impairment is the main complication since 80% of longitudinal growth occurs at the proximal epiphysis.

4. Usually treated with sling and swathe with follow-up with orthopedics within 24 hours.

- **Proximal humeral metaphyseal fractures**
  1. More common than epiphyseal fractures in 5–11-year-old group and may be torus, greenstick, or transverse fractures.
  2. **Management:** same as epiphyseal fractures.

- **Humeral shaft fractures**
  1. Usually due to direct or indirect trauma.
  2. Spiral fracture suggests twisting force, especially in young children—may be the result of child abuse.
  3. **Diagnostic findings:**
     a. Swelling, pain, and some deformity.
     b. Radial nerve is vulnerable for injury: anesthesia of the dorsum of the hand between the 1st and 2nd metacarpals and weakness of the wrist and the finger extensors suggest injury to the radial nerve.
  4. **Treatment:**
     a. Immobilization in a splint to prevent neurovascular compromise during evaluation.
     b. Sling and swathe may be sufficient for young children, otherwise long arm splint in older children with follow-up within 24 hours with orthopedics.

▶ **Elbow**
- **Supracondylar fractures**
  1. Most frequent elbow fractures in children between 3–10 years of age.
  2. Usually from hyperextension injuries.
  3. Considered an acute emergency because of the possibility of brachial artery entrapment resulting in necrosis of the muscle causing "Volkmann contracture", which consists of fixed flexion of the elbow, pronation of the forearm, flexion of the wrist, extension of metacarpophalangeal (MCP) joints, and flexion of interphalangeal (IP) joints.
  4. Six ossification centers appear at different ages:
     a. Capitellum < 1 year
     b. Radial head = 4–5 years
     c. Medial epicondyle = 4–6 years
     d. Trochlea = 8–10 years
     e. Olecranon = 8–9 years
     f. Lateral epicondyle = 9–11 years

5. **Diagnostic findings:**
   a. Tenderness and pain with flexion of the elbow and the arm is usually held in pronation.
   b. Evaluation of neurovascular (including the motor and sensory functions of the radial, medial, and ulnar nerves) status is more important than examination of the fracture site.
      - Assess the "five P's":
         1. pain
         2. poor perfusion (coolness, prolonged capillary refill >2 seconds)
         3. pulselessness: radial
         4. paresthesia
         5. paralysis of the forearm suggests ischemia
   c. Exacerbation of pain with extension of the fingers is suggestive of vascular compromise.
   d. Changes in carrying angle can result from incomplete reduction.
   e. Fat-pad sign is a nonspecific finding with injury, but a visible posterior fat-pad is suggestive of fracture.
   f. Another useful tool is the anterior humeral line which is drawn down the anterior humerus on lateral view and it should intersect the capitellum in the middle or posterior third.

6. **Treatment:**
   a. Elbow should be secured in 20–30 degrees of flexion for splinting.
   b. If the fracture is displaced or there is significant soft-tissue swelling, patient should be admitted with prompt reduction (open or closed).

- **Lateral epicondylar fractures**
   1. Lateral is more common than medial and occurs as a result of an indirect force, such as falling on an outstretched hand with the forearm abducted, transmitting the energy throughout the radius to the lateral condyle.
   2. **Diagnostic findings:** significant swelling and pain in the lateral aspect of elbow, which increases with rotation. They are usually Salter-Harris type III or IV.
   3. **Complications:** cubitus valgus resulting from growth arrest of the lateral condylar physis is not uncommon and could lead to stretching the ulnar nerve around the

medial condyle resulting in ulnar neuritis and delayed ulnar nerve palsy.

4. **Treatment:**
    a. Displaced lateral condylar fractures are unstable and require immediate attention by orthopedics for open reduction.
    b. Nondisplaced fractures are treated with a long arm cast with elbow at 90 degrees flexion and forearm supinated.

- **Medial epicondylar fractures**
    1. Usually occur from valgus stress
    2. More common in patients 7–15 years of age
    3. Concurrent elbow dislocation: 50% of cases
    4. Elbow held in partial flexion for comfort
    5. Ulnar nerve often injured
    6. Proximal radius often fractured
    7. **Treatment** with long arm cast or open reduction depending on degree of displacement, which should be determined by the orthopedic surgeon.

- **Intercondylar and transcondylar fractures**
    1. Occur more often in older children
    2. Often unstable: require immediate orthopedic consultation
    3. Can be complicated by avascular necrosis of the trochlea
    4. Admission for monitoring of the distal circulation usually recommended

- **Elbow dislocation**
    1. Most commonly dislocated joint in childhood: usually from a fall on outstretched hand
    2. Pure dislocation without fracture rare in children
    3. Elbow is often flexed and held by the other hand: associated with shortening, pain, swelling, and restricted elbow ROM
    4. Evaluate for neurovascular compromise: may be complicated by Volkmann contracture
    5. Reduce by placing the patient in a prone position with the arm hanging down then applying countertraction and direct pressure with the thumbs on the olecranon pushing downward and anteriorly
    6. Hospital admission for observation for vascular compromise recommended

- **Radial head subluxation (nursemaid's elbow)**
  1. Accounts for 22% of upper extremity injuries usually between 6 months–5 years; left elbow is more common than right.
  2. Due to direct traction on a pronated hand or wrist.
  3. Often diagnosed by history of a pull (only present in 50% of cases) or a child holding the arm partially flexed, pronated, and close to the body.
  4. Reduction of the radial head with supination and flexion is usually successful. May take 10–15 minutes before the child will start using elbow again.
  5. Consider imaging if unsuccessful after 2–3 attempts.
- **Olecranon fractures**
  1. Usually by direct blow or fall on extended hand and elbow
  2. Patient will have localized tenderness and restricted motion of the elbow
  3. Fat-pad and joint effusion often visible on x-rays
  4. **Treatment:**
     a. Nondisplaced fractures: long arm cast with 90 degrees of flexion for 4 weeks
     b. Displaced fractures: require an orthopedic surgeon

▶ **Radius and Ulna**
- **Radial head and neck fractures**
  1. Common after 5 years of age.
  2. Due to a fall on outstretched hand with valgus angulation.
  3. May be associated with injury to the medial epicondyle or medial collateral ligament.
  4. Patient will hold arm in flexion with restricted flexion, extension, and supination.
  5. Radial nerve function should be evaluated.
  6. **Treatment:**
     a. Incomplete and minimally displaced fractures may be treated with a long arm cast at 90 degrees of flexion.
     b. Displacement requires orthopedic consultation.
- **Monteggia fracture and radial head dislocation**
  1. Ulnar fracture with radial head dislocation (isolated dislocation of the radial head is rare).
  2. Elbow will be held in flexion with pronation with pain and restricted range of motion.

3. Unrecognized: may result in chronic dislocation and impairment of elbow function.
4. Normally a line along the axis of the radius should pass through the capitellum in all views.
5. Reduction of the radial head dislocation and ulnar fracture should be accomplished by orthopedics (supination, traction, and direct pressure on the radial head with the elbow at 90 degrees will help reduce the dislocation).
6. Elbow should be splinted in flexion and repeat x-rays should be completed.
- **Radial and ulnar diaphyseal and metaphyseal fractures**
    1. **Galeazzi** fracture: radial or ulnar fracture with dislocation of the distal radioulnar joint.
    2. **Colles** fracture: transverse fracture of the distal radius with dorsal angulation and loss of volar tilt to the distal radial articulating surface; often associated with a fracture of the ulnar styloid process.
    3. **Barton** fracture: marginal fracture of the dorsum or volar surface of the radius with corresponding dorsal or volar dislocation of the carpal bones.
    4. **Hutchinson** fracture (chauffeur fracture): involves the radial styloid process secondary to direct trauma or impact of the styloid process.
    5. Patient will have point tenderness.
    6. Compartment syndromes are uncommon.
    7. **Treatment** depends on the type of fracture, rotational deformities must be corrected.
    8. Angulated fractures of > 15 degrees must be corrected to prevent functional limitation.
    9. Usually can be splinted after reduction for 4–6 weeks.

Hand and Wrist

▶ The hand is the most frequently injured body part in children.
▶ **Physical Examination:**
- Observation: watch how the child moves and uses the hand, also for any discoloration
- Palpation: should be systematic starting with the wrist, scaphoid bone, metacarpals, phalanges, and interphalangeal (IP) joints.

- **Sensation:**
  1. **Radial nerve:** supplies the dorsal surface of the thumb, index, and middle finger as far as the distal IP joints. It also innervates the whole dorsum of the hand lying on the radial side of the third metacarpal, therefore, the best place to assess sensation is between the thumb and index finger (dorsal surface of the web).
  2. **Median nerve:** mirrors the radial nerve but on the palmar surface in addition to the dorsal surface of the distal phalanges of the thumb and first two digits. The best place to assess sensation is the palmar surface of the tip of the index finger.
  3. **Ulnar nerve:** supplies the ulnar surfaces including the dorsal and palmar surfaces of the terminal two digits and metacarpals. The tip of the little finger is the best place to assess function.
- **Motor function:**
  1. **Extrinsic muscles:** lie in the forearm
  2. **Intrinsic:** in the hand (may be individually assessed).
  3. **Radial nerve** is assessed at the wrist with dorsal and palmar motion actively and then against resistance.
  4. **Median nerve** is assessed by testing the flexion of the proximal interphalangeal (PIP) joints and thenar (thumb adduction toward fifth digit).
  5. **Ulnar nerve** is assessed by asking patient to hold his or her extended fingers together while the examiner attempts to push the fingers together and hypothenar (fifth digit flexion toward thumb).
- **Tendons:** evaluate by checking each joint individually for both extensor and flexor function.
- **Vascular integrity:** radial and ulnar arteries (feel pulses) at the wrist. The Allen test is the formal test for arterial supply. This test consists of:
  1. Examiner simultaneously compress both radial and ulnar arteries.
  2. Patient elevates hand and repeatedly clenches and opens the hand (to facilitate venous drainage).
  3. Examiner releases the radial artery which results in flushing of all five digits (if the artery is intact).
  4. The same method can be used to examine the ulnar artery.

▶ **Fractures**
- Carpal bone fractures are rare in children because they are mostly cartilaginous.
- **Scaphoid (navicular) fractures**
  1. Most commonly fractured carpal bones caused by falling on an outstretched hand.
  2. Pain in the anatomic "snuff box" with a decreased ROM and strength in the wrist.
  3. Radiologic evaluation should include scaphoid series. It is not uncommon for the initial x-rays to be negative.
  4. **Treatment:**
     a. The wrist should be immobilized regardless of radiographic findings for 10–14 days with repeat films at that time.
     b. Thumb spica splint/cast should include the thumb and extended upward covering the elbow.
     c. Consult orthopedics for displaced fractures: requires reduction and possible internal fixation.
- **Metacarpal bone fractures**
  1. Uncommon: but usually result from a direct blow to the hand.
  2. Symptoms: pain, swelling, lack of knuckle prominence at the site.
  3. Assess deformity and angulation with the fingers in flexion.
  4. The 5th metacarpal is the most common fractured (boxer's fracture), usually affects the neck of the metacarpal.
  5. **Bennett fracture:** involves the thumb metacarpal at the base into the joint:
     a. Usually heals with closed reduction and immobilization with the wrist in mild extension and the MCP joint at 45–90 degrees of flexion.
  6. Angulation > 30 degrees or neck fractures of the 2nd or 3rd metacarpal with angulation > 20 degrees reduction is required with orthopedic consultation.
  7. Ulnar displaced fractures are unstable and need weekly follow-up.
  8. Open reduction and fixation is required if closed methods fail.

- **Phalangeal fractures**
  1. The most common.
  2. Result from a direct blow.
  3. Pain and swelling is present over the site.
  4. Only 10% require open reduction.
  5. Any open, intraarticular, or rotational deformity should prompt orthopedic consultation.

▶ **Dislocations and Ligamentous Injuries**
- **Wrist**
  1. Very rare.
  2. Results from a fall on an outstretched hand.
  3. Usually has pain and minimal swelling.
  4. Diagnosed after ongoing problems have occurred: suspect if there is a "clicking" sound with certain wrist movements.
  5. Normal alignment is with the metacarpal, capitate, lunate, and radius in a straight line and the lunate and navicular should form an angle no > 50 degrees (alignment disruption is consistent with a dislocation).
  6. Dislocations and subluxation injuries require referral.
- **Hands and fingers**
  1. Uncommon, because in children fractures usually occur before ligamentous injuries.
  2. Usually result from a direct longitudinal blow.
  3. Most commonly involve the thumb with dorsal subluxation.
     a. Easily reduced
     b. A thumb spica cast should be applied for 6 weeks
     c. May be unstable and should have close follow-up with orthopedics
  4. MCP joint sprains are usually of the radial collateral ligament of the fifth digit and may be immobilized if only first- or second-degree sprains. Unstable sprains should be referred.
  5. MCP dislocations are usually dorsally displaced.
     a. Closed reduction is difficult, often requires general anesthesia.
     b. Forceful manipulation should be avoided to prevent epiphyseal injuries.
  6. Proximal IP dislocations may be posterior or anterior.

    a. Reduced with extension of the joint and pushing the distal bone into location from above.

    b. After reduction, check for lateral instability.

    c. It should be splinted for 7–10 days: if unstable, 3 weeks.

    d. If the dislocation is anterior: there is tendon damage and requires consultation.

  7. DIP dislocations may also be easily reduced.

- **Gamekeeper's or skier's thumb**
  1. Instability of the ulnar collateral ligament of the thumb.
  2. Occurs with fall on an outstretched hand while holding a pole.
  3. Usually accompanied by a Salter-Harris III of the proximal phalanx.
  4. Pain and swelling are usually present with radial deviation exacerbating the pain.
  5. Always evaluate for avulsion fractures with this dislocation if present; requires open reduction and pinning.
  6. Thumb spica should be placed for 6 weeks with the thumb in extension.

▶ **Tendon Injuries**

- **Mallet finger**
  1. Injury to the extensor tendon at the attachment to the distal interphalangeal (DIP) joint: often associated with a fracture of the dorsal lip of the base of the distal phalanx.
  2. Occurs with forcible flexion or laceration.
  3. Finger cannot be extended at the distal phalanx (usually held in flexion).
  4. **Treatment:** may splint in hyperextension if there is a fracture involving < 25% of the joint surface and there is no subluxation. Dorsal or volar splint is appropriate with close follow-up with orthopedics.

- **Boutonnière deformity**
  1. Disruption of the central slip extensor tendon at the PIP joint with volar subluxation of the lateral bands of the tendon.
  2. It occurs with a direct blow or open injury.
  3. The DIP joint is in extension with the PIP joint in flexion with tenderness and swelling.

4. **Treatment:**
   a. If there is no associated fracture, finger should be splinted in extension with close follow-up with orthopedics.
   b. Some patients require surgical reattachment of the tendon particularly if there is delay in the initial treatment.

- **Jersey finger**
  1. Avulsion of the flexor digitorum profundus.
  2. Usually involves the ring finger.
  3. Hyperextension injury (finger catching on a jersey).
  4. Symptoms: inability to flex the DIP joint (do not assume that this inability is secondary to swelling and pain at the DIP joint).
  5. **Treatment**: surgical repair.

▶ **Nerve Injuries**
- Usually with laceration or crush injury.
- Evaluation should include two-point discrimination and sharp and dull touch. Young children may not understand and you may have to look for the lack of sweating or absence of skin wrinkling in water.
- Referral to appropriate subspecialty.

▶ **Soft-Tissue Injuries and Infection**
- **Lacerations**
  1. Always require exploration for the extent of injury as well as testing for sensation, motor, and vascular sufficiency.
  2. Radiographic studies are not necessary unless there is a suspicion of a foreign body.
  3. Apply pressure for bleeding then anesthetize with lidocaine before cleaning and irrigation.
  4. May be repaired if < 8 hours old with 4-0 or 5-0 suture. Deep sutures should not be used.
  5. Tetanus if necessary.

- **Fingertip injuries**
  1. Subungual splinters are common and are usually wooden and have pain and swelling if present for a longer period of time (also concern of infection).
  2. Should trim the nail as short as possible to attempt removal. The nail can be carefully shaved away to reach the splinter if necessary.

    3. The hand should be soaked 3 times per day until well healed to prevent infection

- **Crush injuries of the fingertip**
  1. Swelling, discoloration, tenderness. Often associated with a subungual hematoma.
  2. X-rays should be done to exclude distal tuft fracture.
  3. Tuft fractures are common and may be managed with a hairpin splint for protection.
  4. Subungual hematomas should be drained to decrease the pain and pressure on the nail bed. This may be accomplished with cautery.
  5. Controversy still remains on whether a nail bed laceration should be repaired when the nail is intact. When repaired should be done with 6-0 absorbable suture.
  6. A splint may be placed for protection and comfort.

- **Amputations**
  1. The amputated part should be kept preserved and cool.
     a. Uncooled tissue can survive 6 hours and cooled up to 12 hours.
     b. A single digit can be preserved and reattached up to 24 hours later.
  2. Tissue is best preserved by placing in gauze soaked with sterile saline or lactated Ringer (LR) solution, then placed in a bag in ice water.
  3. X-rays should be done to assess the bones.
  4. Fingertip amputations usually heal well and hand surgeon should be consulted before repair.
  5. Amputations distal to the insertion of the extensor or flexor tendons can be managed nonoperatively with cleaning and debridement. If proximal to the insertions, the tissue should be preserved and hand surgery consulted.

- **Wringer or degloving injuries**
  1. Usually from crush injury with shearing forces
  2. Clean and dress with sterile material and keep elevated
  3. Hospitalize for 24 hours to watch for compartment syndrome
  4. Fasciotomy may be necessary for neurovascular compromise

- **Ring on a swollen finger**
  1. There are several possible approaches to remove the ring:

    a. ↓ Swelling in cool water for 30 minutes then use a lubricant to slide the ring off.

    b. Sliding a string under the ring then looped distally around the finger. Once wrapped the proximal end of the string should be grasped and pulled to allow the ring to slide off the finger.

    c. Ring cutter.

- **Frostbite**
  1. Occurs when tissue is exposed to excessive cold and often includes fingertips.
  2. Superficial frostbite appears white and doughy then red with re-warming.
  3. Deep frostbite is cyanotic, hard, insensate. Re-warming produces a mottled appearance—pain and swelling occur afterward.
  4. The areas should be rapidly re-warmed with warm water for 20–30 minutes (the last minutes may be extremely painful). Be certain extremity is not exposed to additional cold injury.
  5. **Treatment:** most are treated as an outpatient unless there is deep-tissue injury.

- **Infections**
  1. **Eponychia:** infection of the cuticle. It should be soaked 3 times/day for 20 minutes and antibiotic ointment applied to the area.
  2. **Paronychia:** Infection along the side of the nail with visible pocket of pus under the nail. **Treatment** includes digital block for pain relief, incision and drainage, followed by topical antibiotic ointment and oral antibiotics.
  3. **Tenosynovitis:** infection extends to the tendon with erythema, swelling, and pain along the tendon sheath.
     a. Extension of the finger causes pain. Usually requires hospitalization with consultation of hand surgeon.
     b. IV antibiotics should be started.
  4. **Herpetic whitlow:** HSV-I infection along the border of the fingernail. Usually acquired by the patient's own oral lesions.
     a. Lesions are usually vesicular or ulcers with pain and inflammation.

    b. Avoid manipulation if possible because it may spread the infection.

    c. Treat with topical antibacterial ointment to prevent secondary infection.

    d. Topical acyclovir may shorten the course.

5. **Felon:** infection of the pulp of the distal phalanx that is painful because of the lack of space and may cause tissue ischemia.

    a. Often requires admission: for incision and drainage under general anesthesia (unless the same can be accomplished with a digital block).

    b. IV/PO antibiotics.

Lower Extremity Injuries

▶ Growth in height is predominantly from the femur.

▶ Pelvic fractures have a mortality of 5% and are more common between 1–8 years of age.

▶ **Hip Fracture:** rare, but 75–80% associated with trauma. The patient may have hip in flexion with external rotation and shortening of the leg. Requires immobilization, a thorough evaluation for other injuries, and management by orthopedics.

▶ **Hip Dislocation:** posterior is the most common and can result from simple falls. Usually adducted, shortened and in internal rotation. Closed reduction is most successful in the first 8–12 hours after injury.

▶ **Congenital Hip Dislocation:** usually noted at birth or soon afterward. The child needs long-term follow-up with orthopedics and serial casting.

▶ **Transient Synovitis:** occurs most commonly between $1\frac{1}{2}$–7 years of age with peak at 2 years of age (refer to Table 6-17)

▶ **Femur Fractures:** There is usually a good history or mechanism for this fracture and there is usually swelling in the location of the femur. The exception is spiral fracture where the swelling may be minimal. This requires immediate reduction with traction and splinting. Hospitalization is common for observation.

▶ **Knee Epiphyseal Fractures:** displacement of the distal femoral or proximal tibial epiphysis is usually associated with an indirect blow to the knee. The knee is usually held in flexion with swelling and inability to bear weight.

▶ **Knee Fracture:** this includes avulsion of the tibial tubercle, the condyles, and dislocation or fracture of the patella. Dislocations are rare, but are more common in adolescent females.
  • Patellar tendonitis (jumper's knee)
  • Prepatellar bursitis (wrestler's knee)
▶ **Osteochondritis Dissecans:** most common in boys in the 2nd decade of life and is characterized by bone necrosis and softening of the cartilage of the proximal tibia. Activity should be limited and orthopedic referral is appropriate.
▶ **Tibia and Fibula Fractures:** these are the most common lower extremity injuries in children. They are either complete or incomplete (greenstick). A **toddler's fracture** (spiral fracture < 6 years of age) may be caused by torsion of the foot. Compartment syndrome is more common in fractures of the proximal tibia.

Ankle Injuries

▶ **Sprains**
  • The ankle is a hinge joint made up of three bones (fibula, tibia, talus).
  • Lateral support is by the anterior talofibular ligament (ATFL), calcaneofibular ligament (CFL), and posterior talofibular ligament (PTFL).
  • Medial support is by the deltoid ligament.
  • Posterior support is by the PTFL.
  • Inversion injury is more common than eversion because the lateral ligaments are weaker.
  • ATFL is the most commonly injured ligament.
  • Classification of sprains:
    1. **Grade I:** minor with little swelling and tenderness. Patient may be able to ambulate without limp.
    2. **Grade II:** partial tear with diffuse swelling and tenderness. Patient will have difficulty walking.
    3. **Grade III:** complete ligament disruption and instability. Patient will be unable to bear weight.
  • Examination is most reliable immediately after the injury before any swelling.
  • The anterior drawer test evaluates stability of the ATFL (positive test has > 3–5 mm mobility or asymmetry between ankles). This test is performed with the ankle at a 90° angle.

The examiner stabilizes the tibia with one hand while the foot is gently, but firmly, drawn forward.

- The talar tilt test evaluates the ATFL and CFL. The examiner stabilizes the leg and firmly inverts the foot to determine the degree of talar tilt. Compared to the non-injured foot, a positive test is ≥ 10° difference.
- Epiphyseal injuries and avulsion fractures may occur with the sprain.
- Management of grade I and II sprains include the RICE (**R**est, **I**ce, **C**ompression, **E**levation) protocol for 24–48 hours.
- Management of grade III sprains should be decided by orthopedics and may require surgical repair.

▶ **Fractures**
- The Salter-Harris classification is used for diagnosis.
- Point tenderness suggests a fracture.
- Neurovascular status should be evaluated.
- Complications of distal tibia fractures include leg length discrepancy, osteoarthritis, and avascular necrosis.
- All fractures that may involve the epiphyseal plate should be referred to orthopedics.
- Nondisplaced fractures may be immobilized for 4 weeks, but displaced fractures should have closed reduction and short leg casting for 6 weeks.

Foot Injuries

▶ **Fractures**
- Usually a result of a twisting injury with marked swelling.
- Talar fractures are uncommon and may be subtle if nondisplaced (these fractures may be seen on a lateral view). Referral to orthopedics after immobilization.
- Calcaneal fractures are the most common tarsal injury and should have orthopedic referral. The patient should be in non–weight-bearing immobilization for 4–6 weeks.
- Metatarsal fractures are usually from blunt trauma and usually involve the 1st and 5th bones. These can usually be immobilized in a walking cast for 3–6 weeks.
- Phalangeal fractures are also usually from blunt injury and do not require reduction unless the fractures are Salter-Harris III. Otherwise may be "buddy" taped (the injured toe

TABLE 6-15
COMMON CAUSES OF FOOT PAIN

Extrinsic	Trauma	Infection	Structural	Tumors
Ill-fit- ting shoes Foreign body	Stress frac- ture Fracture Sprain Achilles ten- donitis Kohler disease	Osteomy- elitis Septic arthritis Juvenile rheuma- toid arthritis (JRA) Rheumatic fever	Flat foot Pes cavus Congeni- tal prob- lems	Osteoid sarco- ma Ewing sarco- ma

is taped to the neighboring toe) for immobilization for 3–5 weeks. The exception is 1st toe fractures which may be unstable and these should be referred to orthopedics.

▶ **Puncture Wounds**
- The plantar surface is usually involved and may lead to cel- lulites, osteomyelitis, and septic arthritis.
- Cellulitis is the most common complication (15%) with *S. aureus* being the most common organism (*Pseudomonas* rare- ly causes cellulitis).
- Obtain a radiograph to evaluate for a foreign body.
- Osteoarthritis and septic joint are less common (2%), but are more commonly *Pseudomonas*.
- Management is dependent on the severity of infection with deep infections requiring IV antibiotics. Prophylactic anti- staphylococcal antibiotics are recommended for these inju- ries and tetanus should be updated.
- Deep foreign bodies should be removed by a surgeon.

Septic Arthritis

▶ More common in children than adults
▶ Highest incidence between 6–24 months of age
▶ **Pathophysiology:**
- Enters joint space through three mechanisms: hematoge- nous spread, direct inoculation, or contiguous extension

TABLE 6-16
SYNOVIAL FLUID LABORATORY FINDINGS

Type of Effusion	Appearance	Leukocytes (cells/mm³)	% PMNs
Normal	Clear	< 100	25
Traumatic	Bloody or clear	< 5000	< 50
Inflammatory	Clear or turbid	500–75,000	50
Bacterial	Purulent	> 50,000	> 75

PMNs, polymorphonuclear leukocytes.

▶ **Etiology**
- *S. aureus* most common organism accounting for > 50% of cases.
- In neonates group B streptococcus and *S. aureus* are most common.
- *N. gonorrhoeae* is important to consider in sexually active adolescents.

▶ **Clinical Findings:**
- Most commonly involved joints in order of frequency: knee, hip, ankle, elbow, shoulder, and wrist
- Pain in affected joint and extremity, pain with passive movement of joint, decreased active movement of joint
- Limp or refusal to bear weight if lower extremity joint involved
- Fever
- Localized erythema, swelling, and tenderness

▶ **Ancillary Data:**
- Plain films of the joint may show widening of joint space and bone destruction, but these are late findings.
- Ultrasound may help show the presence of a joint effusion.
- Erythrocyte sedimentation rate (ESR) and C-reactive protein (CRP) are usually elevated.
- CBC and blood cultures should be obtained.
- Analysis of synovial fluid from affected joint is essential.

Synovial Fluid Laboratory Findings

▶ Table 6-17 details the synovial fluid laboratory findings.

Osteomyelitis

▶ *Salmonella* is the most commonly reported cause of osteomyelitis in children with sickle cell disease and accounts for up to 50% of cases in children with sickle cell disease.

TABLE 6-17
JOINT PAIN IN CHILDREN

Cause of Arthralgia	Joints Involved	Associated Findings
Traumatic Sprain Fracture Overuse injury	Monoarticular	History of injury, swelling, tenderness, reduced movement.
Degenerative Slipped capital femoral epiphysis (SCFE)	Unilateral or bilateral hips	Limited ROM hip, obese child, age 8–10 years, M:F 2:1; x-ray shows displacement of femoral head.
Legg-Calvé-Perthes	Hip	Limited ROM, 4–10 years; M:F 5:1; x-ray shows avascular necrosis
Osgood-Schlatter	Knee	Pain over quadriceps tendon insertion, x-ray may be normal or have elevation of the tibial tuberosity.
Congenital Hemophilia	Monoarticular	History of bleeding, trauma, swollen tender joints.
Inflammation/ Infection Septic arthritis	Monoarticular	Fever, local signs of infection, x-ray (effusion), joint aspiration.
Osteomyelitis	Monoarticular	Fever, local signs of infection, x-ray (lytic lesion); ↑ uptake on bone scan.
Transient synovitis	Hip	History of viral illness and limp, aspiration to rule out infection; CBC and ESR can be mildly elevated, but are usually normal.
Juvenile rheumatoid arthritis (JRA)	Polyarticular	Rash, fever, GI involvement (liver, spleen) heart.
Henoch-Schönlein Purpura	Variable (mainly ankles and knees)	Fever, rash, conjunctivitis, stomatitis, coronary artery vasculitis, lymphadenopathy.
Kawasaki	Generalized arthralgias	

continued

TABLE 6-17
JOINT PAIN IN CHILDREN (CONTINUED)

Cause of Arthralgia	Joints Involved	Associated Findings
Neoplasm	Variable joints	X-ray findings of bone involvement, abnormal CBC; osteogenic sarcoma: peak age in adolescence, with distal femur and proximal tibial involvement.
Functional	Polyarticular	Tender but no edema or erythema.

CBC, complete blood count; ESR, erythrocyte sedimentation rate; GI, gastrointestinal; WBC, white blood cell; RF, rheumatoid factor; ANA, antinuclear antibodies; HLA, human leukocyte antigen; ROM, range of motion.

▶ *S. pneumoniae* is more common in children < 24 months of age.

▶ *S. aureus* is the most common cause overall.

PAIN CONTROL, ANALGESIA, AND SEDATION

▶ **Background:**
- Pain is defined as "an unpleasant sensory and emotional experience associated with actual or potential tissue damage, or described in terms of such damage."
- Pain assessment in children can be very difficult due to fear of the child of outsiders.
- Pain assessment: face scale most commonly used in pediatric population.

▶ **Types of Sedation Options:**
- **Conscious sedation:** a minimally depressed level of consciousness that retains the patient's ability to maintain a patent airway independently and continuously, and respond appropriately to physical stimulation or verbal command.
- **Deep sedation:** controlled state of depressed consciousness or unconsciousness from which the patient is not easily aroused, which may be accompanied by a partial or complete loss of protective reflexes and inability to maintain patent airway independently and respond purposely to stimulation or verbal command.

- **Procedural sedation and analgesia (PSA):** technique of administering sedatives or dissociative agents with or without analgesics to induce a state that allows the patient to tolerate unpleasant procedures while maintaining cardiorespiratory function. It is extremely important to have adequate equipment to perform PSA in a safe manner. This includes positive-pressure oxygen delivery system, capable of delivering > 90% oxygen, functional suction apparatus with Yankauer tip, equipment for noninvasive cardiorespiratory function and oxygen saturation. In addition, it is imperative to adhere to the specific facility protocol in assessment, monitoring, and documentation guidelines for PSA.
- **Discharge criteria** after sedation should include the ability to maintain airway, move all limbs, respond to verbal commands, sit on the stretcher unassisted for 5 minutes or longer, and hydration possible and adequate. For a very young or handicapped child, the pre-sedation level of responsiveness is achieved.

▶ **Sedatives**
- Sedatives ↓ activity and blunt responsiveness. Therefore, it is useful in procedures that require cooperation. Painful interventions require a combination of sedatives plus analgesics.

▶ **Narcotic Analgesics**
- The actions of narcotics are mediated through binding to specific opioid receptors in the spinal cord and brain.
- In general, monitoring for hypoventilation, oxygen desaturation, and cardiorespiratory depression is essential.

▶ **Other Agents**
▶ **Reversal Agents**
- **Naloxone:** narcotic antagonist
  1. Can be given IV, IM, sublingual, and subcutaneous routes
  2. Dose: 0.1 mg/kg IV for children weighing < 20 kg and 2 mg for children > 20 kg
- **Flumazenil:** benzodiazepine antagonist
  1. Dose: 0.02 mg/kg IV up to 0.2 mg as an initial dose. Can be repeated every minute to maximum of 3 mg.
  2. It is possible for patients who had received flumazenil for termination of sedation to become re-sedated → observation for at least 2 hours after flumazenil use.

TABLE 6-18
AGENTS USED FOR PAIN RELIEF AND SEDATION

Medication	Route	Dose (mg/kg)	Onset/Duration (min)	Advantages	Side Effects
Benzodiazepines					
Midazolam	IV	0.05–0.1	2–3/45–60	Reduces stress and anxiety, and has amnestic and anticonvulsant properties.	Cardiorespiratory depression or apnea. Paradoxical agitation and disinhibition phenomena which could follow, otherwise effective sedation self-limited (about 15 min).
	IM	0.1–0.15	10–20/60–120		
	PO	0.5–0.75	15–30/60–90		
	IN	0.2–0.5	10–15/60		
	PR	0.25–0.5	10–20/60–90		
Diazepam	IV	0.05–0.2	4–6/120–180		
	PR	0.5–0.7	10–20/60–120		
Barbiturates					
Pentobarbital	IV	1–5	1–2/15–45	Excellent sedation choice for radiologic imaging procedures due to its rapid onset of action.	Respiratory depression and hypoxia.
	IM	2–6	10–15/50–120		
	PO	1.5–3	15–30/60–240		
	PR	1.5–3	15–30/60–240		
Thiopental	IV	3–5 (Start with 1 mg/kg)	0.5/10–15	It produces profound hypnosis and sedation within 30 s.	Apnea, hypotension, erythema, edema, and severe tissue necrosis (highly alkaline solution). Histamine release: caution use in asthmatics.
Methohexital	IV	1	0.5/15–30	Similar to pentobarbital.	Myoclonic jerking of the musculature. Seizure induction in patients with temporal lobe epilepsy. Respiratory and airway compromise.
	PR	20	10–15/60		

TABLE 6-19
NARCOTIC ANALGESICS

Medication	Route	Dose (mg/kg)	Onset/Duration (min)	Advantages	Side Effects
Morphine	IV IM	0.1–0.2 0.1–0.2	4–6/120–240 10–20/240–360	Analgesic, sedative, anxiolytic, and euphoric effects.	Respiratory depression especially in children < 2 mos of age. Hypotension, miosis, nausea, emesis, and constipation.
Fentanyl	IV	0.001–0.002 (slowly)	2–3/30–60	Potency 100x that of morphine without hemodynamic compromise, histamine release, or bronchospasm.	Chest wall rigidity, vomiting, seizure, facial pruritus. Risk of hypoxemia and apnea ↑ when fentanyl used in conjunction with midazolam.
Lorazepam Chloral hydrate	IV PO PR	0.02–0.05 50–100 50–75	3–5/180–240 20–30/60–120 15–20/60–120	One of the most common pediatric sedatives for radiologic imaging. Poor choice in a busy ED due to its erratic absorption, slow onset, and prolong duration of action.	The unmonitored use and postprocedure discharge before patient is back to baseline can lead to aspiration and death.

TABLE 6-20
OTHER AGENTS

Medication	Route	Dose (mg/kg)	Onset/Duration (min)	Advantages	Side Effects
Ketamine	IV IM PO	1–2 4–5 5–10	1/45–60 3–5/90–150 120–240	Dissociative anesthetic = "lights on, nobody home" appearance. Excellent safety in children. It has mild sedation, amnesia, inotropic, and bronchodilatory effects.	Hypersalivation, hypertension, tachycardia, ↑ intracranial pressure, vomiting, emergent reactions, nightmares, and laryngospasm. *Atropine 0.01 mg/kg reduces secretions.* **Do not** use in head trauma or globe injuries.
Propofol	IV	0.5–1 boluses or 25–150 µg/kg/min	Its onset is immediate and is so rapidly cleared that IV infusion is required to maintain effects.	Antiemetic, antipruritic, anticonvulsant, anxiolytic, hypnotic, and analgesic properties.	Pain at the site of injection and involuntary movements. Others include loss of consciousness, hypotension, and apnea.
Nitrous oxide	Inhalation	30–60% concentration	3–5/3–5	It is particularly useful in poorly cooperative children (noninvasive).	Drowsiness, nausea, and emesis. **Do not** use in altered level of consciousness, severe maxillofacial injuries, chronic obstructive pulmonary disease, pulmonary edema, pneumothorax, bowel obstruction, and major chest injuries.

3. Flumazenil is useful in terminating paradoxical reactions to midazolam.

▶ **Local Anesthesia**
- **Topical anesthesia**
  1. Use of restraints and sedation in children with lacerations.
  2. TAC (**t**etracaine, **a**drenaline, and **c**ocaine): side effects include systemic absorption of cocaine, seizures, and death mostly due to inappropriate application to mucous membranes. It is largely replaced by LET.
  3. LET (**l**idocaine, **e**pinephrine, **t**etracaine): the same advantages of TAC without the cocaine.
  4. Lidocaine infiltration of wounds: can add bicarbonate, use the smallest needle, gentle pressure, and slow infiltration can reduce infiltration pain. Doses are: 3–5 mg/kg to which can be ↑ to 5–7 mg/kg if lidocaine is used with epinephrine (epinephrine causes vasoconstriction, therefore higher doses can be used).
  5. Eutectic mixture of local anesthetics (EMLA) cream is composed of 2.5% lidocaine and 2.5% prilocaine, both amide anesthetics. It has been used for minor procedures including venipuncture, lumbar puncture, as well as for lacerations. Although the compound does provide adequate analgesia, delay of onset makes it impractical for laceration repair in the ED (unless the cream was applied in the triage area).
- **Regional anesthesia:** digital blocks; minidose Bier block for fracture reduction: uses half the dose of lidocaine used in regional anesthesia. Requires specific precaution, two IVs and monitoring.

PSYCHIATRIC AND BEHAVIORAL DISORDERS
Enuresis

▶ **Primary**
- Never has been toilet trained
- May be constitutional delay
- May be anatomic/physiologic abnormalities:
  1. Ectopic ureter
  2. Sickle cell disease

3. UTI
4. Nervous system lesions
▶ **Secondary**
   • Previously continent for 1 year
   • May be due to diuretics (medications, hyperosmolality) psychogenic (abuse, depression), UTI/vulvovaginitis, constipation, pinworms, spinal cord tumors
▶ **Nocturnal enuresis** occurs in 15% of 5-year-olds, 7% of 8-year-olds, 3% of 12-year-olds

Encopresis

▶ Repeated, involuntary defecation into clothing, in children age *4 years and older,* lasting at least *1 month*
▶ **Pathophysiology:**
   • Constipation in first 2 years of life causes withholding (fear of pain, anxiety).
   • May be due to problems with rectal motility or sphincter control; retention causes rectal enlargement, decreased sensation, and overflow diarrhea, eventual inability to sense or control bowel movements.
▶ **Diagnosis:** history including toilet training, stool pattern (if no stool by day 2 of life and retention from birth, consider Hirschsprung), examination (anterior anus, CNS disorders)
▶ **Management:** immediate bowel clean out (including enemas and laxatives), bran/fruit/vegetable diet, sit on toilet for 10 minutes twice a day regularly, long-term follow-up needed

Sleep Disturbances

▶ **Amount of Sleep:**
   • 3–6 months of age: sleep is mostly at night, total 14–15 hours a day including naps
   • 12-month-old needs 11.5 hours of sleep
   • 5 years: needs 11 hours
   • 9 years: needs 10 hours
   • Naps until 3–5 years old
▶ **Night Awakenings:** unable to fall back asleep without parents, parents reinforce
▶ **Night Terrors:** occur in first $1/3$ of sleep, screaming, difficult to arouse, lasts 15 minutes, amnesia

► **Sleepwalking:** first $1/3$ of sleep, walking/more complex, difficult to arouse, few minutes, amnesia
► **Nightmares:** rapid eye movement (REM) sleep disturbance, last $1/3$ of sleep, wakening easy
► **Management:** set firm bedtimes, if wakens, comfort child but leave while awake, comfort if nightmares

Irritability

► May be due to: ENT (OM, foreign body, corneal abrasion), cardiopulmonary (hypoxia, CHF, dysrhythmias), GI (gastritis/esophagitis), GU (UTI), musculoskeletal (fractures, contusions, tourniquet syndrome, dermatitis), neurologic (hematomas, meningitis), endocrine (Na/Ca/Mg disturbances, hypoglycemia, intoxication, cocaine withdrawal), or psychosocial causes.
► **Colic:** irritability, fussiness in an infant < 3 months old, for over 3 hours a day for 4 or more days a week. Parental reassurance is imperative. Colic resolves by 3–4 months of age.

Depression

► **Diagnosis:** depressed mood, loss of interest/pleasure, ± sleep disturbances, lack of energy, change in weight/appetite, less energy, inability to concentrate, feelings of worthlessness, agitation/lethargy, preoccupation with/plans of death
► **Major Depressive Episode:** 4 or more of latter + one of former for 2 weeks
► **Major Depressive Disorder:** 1 or more episodes
► **Dysthymic Disorder:** depressed mood, + 2 of: change in appetite, sleep habits, fatigue, diminished self-esteem, hopelessness, poor concentration for the majority of 1 year without major depression
► **Differential:** brain tumors, drug abuse, ingestions, abuse/neglect, conduct disorder, separation anxiety, schizophrenia
► **Management:** psychiatric consultation

Bipolar Disorder

► **Manic Episode:** period of abnormally and persistently elevated, expansive or irritable mood, markedly impairing function, lasting at least a week, associated with three of the following:

increased self esteem, decreased need for sleep, garrulousness, flight of ideas, distractibility, agitation, risk-taking
▶ **Hypomanic Episode:** mood different but not abnormal, functioning changed (not impaired)
▶ **Diagnosis:**
  • **Bipolar I disorder:** at least one manic episode, usually with major depressive episodes
  • **Bipolar II disorder:** at least one hypomanic episode with major depressive episode
  • **Cyclothymic disorder:** hypomanic episodes with episodes of depressed mood
▶ **Differential:** attention deficit hyperactivity disorder (ADHD), conduct disorders, schizophrenia (bipolar may have hallucinations/delusions), depressive disorders
▶ **Management:** psychiatric consultation, psychotherapy, pharmacologic therapy

Separation Anxiety Disorder (includes school phobia)

▶ **Diagnosis:** new school, physical symptoms (abdominal pain, headache, nausea, vomiting) with clinging or chaotic families
▶ **Differential:** over-anxiety disorder, depression, truancy
▶ **Management:** firm insistence that the child attend school

Phobias

▶ **Specific:** more persistent, interfere with routines, produce anxiety, avoidance of stimulus
▶ **Social Phobia:** afraid of scrutiny of others/acting in an embarrassing fashion
▶ **Management:** follow-up and parental reassurance

Conversion Disorder

▶ **Diagnosis:** as early as 7 years old, more in adolescence, girls > boys, any body system involved (alteration in sensation, tremors/paralysis, limb pain, headache, abdominal pain, hyperventilation, vomiting, visual symptoms). Need to ask about stresses, family member with symptoms/stresses/secondary gain. Unconscious purpose for the patient.
▶ **Management:** history, physical and minimal labs to exclude organic pathology; treat with reassurance, decrease attention

and secondary gain from symptoms. Medical and psychosocial follow-up.

Attention Deficit Hyperactivity Disorder (ADHD)

▶ Inattention, hyperactivity, and impulsivity.
▶ **Diagnosis:** difficulty sitting still, won't wait their turn, interrupt and blurt out answers, often engage in dangerous activities without considering consequences.
▶ **Differential:** personality, anxiety, and mood disorders; may coexist with mental retardation (MR), autism, deafness, Tourette syndrome, substance abuse, child abuse.
▶ **Management:** do not start pharmacotherapy in the ED, refer to pediatrician, help parents set limits and focus on good behavior.

Conduct Disorder

▶ Persistent and repetitive pattern of aggressive, noncompliant, intrusive, and poorly self-controlled behaviors that violate the rights of others or age-appropriate societal norms
▶ **Diagnosis:** intimidation, physical threats, assaults, cruelty, theft, destruction, lying, law breaking; associated with impairment of function in academic/social settings
▶ **Differential:** ADHD, lying/disobedience in preschoolers, **oppositional-defiant disorder** (hostility and negativity but does not violate societal norms, usually over 36 months old)
▶ **Management:** admission/incarceration if required, longitudinal follow-up

Eating Disorders

▶ **Pica** can occur due to iron deficiency, MR, autism, schizophrenia or without organic cause.
▶ **Rumination Disorder:** may be due to disordered mother-infant relationship or self-stimulation.
▶ **Bulimia** and **Anorexia Nervosa** mostly in adolescents, multifactorial; increased in twins, cultural ideals of beauty and parental expectations involved as well as medical illness, body image, and difficulties in autonomy.
▶ **Diagnosis:**
  • **Pica:** ingestion of non-nutritive substances (hair, paint chips, dirt, paper).

- **Rumination:** regurgitation with re-chewing and re-swallowing or ejection, starts between 3–12 months of age (later if MR), no distress (may seem pleasurable).
- **Anorexia nervosa:** inability to maintain body weight > 15% below predicted, with fear of gaining weight/being fat and distorted self-image. Females account for 95%, may have amenorrhea, mortality is 5–18%.
- **Bulimia nervosa:** recurrent binge eating with feelings of loss of control, accompanied by acts to prevent weight gain (forced vomiting, laxative purging, fasting); must have had on average at least 2 episodes per week for 3 months; over concern with body shape and weight, females predominate.

▶ **Differential:** pica due to nutritional deficiencies; rumination may be organic causes of vomiting; anorexia differs from bulimia in body weight; consider organic causes of weight loss.

▶ **Management:** exclude organic causes in ED, manage dehydration and electrolyte disturbances, arrange close follow-up.

Tic Disorders

▶ 4–10% children, Tourette syndrome is autosomal dominant, dysfunction of dopaminergic, adrenergic, serotonergic, and cholinergic neurotransmitter systems as well as environmental factors

▶ **Tourette Syndrome:** multiple motor/vocal tics for over a year; if vocal only then = **vocal tic disorder**, if the tics are motor only then is this called **chronic motor disorder**

▶ **Transient tic disorder:** symptoms for at least 2 weeks but < 1 year

▶ **Diagnosis:** simple (eye blinking, nodding) and complex (echokinesis, echolalia, etc.); disappear during sleep or with intense concentration, worsen with stress

▶ **Differential:** myoclonus, chorea, athetosis, hemiballismus; intentional behaviors (rocking, bruxism, breath holding, nose-picking)

▶ **Management:** reassurance and neglect

Disorders with Psychotic Features

▶ **Psychosis:** altered contact with reality

▶ **Pervasive Developmental Disorders (Autism, Rett Disorder, Asperger Disorder, Childhood Disintegrative Disorder, PDD-NOS):** impairment in social reciprocity, communication skills, onset in infancy/childhood, do NOT have delusions, hallucinations, loosening of associations.

▶ **Schizophrenia:** presence of two of the following: (1) hallucinations, delusions, catatonia, inappropriate/flat affect, loosening of associations; (2) bizarre delusions; (3) prominent hallucinations involving voice(s) discussing the person's actions or thoughts. Must be present for longer than 6 months.

▶ **Diagnosis:**
- **Pervasive developmental disorder:** onset before 36 months, aberrant and delayed development, impaired communication (expressive and receptive) and social skills, unusual reactions to external stimuli, self-stimulatory behaviors, stereotyped body movements, preoccupation with unusual details.
  1. **Autism:** all areas affected
  2. **Asperger** has normal language/cognition
  3. **Rett** occurs only in females who are normal until at least 5 months old, followed by deceleration of head growth and loss of developmental skills, onset of psychomotor retardation
  4. **Childhood disintegrative disorder:** at least 2 years of normal development, followed by all abnormalities
- **Childhood schizophrenia:** onset after 5 years of age, delusions (often of external control), hallucinations (frequently auditory), blunted or inappropriate emotional reactions, disinterest in normal activities. May also have bizarre movements, social isolation, impulsiveness, loss of identity. **Paranoid schizophrenia** is seen only in adolescence.

▶ **Differential:** organic causes much more common reason for psychosis, such as toxic (drugs of abuse, prescription drugs including TCAs, phenobarbital, phenytoin, INH, benzodiazepines, captopril, digoxin, OTC drugs such as antihistamines), metabolic (electrolytes, thyroid dysfunction, Cushing and Addison diseases, vitamin deficiencies, liver dysfunction, DKA, hypoglycemia), traumatic (subdural hematoma, cerebral contusion), infectious (meningitis, encephalitis, pneumonia, typhoid, Rocky Mountain spotted fever, syphilis, malaria, sepsis), and other causes (hypoxia, anemia, shock, collagen vascular disease); also consider other psychiatric causes (mood disorders, brief reactive psychosis if < 1 month, schizophreniform disorder if < 6 months).

▶ **Management:** exclude organic causes, consider diphenhydramine, lorazepam, chlorpromazine, thioridazine; consult psychiatry, admit for observation and treatment.

Suicide

▶ **Suicide Attempt:** nonfatal self-injury with intention to harm or call attention to oneself

▶ **Diagnosis:** risk factors include psychiatric illness, substance abuse, prior attempts (especially in last 3 months), personality traits (hopeless, hostile, impulsive, perfectionist, poor social skills), environmental (abuse, neglect, parental absence/discord, exposure to suicide, stress), seizure disorder; older age, female gender

▶ **Evaluate:** lethality, chance of discovery, planning and patient intent

▶ **Management:** medical and psychiatric treatment as necessary, admit for observation usually necessary

RESPIRATORY DISORDERS
Signs and Symptoms

▶ **Apnea**
  - **Apnea:** cessation of breathing > 20 seconds, shorter if cyanosis, bradycardia, or pallor. Can be central (absence of effort/muscle activation), obstructive (normal effort, airflow ceases), or mixed (obstructive then central).
  - **Periodic breathing:** normal newborns, pauses > 3 seconds then normal breathing 20 seconds repeated at least 3 times.
  - **ALTE** (apparent life-threatening event): apnea, color change, muscle tone change, and choking/gagging.
  - **Pathophysiology:**
    1. Respiration controlled by pons/medulla; responds to hypoxia (carotid/aortic), PCO_2/pH (central medullary chemoreceptor).

a. During REM sleep ventilatory response to hypercarbia/hypoxia ↓ and arousal response is depressed.

b. Immature responses in neonates (hypoxia causes brief ↑ in RR, then depression of respiratory drive, hypoventilation, apnea).

- **Differential of apnea of infancy:**
  1. Infection: bronchiolitis, pneumonia, respiratory syncytial virus (RSV) (central apnea), pertussis, sepsis, meningitis, encephalitis
  2. CNS: seizure, intracranial hemorrhage (shaken baby), increased ICP, Ondine curse (congenital central alveolar hypoventilation)
  3. GI: gastroesophageal reflux disease (GERD), tracheoesophageal fistula
  4. Cardiopulmonary: respiratory distress syndrome, pulmonary edema or hemorrhage, hypoplastic lungs, congenital heart disease, shock, dysrhythmias
  5. Metabolic: inborn errors
  6. Other: neuropathies, myopathies (Guillain-Barré), ingestions, child abuse, idiopathic
- **Differential of obstructive apnea:**
  1. Structural: adenoids/tonsils, choanal atresia, septal deviation, laryngo/tracheomalacia, vascular anomalies
  2. Hypotonia: Down syndrome, cerebral palsy
  3. Hypothyroidism, Prader-Willi, obesity, airway infections.
- **Diagnosis:** CBC, glucose, electrolytes, calcium, magnesium, chest x-ray, ECG, RSV and pertussis in infants; consider EEG, barium swallow, full septic workup (including LP in infants less than 1–2 months of age)

▶ **Cough**
- **Differential:**
  1. Infants: *Chlamydia* (1–4 months, staccato cough), cytomegalovirus, *Ureaplasma, Pneumocystis carinii* pneumonia, pertussis (paroxysmal), bronchiolitis, cystic fibrosis (chronic wheeze, pneumonias, abnormal stools), congenital anomalies (tracheoesophageal fistula, tracheomalacia), foreign body
  2. Preschool: asthma, upper respiratory infection, pneumonia, if > 7 days consider sinusitis

3. School: asthma, *Mycoplasma* pneumonia, tuberculosis (immigrants, HIV-exposed), mediastinal mass, psychogenic (absent during sleep); hemoptysis consider Group A strep pneumonia, tuberculosis, pertussis, abscess, pseudohemoptysis (epistaxis)

- **Diagnosis:** history and physical exam, chest x-ray, consider decubitus views if foreign body suspected, bronchoscopy, spirometry if > 5–6 years

▶ **Cyanosis**
- Present when > 5 g deoxygenated hemoglobin/100 mL blood (O_2 saturation < 85%)
- **Central:** tongue/mucous membranes affected, arterial blood deoxygenation, usually improves with 100% O_2 unless abnormal hemoglobin (methemoglobin, sulfhemoglobin)
- **Peripheral:** less blood flow, ↑ O_2 extraction (shock, vasomotor instability)
- **Differential:**
  1. Cardiac: congenital with R-L shunting or mixing, usually associated respiratory distress; intrapulmonary shunting due to congestive heart failure, pulmonary hemorrhage, hypertension, or embolism
  2. Upper airway: croup, epiglottitis, tracheitis, retropharyngeal abscess, foreign body
  3. Lower airway: pneumonia, asthma, bronchiolitis, aspiration, foreign body
  4. CNS: via respiratory depression
  5. Infection: meningitis, sepsis
  6. Trauma: CNS, chest, shock
  7. Congenital: cardiac, choanal atresia, laryngomalacia
  8. Intoxication: methemoglobin of > 15% due to benzocaine/nitrites/antioxidants or congenital; sulfhemoglobin due to sulfonamides and phenacetin
- **Diagnosis:** pulse oximetry, ABG, methemoglobin level, hematocrit, chest x-ray

▶ **Respiratory Distress**
- **Pathophysiology:** neonates have immature respiratory control centers, compliant chest wall, small residual capacity, easy fatigue; small diameter of airway in all children predisposes (resistance α 1/radius^4)

- **Differential:**
  1. Upper airway: **inspiratory stridor = supraglottic; expiratory/biphasic = below larynx; abnormal voice = glottic;** pharyngeal or supraglottic; due to croup ("seal-bark" cough, fever), epiglottitis (*H. influenzae*, stridor, high fever, anxious, toxic, drooling), bacterial tracheitis (*S. aureus* or *H. influenzae*, purulent sputum), retropharyngeal/peritonsillar abscess, diphtheria, foreign body, trauma, anatomic anomaly [vascular rings, laryngeal webs, vocal cord paralysis, micrognathia (Pierre Robin), glossoptosis (Down syndrome, Beckwith-Wiedemann, hypothyroid)], allergic
  2. Lower airway: pneumonia (*S. pneumoniae, H. influenzae, S, aureus;* atypical), bronchiolitis (RSV, parainfluenzae), pleural effusions, pulmonary edema (hepatic/renal disease), asthma (recurrent episodes or airway obstruction responsive to bronchodilators), congestive heart failure, pulmonary embolism, polycythemia, anemia, trauma, foreign body, smoke inhalation, cystic fibrosis, neoplasms
  3. CNS: altered level of consciousness causing upper airway obstruction, infection (meningitis, encephalitis), raised ICP, ingestion, seizure, progressive neuropathies (Guillain-Barre, botulism, Werdnig-Hoffman, muscular dystrophy, myasthenia gravis)
  4. Metabolic: acidosis (dehydration, DKA, sepsis, salicylate ingestion), fever
- **Diagnosis:**
  1. History and physical exam, pulse oximetry; chest x-ray and labs dependent on amount of distress
  2. ABG if stable (respiratory failure = $PCO_2 > 50$ mm Hg *or* $PO_2 < 50$ mm Hg; $PCO_2 > 40$ in a child with asthma and distress shows impending failure)
  3. Consider CBC, culture; soft-tissue neck films for upper airway
  4. Consider ECG if cardiac suspicion, other tests focused
- ▶ **Stridor**
  - **Pathophysiology:** turbulent airflow from laryngeal/tracheal obstruction + dynamic tracheal compression
  - **Differential:**
    1. **Acute**
       a. Infectious: croup, tracheitis, epiglottitis, retropha-

ryngeal abscess (< 6 years, drooling and hyperextended neck, β-hemolytic strep), peritonsillar abscess (> 12 years, ± drooling, upright with neck pain, Group A strep), infectious mono, diphtheria

b. Inflammatory: angioneurotic edema

c. Traumatic: foreign body, laryngeal fracture, postintubation, corrosive ingestion

d. Metabolic: hypocalcemia

e. Psychogenic

2. **Chronic/Recurrent**

a. Nasopharynx (choanal atresia, macroglossia, craniofacial anomalies, thyroglossal duct cyst)

b. Larynx (laryngomalacia *most common*, laryngeal web/cleft, laryngocele, subglottic stenosis)

c. Trachea (web/cyst), vascular (ring, hemangiomas), neoplasm (neck/chest), traumatic (postintubation), neurologic (poor pharyngeal tone, laryngeal paralysis, e.g., in Arnold-Chiari)

- **Diagnosis:**
  1. Ensure airway stable
  2. Observe child for preferred position, hyperextension, drooling, trauma, voice quality (muffling = supraglottic, hoarseness = laryngeal), level of consciousness
  3. NO LABS until child stable
  4. Admit unstable; chest x-ray in most (R-sided aortic arch = vascular ring/sling; mediastinal mass, tracheal compression and shift to the left), neck films; pulse oximetry

- **Management:** if distress, minimal disturbance, blow by O_2, intubation with smaller endotracheal tube than usual (neonate = 2.5 mm; < 6 month = 3.0 mm; 6 months–2 years = 3.5 mm; 2–5 years = 4.0 mm; > 5 years = 4.0–5.0 mm)

▶ **Wheezing**

- **Pathophysiology:** air-flow turbulence due to increased velocity from airway narrowing; usually from larger bronchi; infants more prone to obstruction due to small airway, peripheral airways narrower, compliant airway and rib cage

- **Differential:**
  1. First episode: bronchiolitis, reactive airway disease
  2. Sudden onset: foreign body aspiration

3. Prolonged wheeze: asthma, missed foreign body, cystic fibrosis, aspiration due to GERD or fistula

4. Recurrent pneumonias: foreign body, immune deficiency, *Mycoplasma*

5. Slow feeding, grunting, borderline weight gain: cardiac disease

6. Stridor: vascular ring, laryngeal webs, stenosis, subglottic stenosis, tracheal webs, bronchial strictures

7. Systemic symptoms: lymphoma, neuroblastoma, mediastinal masses

- **Diagnosis:** pattern of symptoms, associated findings, degree of respiratory distress and stabilize, examine for associated findings to narrow diagnosis; pulse oximetry, ABG if severe distress, measure peak expiratory flow rate (PEFR) if > 5 years, chest x-ray to exclude diagnoses and for all first-time wheezing

- **Management:** inhaled bronchodilators initially until diagnosis established

Diagnostic Entities

▶ See **Tables 6-21, 6-22, and 6-23.**

TABLE 6-21
DIAGNOSTIC ENTITIES

Disease	Epidemiology/Pathophysiology	Clinical/Lab Findings	Complications/Differential	Management
ASTHMA	5–10% children Onset < 3 y tends to be more frequent attacks **Risks:** bronchiolitis, atopy Recurrent, reversible airway disease Bronchospasm, edema, secretions **Triggers:** infection, allergens/irritants, exercise, weather, stress, β-blockers, aspirin	Dry cough, exercise intolerance, acute wheeze Tachypnea, respiratory distress, pulsus paradoxus, wheeze **Severe:** lethargic, diaphoretic, unable to speak **Status asthmaticus:** no response to multiple β-agonists (see severity table below) Pulse ox, ABG if severe, PEFR (>5 y), ± CXR	**Complications:** respiratory failure, atelectasis, mediastinal emphysema, pneumothorax/mediastinum, dehydration, death **Differential:** *M. pneumoniae*, bronchiolitis, pertussis, chemical pneumonitis, cystic fibrosis, cardiac	O_2 **β-agonists:** inhaled peak 30–60 min; terbutaline SC 0.01 mg/kg (max: 0.25 mg) q15–20 min; epinephrine 1:1000, 0.01 mg/kg SC (max: 0.35 mg) **Ipratropium:** 500 μg/dose with each albuterol; peak 30–120 min **Steroids:** prednisone 2 mg/kg PO; methylprednisolone 1–2 mg/kg q6 IV **Theophylline:** not routine

TABLE 6-22
ASTHMA SEVERITY TABLE

Sign/ Symptom	Mild	Moderate	Severe
PEFR	70–90%	50–70%	< 50% predicted
Respiratory rate	Normal: 130% mean	130–150% mean	> 150% mean
Alertness	Normal	Normal	May be ↓
Dyspnea	- / Mild	Moderate, ↓ cry/ speech/suck	Severe, little speech/ cry/suck
Pulsus paradoxus	< 10 mm Hg	10–20 mm Hg	20–40 mm Hg
Accessory muscle	None: mild	Moderate, + hyperinflation	Severe, ++ hyperinflation
Color	Good	Pale	± cyanotic
Auscultation	Expiratory wheeze	Expiratory/ Inspiratory wheeze	Inaudible
O_2 saturation	> 95%	90–95%	< 90%
PCO_2	< 35 mm Hg	< 40 mm Hg	> 40 mm Hg

TABLE 6-23
SPECIFIC PEDIATRIC RESPIRATORY DISORDERS

Disease	Epidemiology/Pathophysiology	Clinical/Lab Findings	Complications/Differential	Management
BRONCHIOLITIS	< 2 years, most < 1 Viral-induced necrosis of epithelium w/ inflammation RSV (90%), also parainfluenzae, influenza, adenovirus, rhinovirus Duration from 7–10 days to 3–4 weeks or longer Mortality ~ 0.5%	Upper respiratory infection symptoms; worsening cough, vomiting, poor PO intake Tachycardia, tachypnea, distress, ± wheeze, crepitations O_2 sat ↓; may be ↑WBC with left shift, CXR (hyper-inflated, atelectasis)	**Complications:** respiratory failure, atelectasis, ↑ mortality if underlying disorders, asthma bronchiolitis fibrosa obliterans **Differential:** viral pneumonia, CF, bronchopulmonary dysplasia, reactive airway disease, aspiration, cardiac, vascular anomalies	Humidified O_2 β-agonists Inhaled racemic epinephrine Ribavirin in severe cases (not in ED or PICU) Ventilation/CPAP IV hydration **Severe:** SaO_2 < 95%, gestational age < 34 wks, RR >70, atelectasis, age < 3 mos
CROUP (LARYNGOTRACHEO- BRONCHITIS)	Nasopharyngeal infection spreads to larynx/trachea Sudden dyspnea, barking cough, stridor Parainfluenza virus type I; also type III, adenovirus, RSV Most 6–36 mos old Lasts 4–7 d	1–2 days coryza, then hoarse/cough, stridor at night, (inspiratory/expiratory) fever Tachypnea = low SaO_2 cyanosis late SaO_2 if ↓ is ominous Neck x-ray: steeple sign absent in 50–60% (not useful)	**Complications:** airway obstruction, pneumonia, bacterial tracheitis, lymphadenitis, otitis media, dehydration **Differential:** epiglottitis (anxious, toxic, immobile, drooling), tracheitis	Keep procedures to a minimum, push PO, child on mom's lap Humidity Racemic epinephrine 0.5 mL of 2.25%, lasts < 2 h; observe at least 3 h Dexamethasone 0.6 mg/kg IM or PO (up to 54 h) IV fluids Consider ENT consult if not responding

EPIGLOTTITIS	Supraglottic cellulitis *H. influenzae* (nontypeable), *S. pneumoniae*, *S. aureus*, GAS, group C strep	Fever, sore throat, poor PO, no prodrome Anxious, mouth open, drooling, respiratory distress No labs! Until airway stable; ↑WBC, cultures usually positive	**Complications:** obstruction, death, co-existing pneumonia, meningitis, septic arthritis, pericarditis **Differential:** tracheitis, retropharyngeal abscess, uvulitis, severe pharyngitis	**Prehospital:** transport, have anesthesiology and ENT ready, humidified O_2 mom's arms **ED:** calm, comfort, O_2 examine throat via ENT/anesthesia, parent takes child to OR, NT/OT intubation; cultures, cefotaxime ± vancomycin Prophylax family if *Hemophilus influenza B*
TRACHEITIS	Membranous laryngotracheobronchitis *S. aureus* most common, *S. pneumoniae*, GAS, *H. influenzae*	Upper respiratory infection for 1–2 wks, then croup, deterioration over hours Fever, toxic, stridor, distress No labs! Secure airway; ↑WBC, tracheal culture XR: subglottic narrowing	**Complications:** obstruction, arrest, death; pneumonia, toxic shock syndrome **Differential:** viral croup, epiglottitis, foreign body	Approach similar to epiglottitis (see above) IV antibiotics: nafcillin + cefotaxime

continued

TABLE 6-23
SPECIFIC PEDIATRIC RESPIRATORY DISORDERS (CONTINUED)

Disease	Epidemiology/Pathophysiology	Clinical/Lab Findings	Complications/Differential	Management
PLEURAL DISEASE	**Exudate:** infection (S. aureus, S. pneumoniae, PCP) or inflammation (neoplasm, lupus, juvenile rheumatoid arthritis) **Transudate:** ↑hydrostatic pressure (CHF), ↓osmotic pressure (↓protein) **Empyema:** para-pneumonic infection	Dyspnea, dry cough, fever, chest pain, nausea/vomiting due to ileus Tachypnea, respiratory distress, ↓breath sounds, dull to percussion over effusion, friction rub CBC, ESR (collagen vascular), electrolytes, creatinine, LFTs, UA CXR ± decubitus Ultrasound or CT to delineate Labs and culture of fluid (see last column)	**Complications:** respiratory failure, bronchopleural fistula, pneumatocele **Differential:** rib fracture, costochondritis, massive atelectasis	Stabilize, analgesics, sedation **Thoracentesis:** postaxillary line, 7th intercostal space (below scapula); 18G angiocath, 3-way stopcock, tubing, 20 cc syringe **Exudate:** *WBC > 10K, glucose < 60 mg/dL, pH < 7.3, LDH > 200 IU/L, protein > 3 gm/dL* **Transudate:** *WBC ~1K, glucose = serum, pH > 7.3, LDH < 200, protein < 3* Chest tube Treat underlying disease

PNEUMONIA

Interstitial or alveolar Most common respiratory diagnosis in hospitalized children **Neonates:** GBS, E. coli, Klebsiella, Listeria, Pseudomonas, RSV, Chlamydia **1–3 mos:** GBS, H. influenzae, S. pneumoniae, GAS, RSV, Chlamydia **3 mo–5 y:** S. pneumoniae, H. influenzae, S. aureus, GAS, RSV, etc., Chlamydia **> 5 y:** S. pneumoniae, H. influenzae, GAS, Mycoplasma	Apnea may be first presentation in RSV Mycoplasma mild Viral insidious; URI symptoms Bacterial more rapid and severe w/ cough, fever, pain, dyspnea; infants w/ poor feeding, fever, ↓activity, vomiting; rales/crackles Chlamydia afebrile; staccato cough SaO_2, WBC > 15K suggests bacterial, blood culture + in ~10% CXR	**Complications:** respiratory failure, effusions, pneumatocele, bacteremia, reactive airway disease (RSV) **Differential:** asthma, foreign body, atelectasis, CHF, hydrocarbon ingestion, aspiration	Humidified O_2 if distress **Respiratory failure:** PCO_2 > 50 mm Hg, PO_2 < 50 mm Hg on room air at sea level → intubate IV fluids Antibiotics after cultures; oral unless inpatient: to cover S. pneumoniae if < 5 y; Mycoplasma if > 5y; admit and add antibiotics if suspect S. aureus. **Admit:** toxicity, distress, dehydrated, effusion, immunocompromised

continued

TABLE 6-23
SPECIFIC PEDIATRIC RESPIRATORY DISORDERS (CONTINUED)

Disease	Epidemiology/Pathophysiology	Clinical/Lab Findings	Complications/Differential	Management
PULMONARY EDEMA	Abnormal accumulation of fluids in pulmonary tissues/air spaces Most common cause in children is CHF from congenital heart disease **Starling equation:** flow across membrane due to: (1) **Hydrostatic:** ↑ Left atrial pressures in CHF, pulmonary thrombus (2) **Osmotic:** nephrosis, hepatic disease, protein-losing enteropathies, burns, malnutrition (3) **Permeability:** infection, aspiration, ARDS, inhalants, toxins (4) **Transpulmonary pressure:** upper airway obstruction (5) **Lymph drainage** (6) **Other:** altitude, CNS	Dyspnea, frothy pink secretions, chest pain, infants may have feeding difficulties Pale, tachycardia, tachypnea, distress, cyanosis, ↓breath sounds, wheeze, signs of CHF CBC (anemia, ↑WBC, TCP), electrolytes, creatinine, LFTs, protein, albumin, ABG, urine (protein) CXR: Kerley A (upper) and B (lower) lines showing interlobular septal edema; ± pleural effusions	**Complications:** respiratory failure, cardiac failure, infection, DIC **Differential:** pneumonia, asthma, anaphylaxis, pulmonary embolism, intrapulmonary hemorrhage	Treat cause O_2 ± intubation Ventilate with PEEP at least 5 cmH_2O IVF ± albumin Monitor CVP with central line Diuretics if cardiogenic: Lasix 1–2 mg/kg q6h Morphine sulfate 0.1–0.2 mg/kg to dilate venous system and ↓pulmonary wedge pressure UNLESS unstable Pressors if cardiogenic shock Afterload reducers (sodium nitroprusside), only if measuring CVP Admit to ICU

URINARY AND RENAL DISORDERS
Signs And Symptoms

▶ **Dysuria and Pyuria**
- These symptoms are a sign of inflammation of the urinary tract, but may also be present with urethritis and vaginitis.
- Differential includes infections (UTI, pinworms, vaginitis, urethritis, balanitis), irritants (bubble baths, soap, and other products), trauma (masturbation, foreign body, abuse, straddle injury), stones, labial adhesions, and hypercalciuria.
- Urinalysis should be obtained by a clean catch or bladder catheterization.
- Urine culture and other appropriate cultures for gonorrhea and *Chlamydia* (particularly in adolescents females with dysuria, pelvic pain, and/or vaginal discharges) should be evaluated.
- **Treatment** includes warm sitz baths, proper hygiene, treatment of associated vaginal pathology or UTI with antibiotics may be curative.

▶ **Hematuria**
- Evaluation includes macroscopic (visible to the naked eye) and microscopic and determining the source.
- Not all red urine contains blood. Other causes include hemoglobinuria, myoglobinuria, drugs, foods (beets, blueberries), and dyes (food coloring).
- Red diaper syndrome: describes a red color on the diaper, which is caused by *Serratia marcescens* in the infant stool, which produces a pigment after incubation in the diaper pail.
- Different categories of causes include:
  1. Extrarenal: coagulation disorders, anticoagulant therapy, sickle cell disease/trait, and factitious
  2. Extraglomerular: UTI, hemorrhagic cystitis, urethritis, hypercalciuria, renal vein thrombosis, tumors (Wilms, bladder sarcoma), foreign body, renal tuberculosis
  3. Glomerular: idiopathic, IgA nephropathy, acute poststreptococcal glomerulo-nephropathy (GN), Alport syndrome and exercise
  4. Systemic: SLE, HUS, HSP, polyarteritis, and Still disease
- Hypercalciuria is an important cause of hematuria. It is a familial autosomal dominant condition characterized by excessive urinary calcium (> 4 mg $Ca^{++}/kg/24$ h urine collection). This could be due to renal tubular leak (best treated

with thiazide diuretics) or excess intestinal absorption of calcium (best treated with limited dietary intake of calcium and sodium to 500–600 mg/d and maintenance of large fluid intake).

- Diagnostic workup:
  1. A thorough history and physical examination are essential to determine the cause of hematuria such as trauma, medications, abdominal pain, bleeding, rash, and joint pain.
  2. Ancillary data:
     a. Urinalysis and culture are essential initial tests.
     b. RBC casts or darker colored urine is usually from the upper urinary tract.
     c. Coexistent proteinuria is indicative of glomerular disease (protein > 2+ cannot be accounted for by blood) and HSP and HUS should be considered.
     d. If a glomerular lesion is suspected then a throat culture, streptococcal antibodies, ESR, C3 and C4, ANA, and hepatitis B serology should be sent.
     e. The patient's sickle cell status should be determined.
     f. Electrolytes, total protein, and albumin are indicated in the presence of proteinuria, edema, or hypertension. BUN and creatinine should be obtained to assess renal function.
     g. Imaging is rarely needed and based on the evaluation a nephrology consultation and a renal biopsy may be obtained.
- Patients with azotemia, edema, or hypertension should be admitted. Obtain a urology consult in the presence of a calculus. UTI should be treated appropriately.

► **Hypertension (HTN)**
- The best evaluation of BP is based on the age, sex, and height of the patient.
- Always be sure the appropriate size cuff is used.
- A normal systolic and diastolic BP is < the 90th percentile, and HTN is considered > the 95th percentile.
- A hypertensive crisis is a severe elevation of BP without other symptoms.
- Hypertensive emergencies occur with associated symptoms and malignant HTN involves end-organ damage.

- In childhood, 79–98% of HTN is secondary to an underlying cause (renal, coarctation, endocrine, neurologic, and ingestion). Essential HTN is more prominent now with the higher incidence of obesity in children.
- In the ED only a few ancillary tests are required in the stable patient. These include: urinalysis, CBC, chemistry, chest x-ray, ECG, urine VMA, and DMSA scan if a renal cause is suspected.
- The retina should be evaluated for signs of long-standing HTN.
- The goal in the ED is to lower the child's BP by no more than 25% initially. Nifedipine 0.25–0.50 mg/kg is the drug of choice and should have maximum effect in 30–60 minutes.
- If acute renal failure (ARF) is the cause, then the patient may be fluid overloaded and require a diuretic.
- Calcium-channel blockers are contraindicated in intracranial hemorrhage.
- Labetalol may be useful, having alpha and beta effects, but should not be used in patients with bronchospasm, bradycardia, or heart failure.
- In severe cases a nitroprusside drip may be used.
- These patients should all have continuous cardiopulmonary monitoring and admission.

▶ **Proteinuria**
- Etiologies include glomerular, tubular, UTI, DM, orthostatics, exercise, reflux, myeloma, polycystic kidney disease, and hydronephrosis.
- Proteinuria in the ED < 3+ requires no further testing, but 3+ and 4+ involve a more thorough evaluation.
- All patients with proteinuria should have their BP measured.
- False-positives may be caused by gross hematuria, alkaline urine, sodium bicarbonate ingestion, and phenazopyridine.
- Ultimately quantification of protein is necessary with 24-hour urine collection.
- Glomerular disease is marked by excretion of large molecular-weight proteins.
- **Treatment** is dependent on the cause.

▶ **Scrotal Pain and Swelling**
- Differentiating various causes of scrotal swelling can be challenging and priority should be given to address the

more serious causes such as testicular torsion, incarcerated or strangulated inguinal hernia, and ruptured testicles.

- The vast majority (96%) of acute scrotal cases are due to either acute torsion of the spermatic cord, torsion of the appendix testis, or epididymitis. It is important to note that the opportunity to save a testicle lasts only 6–10 hours from the onset of pain in testicular torsion.

- Causes of scrotal swelling are divided according to its association with pain:

  1. Painful swelling of the scrotum:
     a. Testicular torsion
     b. Torsion of the appendage testis
     c. Orchitis (mumps)
     d. Epididymitis
     e. Incarcerated hernia
     f. Tumor, acute hemorrhage
     g. Trauma (contusion, hematocele, hematoma)

  2. Nonpainful swelling of the scrotum
     a. Hydrocele
     b. Reducible hernia
     c. Varicocele
     d. Testicular tumor/leukemia
     e. Testicular cyst
     f. Idiopathic scrotal edema
     g. Systemic edema states (HSP, Kawasaki disease, nephrotic syndrome)
     h. Testicular torsion in the prenatal period
     i. Others: fat necrosis, hypertriglyceridemia and sarcoidosis

- When the diagnosis is difficult or unclear then further imaging studies are warranted such as ultrasound with perfusion.

- A varicocele manifests as a bag of worms palpated superior and posterior to the testis. It is more common on the left as a result of incomplete spermatic vein valves. The left spermatic vein empties directly into the left renal vein and the right into the inferior vena cava (IVC), explaining the left-sided preponderance of varicoceles. A right-sided varicocele should prompt search for intra-abdominal process/tumor that is compressing on the IVC and a new onset left-sided varicocele may reflect the development of renal cell carcinoma obstructing the left renal vein.

- Inguinal hernia:
    1. Indirect inguinal hernia is the invagination of abdominal contents into a peritoneal sac, the processus vaginalis, which then traverses the inguinal canal causing swelling of the scrotum.
    2. Persistent incarceration may result in ischemia of the entrapped bowel and present as an acutely painful inguinoscrotal mass.
    3. Using ice packs, analgesia, and steady manual pressure, 80–95% of incarcerated hernias are reduced.
    4. Testicular compromise can be found in 3–5% of cases with incarcerated inguinal hernias. Consult surgery if reduction fails or in the presence of any signs or symptoms of obstruction.
- Hydrocele:
    1. Fluid accumulation in the tunica vaginalis.
    2. Communicating hydrocele occurs with failure of the upper process vaginalis to obliterate, resulting in conduit between the peritoneum and the scrotum.
    3. Noncommunicating hydrocele: occurs when the upper processus vaginalis is closed.
    4. A painful hydrocele could represent an intra-abdominal pathology such as a ruptured appendix, meconium hydrocele from prenatal rupture of viscus, or associated incarcerated hernia. All these conditions necessitate surgery consultation.
- Trauma: large scrotal hematomas require surgical evaluation because of the higher incidence of other associated injuries.
- Tumors: account for < 2% of all pediatric solid tumors with a peak at 2 years of age and again during puberty.

Diagnostic Entities

▶ **Circumcision Complications**
- Initially hemorrhage is the most common problem, followed by infection, which usually occurs a few days after circumcision.

- Other complications include meatal stenosis and ulcers.
- Excessive prepuce removal may lead to a concealed penis.

▶ **Epididymitis**
- Uncommon in prepubertal males and should be differentiated from torsion. These patients should be evaluated for a UTI or STDs.
- The patient may have a boggy prostate or urethral discharge.
- Prehn sign (relief with elevation) is unreliable.
- Urine culture may be helpful for appropriate antibiotic treatment.
- **Treatment** includes antibiotics (STD treatment when urethral discharge is present), rest, and scrotal elevation.

▶ **Acute Poststreptococcal Glomerulonephritis (AGN)**
- Most common between 3 and 7 years of age and may be related to immune complexes that deposit on the basement membrane of the glomerulus.
- History usually reveals a preceding infection 1–2 weeks prior and then often present with dark brown urine. In addition, patient may develop edema, hypertension, malaise, and abdominal pain.
- Laboratory evaluation should include urinalysis, culture, serum complements (C3, C4), ASO, CBC, chemistry.
- 80–90% recover without problems and most may be managed at home, unless there is significant renal compromise, or severe hypertension.
- **Management** involves fluid, salt restriction, and diuretics.
- Hypertension may need acute and chronic control.
- Hospitalization is necessary in the presence of uncontrolled hypertension, CHF, or azotemia.

▶ **Hemolytic-Uremic Syndrome (HUS)**
- Most frequently occurs in children < 5 years of age with a peak at 3 years.
- Usually associated with *E. coli* (O157:H7) that produces a cytotoxin and causes a microangiopathic hemolytic anemia.
- Symptoms include abdominal pain and watery diarrhea followed by grossly bloody diarrhea, emesis, and low-grade fever. Later development includes ARF with hematuria, petechiae, GI bleeding, and CNS deterioration (absence of GI symptoms is associated with poor prognosis). Hypertension is present in 40–50% of the patients, and may contrib-

ute to the encephalopathy and cardiac failure. Seizures occur in 40% of cases, particularly in the presence of hyponatremia or azotemia.

- Evaluation should include electrolytes, BUN and creatinine, CBC, reticulocyte count, PT, PTT, urinalysis, and serology for *E. coli*.
- **Management** is supportive. Close evaluation of the electrolytes, transfusions, management of hypertension, and seizures.
- Early initiation of peritoneal dialysis may be helpful.
- Hyperkalemia is common and may require emergency management.
- Seizures may be managed with diazepam or phenytoin with particular attention to correction of any electrolyte abnormalities.
- RBCs and platelets should be replaced if necessary.
- Patients should be admitted. HUS usually resolves in 1–3 months with 80–85% having no residual complications.

▶ **Henoch-Schönlein Purpura (HSP)**
- More common in the winter and males are affected more frequently than females.
- HSP is a vasculitis, which is associated with abdominal pain, arthritis, and purpura.
- Skin lesions are pathognomonic: purpura in the gravity-dependent areas of the legs and buttocks.
- Symptoms usually include colicky abdominal pain and diarrhea (may be bloody). Others include migratory polyarthritis and CNS changes.
- Intussusception should be considered and nephritis may develop (renal involvement is determinant of outcome).
- Evaluation should include a CBC, urinalysis, PT, and PTT.
- Care is supportive. If there are significant GI symptoms then prednisone may be beneficial.

▶ **Nephrotic Syndrome**
- Etiology is usually idiopathic.
- Minimal change form is the most common form and affects males > females.
- Presenting symptom is usually edema and BP is usually low to normal, but may be elevated in 5–10%.
- Other findings include proteinuria, hypoproteinemia, hyperlipidemia, and edema.

- Complications include ARF, renal vein thrombosis, severe hypertension, and hypovolemia.
- Evaluation should include a urinalysis, electrolytes, serum protein, lipid studies, C3 and C4, CBC, and radiographs (chest and abdomen to rule out pleural effusions, pulmonary edema, and ascites).
- **Management** goal is to restore the intravascular volume and treat symptomatic edema. The mainstay of management is steroids.

▶ **Orchitis**
- More common in adolescence due to bacterial or viral agents. Although mumps is the most common cause of primary orchitis, coxsackievirus, adenovirus, and enteroviruses are other viral causes.
- Patient will have gradual onset of pain and swelling.
- Acute testicular torsion needs to be excluded.
- Fertility is usually maintained because it is usually unilateral.
- Evaluation may include a CBC, monospot, and urethral cultures.
- This is usually self-limited but can be very painful.
- **Management** includes rest, scrotal elevation. Analgesics, and antibiotics are limited unless there is epididymitis.

▶ **Phimosis and Paraphimosis**
- Phimosis:
  1. Occurs when there is marked constriction of the distal prepuce, preventing easy passage of the foreskin over the glans.
  2. Retractable prepuce is present in 25%, 50%, and 90% at 6 months of age, 1 year, and 4 years, respectively.
  3. Patient may have a ↓ urine stream, hematuria, or pain.
  4. Classically, circumcision is the definitive management, but in the ED may require careful attempt at reduction and dilation of the urethra to empty the bladder.
- Paraphimosis:
  1. Occurs when a tight prepuce becomes retracted over the glans and fixed in position.
  2. Pain may be managed with general sedation or local nerve block. Sometimes cooling the area or lubrication with lidocaine jelly may help with reduction.

3. "Turning a sock inside out" method is used for reduction: pushing gently on the glans through the edematous prepuce while traction is on the prepuce.

4. Patient may be discharged after voiding and follow-up with the urologist.

► **Priapism**
- A persistent, painful erection.
- Most commonly associated with sickle cell disease in childhood.
- **Management** involves pain relief, monitoring of urinary retention.
- Patients may require exchange transfusions and hematologic consultation.

► **Prostatitis**
- Rare in children both pubertal and prepubertal.
- Organisms include *E. coli, Klebsiella, Enterobacter, Proteus, Pseudomonas, Staphylococcus, N. gonorrhoeae,* and *Chlamydia.*
- Symptoms are similar to cystitis or urethritis.
- Complications include obstruction with urinary retention and bacteremia.
- Evaluation should include urethral culture, urinalysis, CBC.
- The anatomy of the GU tract should be evaluated after the acute infection.
- Infants and children should be treated as though they have sepsis and adolescents as though they have an STD.

► **Acute Renal Failure (ARF)**
- Children usually present with ↓ urine output and ↑ solute retention.
- A urine output of 1 cc/kg/h is considered normal. In the dehydrated patient, it may ↓ to 0.5 cc/kg/h.
- ARF is divided into three classes:
  1. Pre-renal: hypovolemia, distributive, and cardiogenic shock, nephrotic syndrome with intravascular depletion
  2. Intra-renal: acute post-streptococcal glomerulonephritis, primary renal disease, systemic disease, nephrotoxins, or neoplasm
  3. Post-renal: posterior urethral valves, stones, crystals, tumor, trauma, or ureterocele

- The five life-threatening complications include severe hyperkalemia, pulmonary edema, hypertension, septic shock, and seizures.
- Evaluation should include CBC, chemistry, urinalysis, culture, ASO, complements, ANA, and total serum albumin.
- Renal function studies include ultrasound, serum BUN to creatinine ratio > 15:1, urine Na < 15 mEq/L, urine osmolarity > 500 mOsm/kg H_2O, urine to plasma creatinine ratio > 40:1, and a fractional excretion of Na < 1 or < 2.5 in neonates. Additional studies include an IVP, VCUG, and chest x-ray.
- **Management** is also supportive with particular attention to the above five complications.
  1. If pre-renal then may require fluid replacement or furosemide once euvolemic.
  2. Intra-renal may require furosemide and possibly dialysis.
  3. Post-renal will require urology consultation and attempt catheter placement to relieve obstruction.
  4. All may require management of hypertension and electrolytes.

▶ **Chronic Renal Failure**

- Defined as renal function between 25–50% of normal and implies an irreversible state for at least 3 months. End-stage renal disease (ESRD) is associated with a GFR < 10 mL/min/1.73 m².
- Congenital renal disease is the most common cause in children < 5 years of age.
- Hereditary causes include Alport disease, juvenile nephritis, and cystic disease.
- Features include hypertension, renal osteodystrophy, growth retardation, electrolyte disturbances, delayed puberty, and progressive anemia.
- Evaluation includes monitoring electrolytes, CBC, and renal function.
- Renal transplantation is the treatment of choice with ESRD, but CRF requires close management to prevent further deterioration. A GFR of < 5% is an indication for dialysis, but also include CHF, hyperkalemia, pericarditis, uremic encephalopathy, and bleeding.
- Recognize that peritonitis may be a complication of peritoneal dialysis.

► **Testicular Torsion**
- Most commonly in adolescence with a peak around 13 years of age.
- Pathognomonic findings include an elevated testicle with a palpable twist, absent cremasteric reflex, abnormal axis of the testis.
- Outcome is dependent on timeliness of intervention, duration of the torsion, and the tightness of the twist.
- Should be evaluated with color Doppler ultrasonography.
- Surgical intervention is recommended for symptoms < 12 hours (best outcome if < 6 hours).
- Complications include hemicastration by infarction and spermatogenesis may be impaired with as little as 4 hours of torsion.

► **Urinary Tract Infection (UTI)**
- Affects 3–5% of girls and 1% of boys (< 3 months of age UTI is more common in males).
- Usually from ascending bacteria unless younger then may be from bacteremia.
- *E. coli* is the most frequent cause.
- Symptoms vary depending on the age of the patient (infants and toddlers often have generalized symptoms with fever whereas older children have more localized symptoms).
- Evaluation should include a urinalysis and culture (in younger children you may also get a CBC and blood culture).
- Collection of urine should be sterile (catheterization or suprapubic tap in infants and clean catch once older. A bag specimen is often contaminated).
  1. Any colony growth from suprapubic tap has > 99% probability of infection.
  2. 10^5 has a 95% probability in catheterization.
  3. 10^4 is a likely infection in a male with clean catch.
  4. 10^4–10^5 is suspicious in a female with clean catch.
- Most patients with a first-time UTI (all males and females < 2 years) should have radiologic evaluation dependent on the practice of the institution (renal ultrasound plus a VCUG or DMSA scan).
- **Treatment** should be initiated before culture results if highly suspicious.

- Culture should be repeated 48 hours after antibiotics have been started (controversial, unless patient continues to have symptoms, particularly fever).
- Pyridium may be used for children over 6 years.
- Hospitalization should be considered depending on age and severity of symptoms and dehydration.

▶ **Urolithiasis**
- Calcium-containing stones (57%) are the most common composition (more common in males with a mean age for diagnosis of 9 years of age), followed in decreasing frequency by struvite, uric acid, and cysteine stones.
- Infectious stones are the second most common and are primarily associated with *Proteus* (urea splitting bacteria).
- Symptoms include pain, fever, hematuria, and UTI.
- Complications include obstruction and deterioration of renal function.
- Evaluation should include a urinalysis and culture, CBC, electrolytes, renal function, serum protein, alkaline phosphatase, and uric acid. Follow-up testing should include parathyroid, first-morning-fasting urine sample for calcium: creatinine ratio, x-ray of the hands.
- **Management** involves analgesia, antibiotic coverage for *Proteus*, adequate fluid therapy, and removal after consultation with urologist.

CHAPTER 7

LEGAL ISSUES

THE DUTY TO TREAT/THE RIGHT TO REFUSE

► **Competence:** the ability to fully appreciate the nature of one's condition, the diagnostic and therapeutic options available, and the consequences of these options including no intervention. There is no drug level or alcohol level that defines a patient as incompetent. Determination requires good documentation and involvement of other staff for a second opinion.

► **Leaving AMA:** a competent parent can sign their child out AMA. In order to do this, documentation should include: determination that the parent is clinically competent, signature of the person who witnessed your warnings, and the nature of the patient/parent's response. However, if necessary, obtain a court order to hold the patient in the ED. Do not withhold treatment (give antibiotics anyway.)

► **The Rights of Minors:** minors are considered incompetent by law and have no right to consent or withhold consent for treatment. Age varies from state to state but you should provide a complaint-related exam on all patients.

  • In loco parentis: in the position of the parent, and there is always someone in this position even if it is the state intervening on the behalf of the child.

  • The ED physician does not have a duty to provide any test that a layman demands and drug testing can only be done for medical reasons.

  • Minors cannot refuse the care requested for them by a competent guardian.

► **Limitations of the Rights of Parents**

  • Parents do not have the right to refuse life-saving therapy for a child and in this case the physician must usurp the position of the parent.

▶ **Emancipated Minors** (varies by state)
- Usually require minor to be married and living independently, pregnant or the primary caretaker of a minor, member of the U.S. military living outside the parent's home, or living away from home and self-sufficient.

▶ **Presumed Consent**
- Patients who are unconscious or minors may be treated without hesitation for an emergency condition. This includes any condition that may be a threat to life, limb, or bodily function.
- If parent or guardian while alert and competent records in writing that he or she does not want to resuscitate a child the choice must be acknowledged. If this is not in the best interest of the child the ED physician should take steps to ensure the family is fully informed and possibly intervene.
- The ED physician has the duty to treat the patient to the extent to which the patient will allow him or her to treat. The patient need not sign out AMA if there is a reasonable alternative for treatment.

▶ **Statutory Liability: Reporting**
- **Abuse:** suspected abuse must be reported and those acting in good faith are protected from liability.
- **Bites:** vary depending on state but usually require reporting of all dog and other animal bites.
- **Wounds:** all gun shot wounds require a report to the local police (including accidental). In addition, any penetrating or nonpenetrating wounds that are acts of violence must also be reported.
- **Deaths:** most deaths occurring in a hospital are reported to the hospital itself. The coroners or ME must be notified of any death occurring outside of medical supervision or death that occurs shortly after arrival to care. (This includes patients with known medical disease and obvious mechanism of death.) The ED physician does not usually sign a death certificate unless the cause of death is obvious (i.e., trauma).
- **Communicable Diseases:** the laboratory is usually responsible for this and includes sexually transmitted diseases. Almost all states have free and anonymous HIV testing.

▶ **Statutory Liability: Civil rights**—the federal Civil Rights Act of 1964 prohibits discrimination and stands above EMTALA (emergency medical treatment and active labor law).

▶ **Statutory Immunity:** the degree of protection for Good Samaritan laws vary by state but protects physicians from liability for damages where assistance is rendered without charge, emergency circumstance, outside of the doctor's usual practice, physician has no preexisting duty to the patient. Two loopholes include that illness may not be the kind of emergency for which this law was developed and the entire hospital may be considered one's usual practice.

▶ **EMTALA:** this started as COBRA (consolidation omnibus budget reconciliation act) passed in 1986 to prevent transfer of patient without funding to another institution and then in order to ensure that EDs serve with equality the EMTALA law developed. This requires three duties: screening, stabilizing, and appropriate transfer if necessary.

- **Medical Screening:** a patient is considered to have come to the ED if he or she is anywhere in the facility or campus, or hospital-owned transport vehicles. They have not come to the ED if they are in a private ambulance on campus. Telemetry or conversation with transport does not trigger EMTALA. Patients can refuse the exam and treatment if they have been appropriately educated and it is all in writing. This includes psychiatric patients and facilities (such patients do not have to accept ambulances in order to be included in the law). The hospital decides who will perform a screening exam and a missed diagnosis is not an EMTALA violation. A registration process may occur if it does not affect the patient's access to care.

- **Further Examination and Stabilizing Treatment Requirement:** the hospital must maintain a list of physicians available routinely to the ED and every service should be represented. The term *stabilize* is based on the safety of patient transfer and includes discharge.

- **Transfer Requirement:** this does not address the transfer of stable patients. In order to be appropriate, there must be signed written consent after being informed of the risks and benefits, or the benefits must outweigh the risks for transfer and the physician must sign. Even if the physician is not present in the ED another individual may sign for the physician but then this must be countersigned. This does not imply that the patient is stable. The transferring hospital must provide qualified personnel and transport equipment during the transfer. All records MUST accompany the patient and a log must be kept for no less than 5 years. An ED must accept patients if it has adequate space, personnel, and equipment and the ability to expand will be considered. Patients cannot be discharged with the intent of proceeding directly to another facility to obtain further care.

- **Enforcement:** civil statute with a $50,000 fine to physicians and hospitals breaking the law and $25,000 for hospitals with fewer than 100 beds. There is no limitation for the number of violations per case. Malpractice does not have to be found to result in a fine. Physicians in the ED treating a patient who requires consultation with a physician on call who does not see the patient and is transferred before being reasonably stabilized are immune and the one on call is at fault.

▶ **Medical Malpractice Actions:** malpractice is medical negligence.
- **Duty:** an ED physician has a duty to all patients present and this duty ends when another physician takes over the case, which may occur in the ED. The ED doctor may be liable if he or she turns the care over to someone who is impaired or represents a clear danger to the patient.
- **Breach of Duty:** a breach in the standard of care. Cannot be determined retrospectively based on a poor outcome.
- **Loss to the Plaintiff:** plaintiff must demonstrate losses (medical expenses, lost wages, future income; pain and suffering; loss of punitive damages). To be found guilty of punitive damages there must be willful or wanton disregard for patient safety.
- **Proximate Cause:** the defendant's actions were a substantial contributing cause to the adverse outcome. Negligence that is not associated with alleged loss is not legal malpractice.

▶ **Risk Management:** designed to reduce the losses associated with being sued and prevent a bad outcome.
- **Protect the Patient:** there is no duty to order tests that are not indicated. It is not usually a failure in knowledge that leads to lawsuits against the ED but failure in diagnostic orientation and therapeutic promptness.
- **Protect Yourself:** documentation because the chart serves to demonstrate the standard of care. This includes the timing and content of conversation with consultants.

HANDY PEDIATRIC FORMULAS AND NORMAL PARAMETERS

1. **Endotracheal Intubation**
   a. Tube size: **(16 + age in years)/4** or **4 + (age in years/4)**
   b. ETT placement: **10 + age in years at the lips or 3×ETT size**
      - 1 kg newborn—7
      - 2 kg newborn—8
      - 3 kg newborn—9
      - 4 kg newborn—10
2. **Estimate of Nasogastric/Orogastric or Foley Catheter Size: 2× ETT size**
   Estimate of Chest Tube Size: 4× ETT size
3. **Estimate of Weight in Kilograms**
   a. (2 × Age in years) + 8
   b. 1-year-old weighs 10 kg
   c. 5-year-old weighs 20 kg
4. **Systolic Blood Pressure Parameters**
   a. PALS: (2 × Age in years) + 70—starting at age 1
      - Remember that this is only the 5th percentile
   b. Preferred formula: **(2 × Age in years) + 90**
      - This is the 50th percentile
   c. Newborn systolic blood pressure: 60
5. **Initial Fluid Bolus**
   a. Newborn: start with 10 cc/kg NS or LR
   b. Child: 20 cc/kg NS or LR
      - 10 cc/kg of PRBCs or fresh frozen plasma
6. **Normal Pediatric Vital Signs (Pulse, Respiratory Rates, and Systolic Blood Pressure)**

Age	Respiratory Rate (breaths/min)	Heart Rate (bpm)	Systolic Blood Pressure (mm Hg)
Newborn (28 days)	30–60	120–160	50–70
Infant (1 month– 1 year)	20–40	80–140	70–100
1–5 years	20–30	80–130	80–110
6–12 years	20–30	70–110	80–120
Adolescents	12–20	60–100	110–120

7. **Correcting Hypoglycemia**

   a. A dose of 0.5 g/kg to 1 g/kg is recommended to raise the blood sugar about 100 mg/dL.

Dextrose Concentration (%)	Bolus Dose (mL/kg) to replace 0.5 g/kg or 50%	To replace 1 g/kg or 100%
10	5 mL/kg	10 cc/kg
25	2 mL/kg	4 cc/kg
50	1 mL/kg	2 cc/kg

   b. For example, in a 20 kg child, 40 cc of D_{25} will raise the blood sugar by 100 mg/dL.

   c. D_{10} for infants and young children, D_{25} for older children, D_{50} for adolescents.

PEDIATRIC PROCEDURES

(Special thanks to Maureen McCollough MD for her assistance in preparing these instructions)

NEEDLE CRICOTHYROTOMY (JET VENTILATION)

► Use when endotracheal intubation with or without rapid sequence induction is not successful
► Replaces the surgical cricothyrotomy used in older children and adults
► Complication rates are 10–40%
► Unclear age limit—probably could be performed on kids > 8–10 yr
► Most procedure texts will discuss the use of a jet ventilator in order to ventilate through a needle cricothyrotomy; unfortunately most EDs do not have access to a jet ventilator; this hand-out describes various oxygen setups that can be utilized in any ED in order to ventilate using a needle cricothyrotomy
► Identify cricothyroid membrane; prepare with Betadine if possible
► Then use a larger 12–14 g angiocath to puncture membrane, directed at a 45 degree angle caudally (toward feet)
► Remove needle from angiocath

Methods for Ventilation (Choose One)

1. Attach a **3 cc syringe barrel** to the angiocath, then attach a **7.0 ET tube adapter,** then attach a BVM bag; turn wall O_2 up to 15 L and attempt to bag through angiocath.
2. Attach a **3.0 ET tube adapter directly to angiocath,** then attach a BVM bag; turn wall O_2 up to 15 L and attempt to bag through angiocath

3. Attach a **3.0 ET tube adapter** directly to angiocath, attach an **"aerosol T adapter"** to the angiocath; attach **wall oxygen tubing**[*] to one side of the "T adapter" and plug this into wall oxygen at 15 L (15 L wall O_2 should equal 40–50 psi); using the other open port of the "T adapter" as an on/off switch, place your finger over the open part to allow air to flow into the angiocath and into the trachea = inhalation (hold for approximately 1–2 seconds); then let go of the port to allow the wall oxygen to take the path of least resistance and flow out of this open port = exhalation (open for 3–4 seconds)

- Some advocate inserting another 14 g angiocath into cricothyroid membrane to allow exhalation (be sure to occlude this 2nd angiocath while squeezing BVM bag or occluding "T adapter" port [inhalation], then un-occlude to allow exhalation)
- Child can be oxygenated, but ventilation (CO_2 exhalation) is limited

Complications:

- ▶ Exsanguinating hematoma
- ▶ Perforation of the esophagus, posterior wall of the trachea, or thyroid
- ▶ Infection
- ▶ Inadequate oxygenation (inadequate ventilation with a rise in CO_2 is inevitable); the goal is good oxygenation
- ▶ Subcutaneous or mediastinal emphysema

LMA—LARYNGEAL MASK AIRWAYS

Technique

- ▶ Completely or partially deflate cuff
- ▶ Apply water-soluble lubricant to the back surface of the cuff and tube
- ▶ Place the child in the sniffing position. The head is held in slight extension by having the nonintubating hand stabilize the occiput.

[*]Wall oxygen tubing can be found on hand-held-nebulizers or on standard oxygen face masks

▶ Use thumb or index finger to slide cuff along the palato-pharyngeal curve (while avoiding the structures of the anterior pharynx) into the hypopharynx (covering the glottis)

▶ Continue to pass into the hypopharynx until resistance is felt

▶ Inflate cuff to minimum pressure that provides a seal.

▶ The LMA will come forward a little after the cuff is inflated

LMA size	Weight	Cuff Vol (cc)	Age
LMA 1	< 5kg	2–5 cc	< 1 month
LMA 1.5	5–10 kg	2–5 cc	< 1 y/o
LMA 2	10–20 kg	7–10 cc	1–5 y/o
LMA 2.5	20–30 kg	14 cc	5–9 y/o
LMA 3	30–50 kg	15–20 cc	
LMA 4	50–70 kg	25–30 cc	

Limitations

▶ Contraindicated in an infant or child with an intact gag reflex

▶ Main disadvantage: not protective of the airway from regurgitated gastric contents

▶ Does not allow for administration of resuscitation medications

▶ May be more difficult than ETT to maintain during patient movement and careful attention is required to make sure proper positioning is maintained.

FOREIGN BODIES CAUSING AIRWAY OBSTRUCTION

▶ Young child's trachea is pliable; airway obstruction can be caused by FB in the stuck in esophagus and pushing trachea from behind

▶ Remember BLS maneuvers!!!
  • infants < 1 yo—5 back-blows and 5 chest thrusts
  • children > 1 yo—5 abdominal thrusts
  • Remember, NO BLIND FINGER SWEEPS!!

▶ Stock ED with pediatric McGill forceps for FB removal

▶ McGill forceps not to be used below vocal cords

▶ After removal of FB, before pulling out laryngoscope, look around for additional FBs; should be able to see clear path to vocal cords

▶ If unable to ventilate child after removal of FB and clear path to cords visualized, then additional FB probably exists below vocal cords

VASCULAR ACCESS
Peripheral Access

▶ Effective for blood samples or administration of fluid or medications
▶ External jugular has low risk of pneumothorax or injury to carotid, and is relatively safe in a child with a coagulopathy
▶ Preferred sites
  • Antecubital
  • Dorsum of hand
  • Basilic / cephalic vein
  • Saphenous vein
  • Scalp veins
  • External jugular
▶ 22 or 24 gauge catheters used primarily in children

Saphenous Vein Cutdown

▶ Location is 1–2 cm anterior to medial malleolous
▶ Externally rotate the leg
▶ 2 cm transverse incision over medial malleolous
▶ Blunt dissection parallel to vein
▶ Tie-off the distal end of the vein
▶ Loosely wrap tie around proximal ends of vein
▶ Incision then made in upper one-third of vein; advance the catheter into the vein
▶ Secure the catheter with the proximal tie already in place
▶ Cutdown complications
  • Bleeding
  • Phlebitis or infection
  • Nerve damage

Central Venous Access

Femoral Vein
▶ Dirty area for central vein access but easiest of central veins to find in small kids

- ▶ Remember, NERVE – ARTERY – VEIN from lateral to medial
- ▶ If a line is drawn between the anterior superior iliac spine and symphysis pubis, the femoral artery runs directly across at the midpoint, and medial to that is the vein
- ▶ When accessing the femoral vein using the needle that advances the guidewire, try finding the vein *without a syringe on the needle*; when the needle advances into the vein, blood will fill the hub of the needle; at this point, insert the guidewire and advance into vein

Subclavian Vein
- ▶ Higher risk of pneumothorax
- ▶ Place child in Trendelenberg and place small rolled towel under thoracic area to open up area
- ▶ Use a tuberculin syringe instead of a large syringe to find the vessel; larger syringe may collapse the vein and make it possible to miss the flash

Internal Jugular Vein
- ▶ Landmarks may be difficult to find in small children; remember, vein tends to lie lateral to artery
- ▶ Risk of puncturing carotid artery
- ▶ Contraindicated if child has a coagulopathy

Complications of Central Vein Access
- ▶ Pneumothorax
- ▶ Bleeding and hematoma secondary to laceration of the vessel
- ▶ Arterial puncture
- ▶ Air or catheter embolism
- ▶ Infection
- ▶ Hemothorax

Intraosseous Line
- ▶ Reserved for situations in which a child in severe shock has failed three attempts at intravenous access or 90 seconds have elapsed in the attempt
- ▶ **New PALS recommendation is to use IO lines as needed in all pediatric age groups
- ▶ Use this vascular access route as FIRST-LINE approach for

pediatric CARDIAC ARRESTS (nearly impossible to achieve peripheral access in a young child in full arrest)
► Absolute contraindications
  • Previous attempt in that bone
  • Ipsilateral fracture
  • ** In both of these cases, any fluid or medication give will flow out of the bone marrow area and into the subcutaneous tissue in the area
► Relative contraindications
  • Osteogenesis imperfecta
  • Local infection
► Preferred sites
  • Proximal aspect of tibia
  • Distal aspect of tibia on malleoli
  • Distal aspect of femur
► Equipment
  • Intraosseous needle or bone marrow needle
  • 10 cc syringe
  • Saline flush
  • 3-way stopcock
  • T-connector intravenous tubing

Procedure
► Clean area with Betadine solution
► Proximal tibia landmarks–
  • 2 finger-breadths distal to tibial tuberosity, on flat part of tibia (medially)
► Insert intraosseous needle perpendicular to the bone using twisting back-and-forth motion with gentle pressure
► If possible, during insertion, angle needle away from epiphyseal growth plate
► Placement is verified by lack of resistance, needle standing erect in bone without support, aspiration of bone marrow, and free flow of fluids

Complications
► Complications are very rare with IO lines; rate of infection higher for peripheral intravenous access compared to IO line placements
► Osteomyelitis <1% or other infections

► Extravasation of fluid, cellulitis, fractures, epiphyseal cartilage
► Fat embolism
► Compartment syndrome
► Skin necrosis

Umbilical Vein Catheterization

► Umbilical vein remains patent for at least 1 week after birth; used for newborns or young neonates who require emergent vascular access and peripheral attempts have been unsuccessful.
► Equipment –
  • Antiseptic solution and sterile gauze pads
  • Sterile drapes
  • Umbilical tape or 3-0 silk suture on a straight needle
  • Small hemostat
  • Sterile scalpel
  • 3.5 or 5F umbilical catheter (can also use 5F feeding tubes)
  • 3 way stopcock
  • 10 cc syringe
  • Saline flush

Procedure

► Place newborn supine and restrain extremities as necessary
► Newborn should be placed on a cardiac monitor and pulse oximeter; also monitor newborn's temperature; use warming bed or lamps if possible
► Attach 5F umbilical catheter (or feeding tube) to the 3-way stopcock an syringe filled with saline
► Flush catheter with saline
► Clean umbilical stump and abdomen from xyphoid to pubic symphysis
► Loosely tie umbilical tape or silk suture around base of umbilical stump
► Cut the cord 1–2 cm from the abdominal wall
► Identify the vessels (the umbilical vein is a single, thin walled, large diameter lumen, usually located at 12 o'clock; the arteries are paired and have thicker walls with a smaller diameter lumen; cut end of cord resembles "Oh no, Mr. Bill" from *Saturday Night Live*)

- ▶ Gently remove any clot from in the umbilical vein
- ▶ Insert the catheter until free return of blood (about 5–6 cm)
- ▶ Confirm catheter placement with abdominal x-ray; catheter should not curve into RUQ—might be entering hepatic portal circulation; x-ray should show placement at or above the diaphragm

Complications
- ▶ Infection
- ▶ Embolization or thrombosis
- ▶ Vessel perforation
- ▶ Hemorrhage
- ▶ Ischemia of extremities or intra-abdominal organs

PEDIATRIC FOREIGN BODY REMOVAL
Ear
- ▶ Round objects—loop curettes
  - • Drop of *CRAZY GLUE* on end of wood end of Q tip—apply to FB, let dry, pull FB out
- ▶ Insects—Alligator forceps
- ▶ Don't forget to check other ear!!

Nose
- ▶ Occlude non-obstructed nostril and have parent blow gently but quickly into child's mouth—warn parent it might result in "snot" on parent's cheek
- ▶ Occlude non-obstructed nostril and blow into child's mouth gently but quickly with an bag-valve-mask
- ▶ Insert 6F Foley past obstruction, gently inflate and pull FB out

Esophagus
- ▶ Foley catheter technique for removal of esophageal FBs:
- ▶ Appropriate patients:
  - • Smooth, round, flat objects in proximal $2/3$ of esophagus
  - • Age > 1 yo and normal level of consciousness with good gag
  - • Duration of < 24–48 hours

- No history of esophageal surgery or esophageal edema on chest xray
▶ No anesthesia—child must be able to protect on airway
▶ Personnel equipped and experienced with pediatric airway management
▶ Equipment needed:
  - Foleys—sized 12, 14 or 16 F that can pass through nares
  - Lubricant
  - McGill forceps
  - Laryngoscope
  - Table that can tilt into Trendelenberg
  - Pediatric crash cart
▶ **Procedure:**
  - Estimate how far down coin is in child based on child's size and location on xray
  - Restrain child supine in papoose board or wrapped bed sheets (use some tape to secure bedsheets)
  - Try oral insertion of Foley first , with balloon deflated (use padded tongue blade as bite block if necessary)
  - Insert Foley catheter into child's esophagus to a distance where the Foley balloon is estimated to be past the coin
  - STOP if you meet resistance **see below
  - Inflate the balloon with 3–5 cc of NS
  - Roll the patient now into a prone position and in Trendelenberg (head down)
  - Gently pull the Foley to move the coin into the mouth
  - If patient starts to cough or tension is released on the Foley, remove the Foley and allow the patient to cough or spit out the coin
  - No follow-up xray is needed in uncomplicated removals
  - Observe patient for 1 hour and be sure patient is tolerating liquids
  - Patient should be instructed to return for fever, pain, or dysphagia
▶ **Failures:**
  - If first attempt fails, but patient is tolerating procedure well, you may try again
  - If patient bites on tube even with bite block, you can pass Foley through nares (may need smaller size)

- If mild resistance is felt at the upper esophagus, try flexing child's neck gently to allow easier passage

Vagina

▶ Try positioning child in knee-chest position if lithotomy position does not give good view of vaginal canal

▶ Alligator forceps (watch sharp tips!)

NEEDLE THORACOSTOMY AND PERCUTANEOUS CHEST TUBES

Diagnosis

▶ Children requiring positive-pressure ventilation in ED are at high risk for pneumothoraces or tension pneumothoraces

▶ Remember pneumonic for sudden deterioration of an intubated patient:

D – dislodgement – check ET tube placement

O – obstruction – suction ET tube

P - tension pneumothorax – diagnosis of exclusion

E – equipment failure – check tubing, O_2 source, ventilator

▶ Tension pneumothorax—sudden desaturation, hypotension, and bradycardia; may also have decreased breath sounds, shift of PMI, decreased chest rise, hyperresonance or tympany of the chest

▶ In young infants, may be able to transilluminate chest wall; do while waiting for xray; true positive follows shape of thoracic cavity, varies with respiration and position, has larger area of light than another normal site; false negative if chest wall is too thick or skin is darkly pigmented, if room light is too bright or if area is obscured by monitor leads or clothing / dressings on infant.

▶ If true tension pneumothorax, child will not be able to wait for an x-ray; but if you do get an x-ray, distinguish pleural air collections from skin folds, thymus, artifacts, or other non-pleural, intrathoracic air collection on x-ray.

Needle Thoracostomy

▶ Prepare skin with Betadine

▶ Connect 3-way stopcock between 18 (or 20) gauge angiocath and syringe; open stopcock to the angiocath

- Insert angiocath at 45-degree angle to skin, directed cephalad, in 4th or 5th intercostal space, just over top of ribs, below breast tissue, in anterior axillary line
- Withdraw on syringe as you are inserting angiocath until you get a rush of air.
- As angiocath enters pleural space, decrease angle to 15-degrees above chest wall, and slide catheter in while removing needle stylet.
- Withdraw the needle stylet from the catheter and reattach the catheter to the stopcock and continue withdrawing air; then close the stopcock to the child and depress the syringe to evacuate the air in it.
- Alternatively, you can use a butterfly needle, inserted at 90-degrees angle to the skin in 2nd or 3rd intercostal space, midclavicular line, attached to stopcock and syringe as above.

Percutaneous Chest Tubes

- Rough rule for chest tube size = 4 × ETT size
- This procedure is similar to percutaneous central line placement using guidewire and dilators.
- Chest tube should be placed in the 4th or 5th intercostal space
- Measure the chest tube length necessary—measure from area of skin insertion to mid-clavicle area.
- Using finder needle to enter pleural air space, insert guidewire into pleural space through the finder needle.
- Remove finder needle; nick skin with blade going directly on top of the guidewire
- Place the first dilator over the guidewire and insert into chest
- Remove first dilator and proceed, in order, with subsequently larger and larger dilators
- After last dilator has been used and removed, tract that has been created should be large enough to accommodate the chest tube chosen.
- Place chest tube over the guidewire and remove guidewire.
- Observe for humidity or bubbling in chest tube to verify intrapleural location.
- Connect tube to drainage system without putting tension on tube.
- Secure chest tube to skin with suture.

Complications

- ► Misdiagnosis with resultant unnecessary chest tube placement
- ► Lung laceration or perforation, puncture of liver, damage to breast tissue, chylothorax
- ► Horner's syndrome due to nerve damage or phrenic nerve injury
- ► Misplacement of tube—in subcutaneous tissue, last side-hole is outside of pleural space, tip of chest tube is across mediastinum
- ► Infection
- ► Subcutaneous emphysema

INFECTIVE ENDOCARDITIS

DUKES CRITERIA FOR INFECTIOUS ENDOCARDITIS

Major Criteria
1. Isolation of organisms from 2 blood cultures:
   Must be typical organisms—Viridans streptococci, *Streptococcus bovis*, HACEK group, or *S. aureus* or enterococci in absence of primary focus
2. Persistently positive blood cultures:
   2 or more positive blood cultures for same organism separated by 12 hours, or, 3 or greater positive blood cultures for same organism with 1 hour between first and last culture
3. Positive echocardiogram for oscillating intracardiac mass at sites vegetations typically occur
4. Intracardiac abscess identified by echocardiogram
5. New partial dehiscence of prosthetic valve as identified by echocardiogram
6. New regurgitant murmur

Minor Criteria
1. Fever greater than 38 degrees Celsius
2. Predisposing heart condition and/or IV drug use
3. Vascular phenomena: Including major arterial emboli, mycotic aneurysms, CNS hemorrhages, Janeway lesions, conjunctival hemorrhages, peripheral necrotic skin lesions
4. Immunologic phenomena: includes elevated rheumatoid factor, immune complex glomerulonephritis, Osler's nodes
5. Echocardiogram findings consistent with endocarditis but not meeting major criterion: nonoscillating masses, nodular valve thickening

CARDIAC CONDITIONS REQUIRING PROPHYLAXIS AGAINST ENDOCARDITIS

Endocarditis Prophylaxis Recommended
  1. High-risk category
    Presence of prosthetic valves

Previous bacterial endocarditis
Complex cyanotic heart disease
Surgical systemic pulmonary shunts or conduits
2. Moderate-risk category
Acquired valve dysfunction
Hypertrophic cardiomyopathy
Other congenital heart malformations
Mitral valve prolapse with regurgitation or thickened leaflets
Endocarditis Prophylaxis Not Recommended
1. Negligible-risk category
Isolated secundum atrial septal defect
History of coronary bypass graft surgery
Mitral valve prolapse without regurgitation
Physiologic, functional, or innocent murmurs
Cardiac pacemakers and implanted defibrillators
History of rheumatic fever without valve dysfunction
History of Kawasaki disease without valve dysfunction
Surgically repaired atrial septal defect, ventricular septal defect,
or patent ductus arteriosus

PROPHYLAXIS FOR ORAL, DENTAL, ESOPHAGEAL, OR RESPIRATORY TRACT PROCEDURES

Situation	Recommended antibiotic	Dosing regimen
Standard prophylaxis	Amoxicillin	50 mg/kg PO 1 h prior to procedure, not to exceed 2 g
Unable to take oral medications	Ampicillin	50 mg/kg IM or IV within 30 minutes prior to procedure, not to exceed 2 g
Allergic to penicillin	Clindamycin	20 mg/kg PO 1 h prior to procedure, not to exceed 600 mg
	Azithromycin or clarithromycin	15 mg/kg PO 1 hour prior to procedure, not to exceed 500 mg
Allergic to penicillin and unable to take oral medications	Clindamycin	20 mg/kg IV within 30 minutes before procedure, not to exceed 600 mg

PROPHYLAXIS AGAINST ENDOCARDITIS FOR GASTROINTESTINAL AND GENITOURINARY PROCEDURES

Situation	Recommended antibiotic	Dosing regimen
High-risk patients	Ampicillin and Gentamicin	Ampicillin 50 mg/kg IM or IV, not to exceed 2 g, plus gentamicin 1.5 mg/kg IV, not to exceed 120 mg. 6 hours later ampicillin 25 mg/kg IM/IV or amoxicillin 25 mg/kg PO
High-risk patients with penicillin allergy	Vancomycin and Gentamicin	Vancomycin 20 mg/kg IV over 1–2 hours, not to exceed 1 g, plus Gentamicin as above.
Moderate-risk patients	Amoxicillin or Ampicillin	Amoxicillin 50 mg/kg PO 1 hour prior to procedure, not to exceed 2 g, or ampicillin 50 mg/kg IV/IM within 30 minutes of procedure, not to exceed 2 g
Moderate-risk patients with penicillin allergy	Vancomycin	Vancomycin 20 mg/kg IV over 1–2 hours, complete within 30 minutes of procedure, not to exceed 1 g

COMMON ABBREVIATIONS

ABCs, airway, breathing, circulation
ACTH, adreno-corticotropin hormone
ADH, alcohol dehydrogenase
ADHD, attention deficit hyperactivity disorder
AED, antiepileptic drugs
AGN, acute poststreptococcal glomerulonephritis
AIDS, acquired immunodeficiency syndrome
ALL, acute lymphocytic leukemia
ALOC, altered level of consciousness
ALT, alanine aminotransferase
ALTE, Acute Life-Threatening Event
AML, acute myelogenous leukemia
AMS, acute mountain sickness
ANA, antinuclear antibodies
ANC, absolute neutrophil count
AO, atlantoaxial
AOM, acute otitis media
AP, anteroposterior
APAP, acetaminophen
APD, afferent pupillary defect
ARDS, acute respiratory distress syndrome
ARF, acute renal failure
ASA, aspirin
ASD, atrial septal defect
ASO, antistreptolysin
AST, aspartate aminotransferase
ATFL, anterior talofibular
AV, atrioventricular

AVM, arterial-venous malformation
CAD, coronary artery disease
CAH, congenital adrenal hyperplasia
CF, cystic fibrosis
CFL, calcaneofibular
CHF, congestive heart failure
CMG, cardiomegaly
CMV, cytomegalovirus
CO, cardiac output
COPD, chronic obstructive pulmonary disease
COHgb, carboxyhemoglobin
CPAP, continuous positive airway pressure
CPP, cerebral perfusion pressure
CRP, C-reactive protein
CVA, cerebrovascular accident
DIP, distal interphalangeal
DM, diabetes mellitus
DMSA, disodium monomethanearsonate
DPG, diphosphoglycerate
EBV, Epstein-Barr virus
ECF, extracellular fluid
ED, emergency department
EF, ejection fraction
EIA, enzyme immunoassay
ELISA, enzyme-linked immunosorbent assay
EMG, electromyogram
EOM, extraocular movement
EPAP, end expiratory positive pressure
ESRD, end-stage renal disease
FB, foreign body
FFP, fresh frozen plasma
FSH, follicle-stimulating hormone
FTT, failure to thrive
GABA, gamma-aminobutyric acid
GABHS, group A beta-hemolytic streptococcus
GAS, group A strep
GERD, gastroesophageal reflux disease
GFR, glomerular filtration rate
HACE, high-altitude cerebral edema
HAPE, high-altitude pulmonary edema

HAV, hepatitis A virus
HBIG, hepatitis-B immune globulin
HBO$_2$, hyperbaric oxygen
HB$_s$Ag, hepatis B surface antigen
HBV, hepatitis B virus
HIV, human immunodeficiency virus
HPV, human papillomavirus
HR, heart rate
HSP, Henoch-Schönlein purpura
HSV, herpes simplex virus
HUS, hemolytic uremic syndrome
IBD, inflammatory bowel disease
ICF, intracellular fluid
ICH, intracranial hemorrhage
IDDM, insulin-dependent diabetes mellitus
IG, immune globulin
IgE, immunoglobulin E
IgG, immunoglobulin G
IgM, immunoglobulin M
INH, isoniazid
IOP, intraocular pressure
I/Os, strict inputs and outputs
IP, interphalangeal
ITP, idiopathic thrombocytopenic purpura
IVGG, IV gamma globulin
IVIG, IV immune globulin
IVP, intravenous pyelogram
JRA, juvenile rheumatoid arthritis
JVD, jugular venous distention
LDH, lactate dehydrogenase
LE, lower extremity
LH, luteinizing hormone
LLQ, left lower quadrant
LLSB, left lower sternal border
LOC, loss of consciousness
LUQ, left upper quadrant
LUSB, left upper sternal border
LV, left ventricle
LVH, left ventricular hypertrophy
MAP, mean arterial pressure

MCP, metacarpophalangeal
MDAC, multidose-activated charcoal
MR, mental retardation
MRSA, methicillin-resistant *Staphylococcus aureus*
NEC, necrotizing enterocolitis
NSAIDs, nonsteroidal antiinflammatory drugs
OCP, oral contraceptive pill
OD, overdose
OM, otitis media
OR, operating room
OTC, over the counter
PCR, polymerase chain reaction
PDA, patent ductus arteriosus
PDDNOS, pervasive developmental disorder not otherwise specified
PEEP, positive end expiratory pressure
PEFR, peak expiratory flow rate
PGE_1, prostaglandin E_1
PICU, pediatric intensive care unit
PID, pelvic inflammatory disease
PIP, proximal interphalangeal
PMN, polymorphonuclear leukocytes
PPD, purified protein derivative
PPS, peripheral pulmonary stenosis
pRBC, packed red blood cells
PRN, as needed
PSA, procedural sedation and analgesia
PTFL, posterior talofibular ligaments
PTH, parathyroid hormone
PTS, Pediatric Trauma Score
PTPI, posttraumatic pulmonary insufficiency
PUD, peptic ulcer disease
PVC, premature ventricular contractions
PVR, peripheral vascular resistance
RDS, respiratory distress syndrome
REM, rapid eye movement
RF, rheumatoid factor
RLQ, right lower quadrant
RPR, rapid plasma reagin
RR, respiratory rate

RSV, respiratory syncytial virus

RTA, renal tubular acidosis

RUQ, right upper quadrant

RV, right ventricle

RVH, right ventricular hypertrophy

SBO, small bowel obstruction

SBP, systolic blood pressure

SCD, sickle cell disease

SCI, spinal cord injury

SCIWORA, spinal cord injury without radiologic abnormality

SCM, sternocleidomastoid muscle

SIADH, syndrome of inappropriate secretion of antidiuretic hormone

SLE, systemic lupus erythematosus

SOB, shortness of breath

STD, sexually transmitted disease

SV, stroke volume

TB, tuberculosis

TBSA, total body surface area

TBW, total body water

TCA, tricyclic antidepressants

Td, tetanus-diphtheria (toxoids, adult type)

TEC, transient erythroblastopenia of childhood

TEN, toxic epidermal necrolysis

TIA, transient ischemic attack

TM, tympanic membrane

TMJ, temporomandibular joint

TORCHS, *Toxoplasma gondii*, O "other" rubella, cytomegalovirus, herpes simplex virus, syphilis

TSS, toxic shock syndrome

TTP, thrombotic thrombocytopenia purpura

UE, upper extremity

URI, upper respiratory tract infections

UTI, urinary tract infection

UVC, umbilical venous catheter

VA, visual acuity

VCUG, voiding cystourethrogram

VIP, vasoactive intestinal peptide

VQ, ventilation perfusion lung scan

VSD, ventricular septal defect
vWD, von Willebrand disease
vWF, von Willebrand factor
V. Fib., ventricular fibrillation
WHO, World Health Organization

INDEX